This special first edition hardcover of
The Whole Health Life
is limited to 2,000 copies.

I hope this book helps you find wellness
on your own health journey.

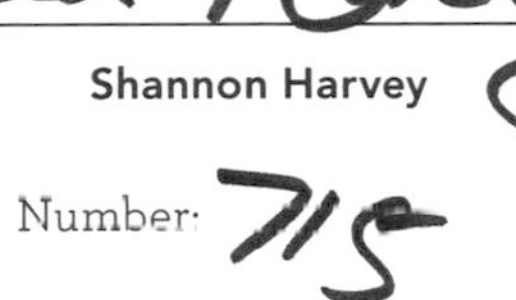

Shannon Harvey

Number: 715

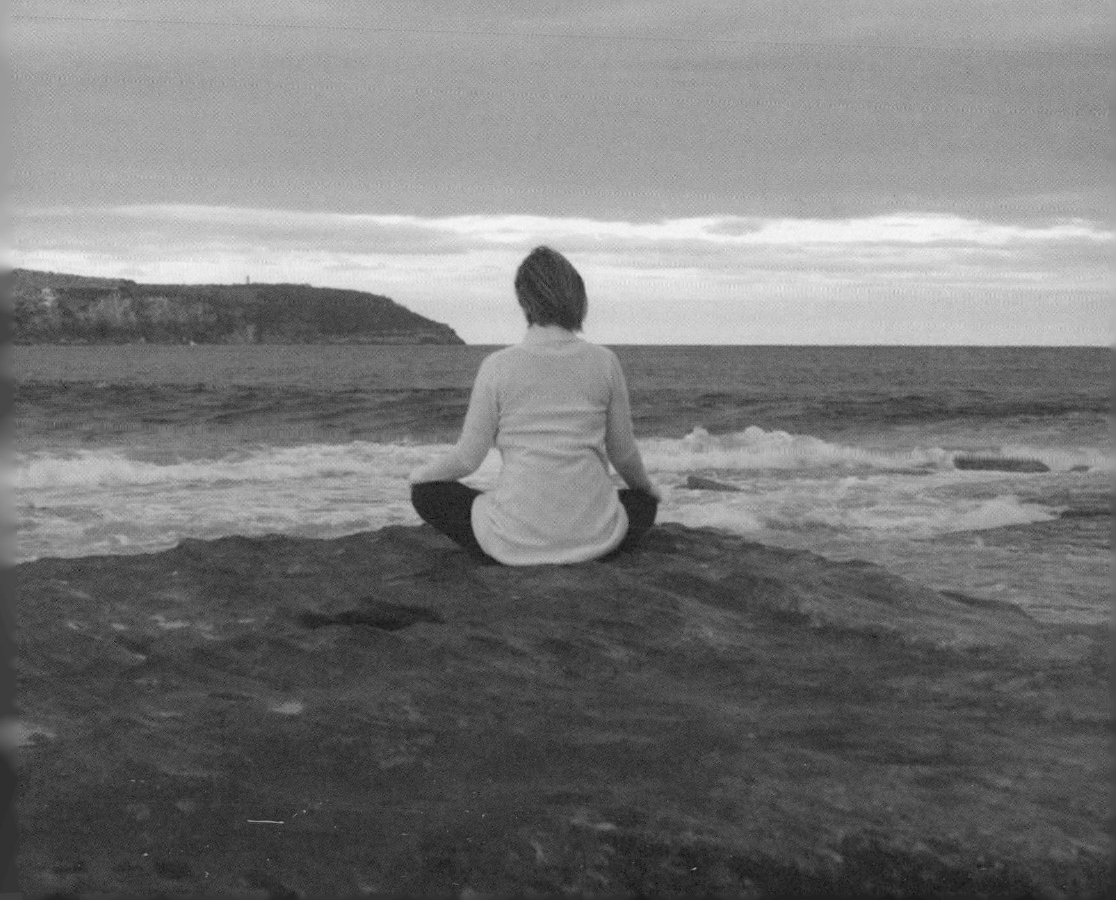

PRAISE FOR *THE WHOLE HEALTH LIFE*

"Written by a journalist who thinks like a scientist, Shannon Harvey's book uses the best available science to explain in simple language why we so often fail to get well, but more importantly, how we can succeed. The science provides a compelling explanation of Shannon's own recovery; her book and her story will inspire countless people on their journeys of recovery from serious illness."

Professor George Jelinek MD, author of *Overcoming Multiple Sclerosis.*

"The Whole Health Life depicts an inspiring personal journey into the expanding field of body mind science. Shannon Harvey generously shares the knowledge and tips for happiness and health she's picked up in her own quest for a fulfilling life after being diagnosed with a chronic disease. A must read."

Lynne Malcolm, Presenter *ABC Radio National, All in the Mind*

"Shannon Harvey's The Whole Health Life provides authoritative science, journalistic rigour, real-life experience and eminently practical strategies to enhance your health, and all in one totally readable package. What a rare combination!"

Craig Hassed MD, author of *The Essence of Health.*

MORE FROM SHANNON HARVEY

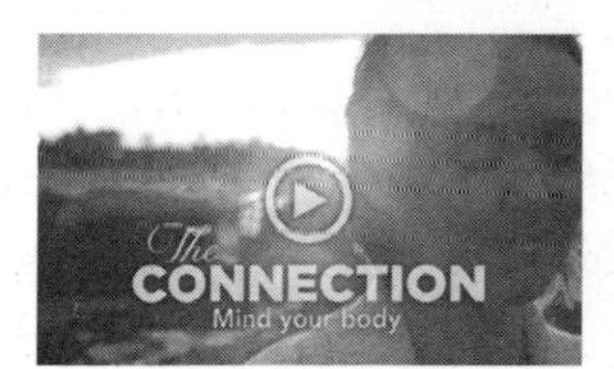

The Connection is a feature documentary that uncovers the latest science in mind body medicine and proves we have much more to say about our health than we thought possible.

www.theconnection.tv

PRAISE FOR *THE CONNECTION*

"If you're a fan of health documentaries such as Food Matters and Super Size Me, you'll eagerly munch (butter-free) popcorn watching the newest film on the block The Connection."

Women's Health Magazine

"There's a very important documentary that you need to see. And I don't want you to miss it. It's called The Connection."

Tom Roston, PBS

First published in Australia in 2016
Whole Health Life Publishing
www.wholehealthlifepublishing.com

Cover design by Blended Creative www.blended-creative.com.au
Internal design by Hieu Nguyen www.thinkbigdesigngroup.com

ISBN 978 0 9946466 0 6 (paperback)
ISBN 978 0 9946466 1 3 (hardcover)

The Whole Health Life

SHANNON HARVEY

Dedication

This book is dedicated to the people who have seen my film or read my blog and taken the time to write to me and share their own story. You fuel my fire.

Contents

Introduction

The Diagnosis

After working my heart out in high school and being accepted into a prestigious journalism school in Sydney, I landed my dream job as a news journalist for the Australian Broadcasting Corporation (ABC). My whole life had been building to this moment and I was finally there. Then I got sick.

In my first year of study at the University of Technology, Sydney, I was told that only two or three of us in a class of over a hundred would actually end up as paid journalists. I was determined to be one of them. I worked casual jobs at night while studying full time and took unpaid internships and extracurricular courses in film editing and photography to give me an edge for future job opportunities. I travelled overseas so I could pitch freelance stories to news organisations back home, hoping to get a lucky break. I was passionate about my craft and about seeking truth and telling stories that would, I hoped, make the world a better place.

The role with the ABC took me to Tasmania where I was responsible for reporting the news for the northwest of the state. It was a key region during elections and a fascinating part of Australia where folks were mostly farmers or miners and the stories I covered were anything and everything from the Prime Minister's visits to the potato crisis that farming families were facing. There were always two pairs of shoes in my car: heels for when the bigwigs were in town and muddied boots for when the story of the day involved presenting to camera from a paddock strewn with cow dung. I loved my job. I was 24 years old and my dreams were finally becoming reality... then the first signs of illness started to appear.

The symptoms came on slowly. After my regular evening runs my muscles were slow to recover. I thought I was just getting older and committed to pushing harder. Then it became difficult to get up in the mornings. I never felt as if I'd had enough sleep. I assumed it was my vegetarian diet and bumped up my supplements. But my symptoms got worse. My joints felt tender and my muscles started spasming, leaving me feeling inflamed and sensitive. Getting out of bed, getting dressed, brushing my teeth – all normal activities I'd never given a thought to – suddenly felt like hard work. The pain turned to agony. It started affecting my sleep and I needed painkillers to get through the day. My mood plummeted. I felt heavy. Exhausted. And worried.

I decided to see a doctor. I assumed she would prescribe some kind of medicine, give me an iron boost, or tell me to start eating meat. Instead she told me that my blood test results showed positive antinuclear antibodies and a positive rheumatoid factor, indicating an autoimmune disorder. The look she gave me said, "This is serious."

It wasn't until I saw a rheumatology specialist in Sydney that I understood why my doctor was worried. The rheumatologist thought I might have systemic lupus erythematosus (known as SLE, or lupus) and explained that my immune system was hyperactive. Instead of attacking only foreign invaders, it had also turned against my normal healthy tissue. He warned me that if the disease progressed I could end up in a wheelchair or with organ failure. He also explained that when the time came, I could have trouble conceiving a baby. There was no known cure and no known cause, though he suggested genetics might play a role. He prescribed immune-suppressing steroidal medication, wished me well, and sent me off to live the rest of my life with a chronic disease.

Because many autoimmune diseases have similar diagnostic markers and symptoms they can be very difficult to distinguish. Over the next six years different doctors I consulted gave my illness different labels (such as Sjögren's syndrome, fibromyalgia, or simply "connective tissue disorder") and I dutifully took their prescribed medications, trying different drugs and different doses. When these medicines did little more than cause weight gain, increase my sensitivity to sunlight, or fog up my head, I turned to alternative therapy. I tried everything – acupuncture, naturopathy, homeopathy, kinesiology, reiki, and every kind of massage. I went on organic food missions, took supplements and vitamins, started eating meat again, and switched to all-natural cosmetics and soaps. I saw psychologists who steered me into thinking I had a subconscious desire to stay sick, or a belief that I didn't deserve to be well. I tried reciting "I am well" mantras and even turned to tarot card readers, numerologists, and intuitive healers. If my doctors didn't have answers, then maybe The Universe did. I handed my money over to anyone and everyone who promised a cure, but I was still sick.

On one especially dismal day while on my lunch break from work, I remember hobbling across a road, taking each step as if I were walking through thick mud. I felt heavy and slow, with ceaseless pain from my inflamed muscles and joints. A frustrated driver waiting for me to cross saw only a young woman dawdling and holding things up. She beeped her car horn to hurry me on. The urgent, sudden noise was like a bomb exploding in my head. My heart raced; my muscles screamed. After I managed to get back to my office, I sat at my desk and started sobbing. In that moment – hopeless, helpless and burdened with arthritic pain no one could see or understand – facing the future was unbearable.

I wish I could travel back in time and tell that young woman what I now know. I would tell her there are many reasons she is sick but merely thinking or saying the words "I am healthy," even a hundred times a day, will not make her better. I would tell her that the answers she needs do not lie in the exploration of past lives or in visualising glowing balls of light. I would tell her that even though she is frustrated with conventional medicine, emerging research that expands mainstream medical understanding offers her a clear path to follow.

I would start by telling her what I have learned about the latest research in mind-body medicine – the scientific line of inquiry to understand how our minds and bodies interact to affect our health. I would tell her how this evidence-based, peer-reviewed academic research coming out of some of the most respected institutions in the world has exploded in the last 5-10 years thanks to advances in modern technology, and that some of this research is so hot off the press that even our doctors haven't had time to absorb it. I would explain that there is research linking the brain to the immune system, and research linking the brain to the gut to the immune system. I would explain that there is research about the importance of group support in improving outcomes for sick people and showing how feeling part of a closely-connected community affects human biochemistry in a way that makes it a keystone in the architecture of health. I would tell her about the research showing that stress reduction techniques (like meditation) can flip the switch on genes that affect disease and the rate of cellular ageing in our bodies. And I would tell her about the research showing that the interaction between a patient and a doctor can significantly alter the way a sick person's body responds to treatment.

I would sit my former chronically-ill self down, hand her this book, and explain that all this research put together predicts a hopeful future; that there are many things she can do for herself at that moment that will make a world of difference to her health. I would tell her in the kindest, gentlest way that she needs to make some changes. I would say, "It won't always be easy, but it *will* be worth it."

A Chronic Life and a Chronic Illness

At the time I got sick, I looked like a health insurer's ideal customer. No red flags. No reason to suggest I was destined to cost my insurer tens of thousands of dollars in medical claims.

Young ✓
Good income ✓
Regular exercise ✓
Healthy diet ✓
No family history of heart disease, cancer, obesity, or diabetes ✓
Non-smoker ✓
Low alcohol consumption ✓

But in reality, I was constantly stressed. I was responsible for feeding ever-hungry radio and television news bulletins that demanded fresh content every hour. The stories were short and fleeting and new ones were needed now. *Now.* NOW. At the end of each day I was frazzled, and as I drifted off to sleep at night, I worried about having to find a whole new set of stories the next day.

It wasn't just work that was worrying me. I was also living away from my family and friends and had been for years. Before getting the job with the ABC, I'd been working in Vanuatu in the South Pacific with a nongovernmental organisation (NGO) that trained local people in documentary production. In the days before social media and FaceTime, my connection with people who knew me well was mostly via text messages and email. Although I made an effort to make new friends, socialise, and take trips home, maintaining close relationships was getting harder and harder. People started forgetting my birthday. I had a deep underlying sense of isolation and loneliness.

When it came to some of the relationships I did hold on to, I was a chronic caretaker, investing enormous amounts of energy into certain friends and family members I thought needed saving. I would take their problems on as my own and fret when they didn't act on my advice. And when I wasn't dealing with other people's problems, I was taking on the problems of the entire world. I was the kind of person who agonised about which was the more environmentally friendly way to dry my hands in a public bathroom – hand dryer or paper towel?

To make up for sleep deprivation, I turned to coffee and caffeinated energy drinks. In a vicious cycle, the anxiety-infused insomnia led to more caffeine, and the caffeine led to more insomnia.

Life as a journalist also often meant eating on the run. While I made an effort to find good food and avoid fast food, I ate a ton of takeaway. I had been a vegetarian for six years and was lactose intolerant at a time when lactose intolerance was seen as a new age, hippie fad. Living in the northwest of Tasmania, an area with a proud tradition of family-owned dairy farms, where the standard evening fare involved variations on meat and three veggies, I was a difficult, odd dinner guest and dreaded explaining my diet to people. The non-dairy, non-meat meal options didn't necessarily mean healthier choices either. I was eating a lot of processed foods. Included in my weekly shopping were products with names like "Not Bacon" (which lived up to its name and tasted more like rubber than the real thing). I would also get crippling stomach cramps on a regular basis, which I now know were caused by an undiagnosed egg allergy. I dealt with these cramps by taking over-the-counter medication, and just pushed through.

On top of all this, despite not having any family history of the big three – cancer, diabetes, and heart disease – chronic disease *does* run in my family. My dad has psoriatic arthritis, a condition where his immune system causes dry skin and inflammation; my grandmother vaguely recalls being diagnosed with lupus when she was in her 30s; and on both sides of my family there is a long history of mental illnesses such as anxiety, depression, and addiction.

The point here is that all these elements of my stress-charged life came together to create the perfect storm in my body, a storm that switched on genes to trigger autoimmune disease. Had I been able to step back and look at my life as a whole, I would have seen that things were way out of balance and that I was actually far from being a poster girl for health insurance.

Constant stress ✓
Poor sleep ✓
Dysfunctional relationships ✓
Loneliness and isolation ✓
Family history ✓
Unbalanced diet, food allergies, and sensitivities ✓ ✓ ✓

An Epidemic

The scary thing about my illness is that I'm no unique snowflake. According to the World Health Organization (WHO), there's a two in three chance you'll end up dying from a chronic disease.[1] In the US alone, 43 percent of *kids* have a chronic health condition[2] and healthcare costs are rising more quickly than incomes.[3] It's the same in Australia, where medical costs are increasing by more than eight percent every year and doubled between 2002 and 2012.[4] Our healthcare systems are drowning under the rising tide. For all the wonders of modern medicine and all our advances in drugs and surgeries, the number of worldwide deaths from chronic diseases is projected to increase from 38 million in 2012 to 52 million by 2030,[5] and the cost of this global burden of disease is predicted to soar beyond $47 trillion by 2030.[6] No wonder WHO has labelled this "an impending disaster"[7] and the United Nations Secretary-General Ban Ki-moon describes the rise in chronic illness as a "global epidemic."[8]

It's highly likely that your great grandparents would never have heard of many of the conditions causing concern among today's health experts[9] – obesity, diabetes, depression. But chances are you know someone, or you are someone who is taking medication or supplements for ailments such as asthma, high blood pressure, arthritis, thyroid conditions, sinus issues, gut problems, migraines, back pain, chronic fatigue, or anxiety. These illnesses are all attributed to, or worsened by, our lifestyles.[10] In fact, in the US alone, one in four adults has two or more chronic health conditions.[11] While we may be living longer than our ancestors, it's arguable that when it comes to our health, many of us are not living any *better*

There is one thing we know for sure about this epidemic of chronic disease: the current approach is not working. I have spoken to countless people who have described the soul-destroying endless loop of tests, drugs, and appointments followed by more tests, drugs, and appointments that inevitably follow a diagnosis of chronic illness. Don't get me wrong; if I were in a serious car accident, the first place I'd want to be is the emergency room of a major hospital. If I had a heart attack, broken bones, a major wound or infection, or if I urgently needed a cancerous tumour removed, I would want to be treated by the best conventionally-trained medical expert I could find. Conventional medicine works wonders when it comes to acute care and life-saving emergency responses. Where conventional medicine is failing us is in dealing with ongoing chronic health issues that don't heal quickly and can worsen over time.

When we see our doctor because of fatigue, aches and pains, an upset stomach, sinus problems, insomnia, or depression, we usually leave with a prescription that treats our symptoms rather than the cause of our discomfort. Have a sore back? Take some painkillers. Chronic arthritis? Try this anti-inflammatory. Feeling blue? Have some anti-depressants. These are bandage solutions that rarely treat the actual causes of these sorts of problems.

As patients we can end up feeling disempowered, leaving each appointment with a prescription, a bill, and a feeling of helplessness. We become afraid. Afraid to plan for the future because we don't know how our illness might progress from one day, month, or year to the next; and afraid of being seen as a burden or killjoy to those around us. The illness stops us from living life to the full, pain weighs us down, discomfort makes us short-tempered, and physical and emotional limitations prevent us from fully embracing life. We're alive. But we're not *living*.

Our doctors and other health care professionals mean well, but many don't know where to start. They don't have the time, money, or resources to invest in keeping up to date with the latest peer-reviewed science that forms the backbone of this book. In the US, demand for physicians continues to grow faster than supply, with a projected shortfall of up to 90,400 physicians by 2025.[12] In a review of the quality of care among patients in the US, only 60 percent of those with chronic conditions received the recommended level of care.[13] Our doctors are drowning; too busy mopping up the flood rather than turning off the tap. They're struggling to keep up with the tsunami of chronic illness patients. This may in part explain why a recent study showed that doctors are at great risk for burnout,[14] and highlights to me that our health care providers need to be given this information just as much as their patients do.

With all this in mind, it's really little wonder that one study showed it takes an average of *17 years* for new discoveries to become part of medical

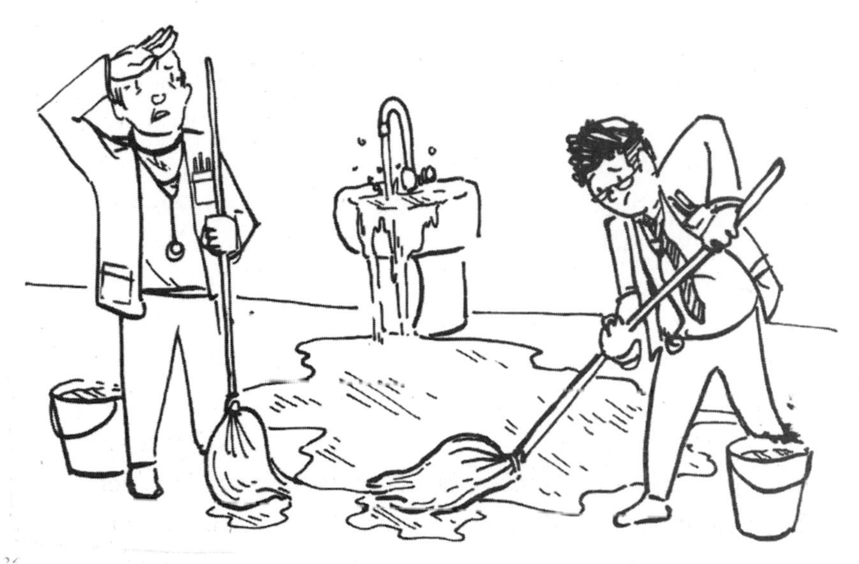

Our doctors are drowning; too busy mopping up the flood rather than turning off the tap.

practices.[15] That's a long time to wait when you're living with a chronic illness. I wasn't prepared to wait around when the directions I needed to put me on the road to recovery were waiting to be uncovered. I decided to use the skills I had developed as a journalist to make my own map.

I scoured countless scientific papers and systematic reviews of the health literature, taking four and a half years to wade through the evidence and interview leading scientists and experts in order to make sense of it. I wanted to go way beyond catchy media headlines in order to understand the science behind the news and interpret how to apply this information to my life and my health. Although the science was often complex, the real-world application was simple: these were things I could be doing for myself, they were inexpensive, and I could get started right away.

Throughout this book you'll learn about some of the critical factors that are often overlooked when we're considering how to get well or stay well in our modern world. I will introduce you to pioneering researchers at the frontier of health and wellness, and I'll share some of the things in my life that made all the difference in my own journey to getting well. But before we dive in, I want to make an important point. This book is not about wishing yourself well or imagining away cancer cells in order to shrink a tumour. While this book does explore the research showing that the state of your mind is extremely important in changing the course of an illness and may even add years to your life, I am not making an argument that tending to your mental state is more important than taking advantage of what modern medicine has to offer. This book has its foundations in evidence-based journalism and throughout you'll notice references to the primary studies and systematic reviews I examined so you can look them up if you'd like to go deeper into the research for yourself.

The Whole-Health Prescription

I write these words 10 years after my diagnosis. My life is completely different now than it was then, not only because my health has done a 180-degree turn, but because of the changes I have made in order for that to happen.

My starting point was a paper written for medical students by an Australian MD named Craig Hassed that I stumbled across in late 2009 on about the twentieth page of a Google search. This paper –"Mind-Body Medicine: Science, Practice and Philosophy" – changed my life.[16] Hassed is an associate professor at Monash University and a prolific author. In this particular paper, he summarised peer-reviewed academic research so that future doctors being trained at the Monash School of Medicine could apply it to their own clinical practice. The paper highlighted the emergence of *evidence-based* mind-body medicine and explained how advances in technology have allowed us to look at the way things like the brain and the immune system interact to affect health. For example, Hassed referred to research demonstrating that the immune systems of medical students became profoundly suppressed before or just after a stressful exam period, but when they were taught relaxation techniques, the students showed significantly better immune function and less illness during exams.[17] He also cited research examining how chronic or long-term activation of the stress response leads to what is called "allostatic load" which is associated with impaired immunity, obesity, hypertension, and atrophy of nerve cells in the brain.[18]

Hassed also referred to the work of Jon Kabat-Zinn, a microbiologist turned mindfulness meditation teacher whose pioneering research, begun in the late 1970s, was instrumental in introducing stress reduction and meditation in medical settings. Kabat-Zinn's early research found that people who meditated while receiving light therapy to treat psoriasis healed four times more quickly than non-meditators.[19] The idea that doing something in the mind could have such a dramatic impact on the scaly, dry skin of these sick people captivated me. What other evidence was there for taking a mind-body, whole-health approach in treating chronic disease? My evidence-based journey to recovery had begun.

I came across a study published in the *Journal of the American Medical Association* that showed that a lifestyle program for people with heart disease resulted in delaying, stopping, or reversing the progression of heart disease.[20] The man behind that study and similar studies is Dean Ornish, a clinical professor of medicine at the University of California at San Francisco, and the founder of the Preventive Medicine Research Institute.[21] I travelled to San Francisco to interview him and learned that, in addition to heart disease, the Ornish program has been effective in treating type 2 diabetes and may slow, stop, or even reverse the progression of early-stage prostate cancer.[22] The Ornish program is a doctor-supervised lifestyle program that includes a healthy diet, exercise, stress management training – including yoga and meditation – smoking cessation, and group support (for which US Medicare covers the cost in hospitals and clinics). Ornish also teamed up with a major health insurer, and not only did the people in the program achieve better health outcomes, when the insurer looked at the dollars and cents, it reported that customers' health care costs were reduced by half in a three-year period.[23] The whole-health approach wasn't just making sense from a patient outcome perspective. It was making financial sense too.

The Ornish program isn't the only one turning the medical paradigm upside down. I travelled to Massachusetts, the heartland of this research, where I interviewed Herbert Benson, a professor of medicine at Harvard University who is known as the father of mind-body medicine. Recently, patients who participated in his programs – which also involve healthy eating, stress management, and exercise – reduced their medical visits on average by 43 percent in the following year.[24] As part of the program, Benson developed a meditation technique called the "relaxation response" that has also been shown to switch off genes affecting disease.[25]

Back home, I met Professor George Jelinek, an Aussie trailblazer making waves in the multiple sclerosis (MS) community by developing a program for this autoimmune disease for which conventional medicine has no cure. Jelinek, who is one of the most respected emergency physicians in Australia, was diagnosed with MS when he was in the prime of his career. This was a crushing blow to a man who witnessed his mother's tragic experience with this inheritable illness that ultimately led her to commit suicide.

Instead of accepting his diagnosis as destiny, he used his academic skills to scour medical literature and developed an evidence-based lifestyle program to treat MS.[26] The amazing thing about Jelinek is that he has not only recovered from MS, but others who follow his *Overcoming Multiple Sclerosis* program have done the same.[27] I like to call them the "OMS All Stars" because, by following the program which involves a healthy diet, exercise, stress management, sunlight, vitamin supplementation and, when needed, medication, they have achieved what conventional medicine says cannot be done: recover from MS.

When you look at the lifestyle changes these programs recommend, they all have something in common. Rather than focusing on just one key aspect of health, such as medication or diet, their foundation is taking a whole-health, whole-life approach to getting better. Those who follow these programs are supervised by conventional medical doctors. They shift their diets to include more whole foods and fresh fruits and vegetables and integrate movement and exercise into their everyday lives. They're taught how to make meditation and mindfulness a habit, not a chore. They're taught about emotional balance, to change the way they view stress, and to work out what really matters in life. Another element these programs share, which I think is at the heart of their success and is perhaps the most underestimated weapon we have in the fight against chronic disease, is that participants become part of a supportive community that encourages them every day to prioritise their health – and shows them how to do so.

The exciting thing about these programs and the new science of mind-body health is that we now have a bridge between the "reductionist" approach to medicine that brought us great advances in modern medicine by breaking down complex processes in our body into smaller component parts, and the "holistic" approach that takes the view that we cannot study the forest by looking at one tree alone. Holism is based on Aristotle's observation that "the whole is more than the sum of its parts," a sensible statement when we consider the human body and how its different systems interact. Unfortunately, the term "holistic medicine" has become tainted in some medical circles and is seen by some conventional medical experts as having been hijacked by alternative therapists. But this new research, which forms the basis of this book, shows us that the two principles can now come together. We can now develop a rigorous, evidence-based, whole-health approach to healing and wellness.

The take-home message is that good health is not just about taking our medicine, eating our vegetables, exercising regularly, and getting enough sleep. Those things are all essential, but we need to take a whole-health approach, and that means also reviewing our mindsets, beliefs and expectations, tending to our stress levels and emotional wellbeing, and nurturing our relationships. In the same way that holism teaches us we cannot study the forest by looking at an individual tree, we cannot just tend to one aspect of our life and expect that our health ecosystem will be in balance. Good health means nourishing each of the components in the system that are dependent on one another. As one part begins to thrive, we can turn our attention to another, and pretty soon what follows is the very definition of health that, as WHO so eloquently says, is "a state of complete physical, mental, and social wellbeing, and not merely the absence of disease or infirmity."

The Whole-Health Life

My own whole-health life transformation involved practising yoga and meditation regularly; changing my perception of work stress; learning to balance my emotions; and fostering deep connections with family and friends to build a supportive community. In time, my insomnia passed. I started exercising regularly again. I overcame my nutritional deficiencies and developed better food habits. Eventually, my arthritic flare-ups became fewer and farther apart. I no longer felt the need to try different prescription medications or search for a label for my disease. The darkness, hopelessness, and despair shifted. I began planning exciting, challenging projects for myself, no longer afraid of what my health might be like in the future. I fell in love, got married, and became a mother. My life is turning out nothing like the medical prognosis I was given.

I felt driven to share what I had learned with others, so instead of paying down the mortgage on our little house on Sydney's northern beaches, my film producer husband, Julian (Jules) Harvey, and I decided to invest the profits from my production company into making a film. The result of three years of work was *The Connection*, a documentary featuring some of the world's leading experts in mind-body medicine as well as people with remarkable stories of recovery from illnesses like heart disease, infertility, chronic back pain, terminal cancer, and multiple sclerosis – despite their medical prognoses.

The film was released in October 2014 through a sold-out worldwide tour. The response was phenomenal. Within months, hundreds of people had hosted their own screenings and held community forums. One of the biggest surprises was the medical community's response. Hospitals, medical centres, and healthcare groups hosted screenings and held public discussions. Doctors started handing DVDs of the film to their patients and showing it in their waiting rooms. The film became essential viewing for medical students at some of the most respected universities in the world. Even health insurers and corporate behemoths got in touch with me, wanting to know more about getting the message out. When I began writing my blog (www.thewholehealthlife.com) people all around the world started following along and writing to me, wanting to know more about my own autoimmune disease recovery and what steps I had taken. From there, the idea for this book was born.

I've written this book partly as a personal journey informed by the scientific evidence, but also as a practical guide so that you can follow along and make slow, sustainable changes in your own life if you wish. It's not just a book for sick people. It's for well people too. I've lost count of the number of times people have told me they wish they hadn't needed to get sick in order to start making the necessary changes in their lives.

This book covers a lot of ground, and while you may be keen to get started making changes in your own life straight away, my experience has shown me that doing too much, too quickly, is a sure-fire way to set yourself up to fail in the long run. I suggest you focus on just one topic per month. Some aspects will be easy to implement, some will be hard. You will have setbacks and you will have monumental breakthroughs. You'll find you're already on top of some things, and others will feel like a mountainous climb to the summit. Most important, if you're reading this and you're sick, I do not recommend waiting 10 or 20 years for the system to catch up with the latest science. Don't rely solely on drugs and surgery or the next medical breakthrough to get you well when there are things you can be doing for yourself *right now* that can make a huge difference. I cannot promise this approach will make you live longer. I cannot even promise that this will cure your ills. But I can promise that focusing on the 10 topics in *The Whole Health Life* will lead to a better life.

Finally, if you're reading this and feeling well, I ask you this – why wait until you experience a personal health catastrophe to take control of your health? There is nothing to lose here and everything to gain.

Chapter 1

Stress

A Turning Point

In 2009 I found myself in the South Pacific island nation of Samoa the day after a 3.5 metre (11.5 foot) tsunami rolled through and killed more than a hundred people.[1] I was there as a video journalist – a one-woman band traveling with a light camera and editing kit in order to get to people and places that conventional crews could not. At the heart of my story were the remarkable people from the Australian Federal Police Disaster Victim Identification team. Their job requires them to be on call 24/7 to respond to any kind of disaster. They worked tirelessly to find and identify the missing tsunami victims so their families could get closure. Telling the story meant getting to know an amazingly resilient group of people that had spent days and days in the morgue of a developing country that was utterly destroyed. Their triumphs were bittersweet; every breakthrough meant sorrowful news for a victim's family. They had to apply meticulous detective skills in the face of cataclysmic grief and find meaning and lightness in the face of devastation.

I dropped everything to tell this story. I left colleagues in the lurch back home and missed important family events. I went days without proper sleep. What's scary is that prioritising work in this way wasn't at all unusual for me. It was the rinse-and-repeat story of my life. I was determined not to let my illness get in the way of my career, so I ploughed on and took new and exciting roles whenever the opportunity arose.

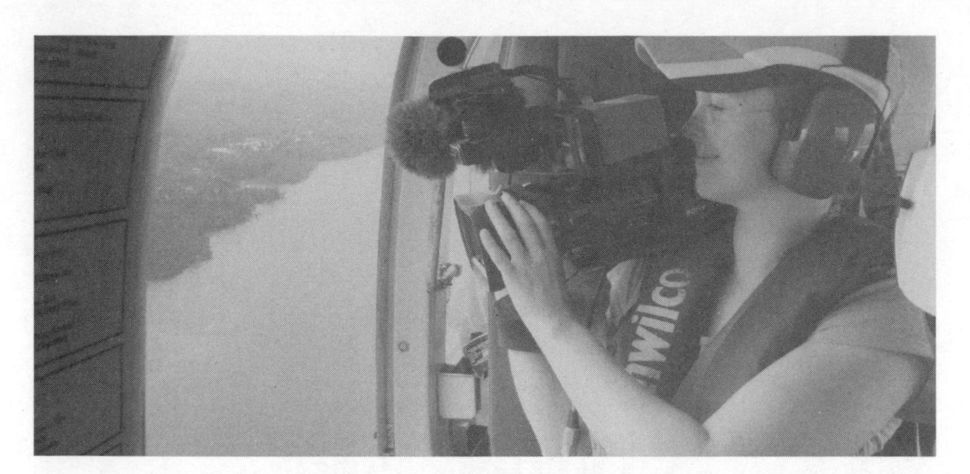

Shannon Harvey filming from a helicopter in the South Pacific, 2009 *Credit: Nathan Long*

In the years since my autoimmune disease diagnosis, I had landed a job in Sydney with Fairfax, one of the biggest media brands in Australia. At a time when digital innovation was the company's focus, I was making a name for myself as a video journalist and had developed skills not only in research and reporting, but also in shooting and editing. I'd taken on new producing roles in television, established my own production company, and started lecturing in television journalism at the University of Technology, Sydney. Work was my number one priority. Weekends were non-existent. I remember more than once wishing the whole world would just stop for few days so I could catch up on my To Do list. When that wish was granted because of a four-day Easter long weekend, I seized the opportunity to bulldoze through while everyone else took a break.

But the Samoa story changed things. Despite my exclusive access, the worthiness of the story, and the compelling accounts from people who opened their hearts to me on camera, the story didn't fit into the program schedule. It never went to air. To this day, no one has seen it. And I paid a costly price. While the story sat on the cutting room floor, my immune system went into overdrive and my disease flared up. I felt as if I'd been hit by a truck. Everything hurt. Every nerve. Every muscle. Every joint. A thick fog descended over me disconnecting my mind and body, perhaps as a way to cope with the ceaseless pain that came from my whole body being inflamed. I was popping painkillers like candy. My relationships were at breaking point. I was stressed out, overwhelmed, and functioning on fumes.

It was a turning point because what came next was a necessary time of self-reflection. I thought about the work I had done over the years and about the stories I had reported. I wondered what difference they really made and realised I could count on one hand the number of times I had actually made any kind of lasting impact. I would give my work everything, above and beyond anything else – and at immeasurable personal expense – all for a lofty ideal that was rarely achieved. I was five years on from my autoimmune diagnosis, had spent more than $30,000 on my health, and I was still sick. Something had to change. The never-to-be broadcast Samoa story was a wake-up call and started me thinking about my work, about my stress, and about my illness. It made me seriously reconsider where my priorities needed to be.

The Stress Epidemic

These days I often see my stressed-out former self reflected back at me when I have conversations with friends and colleagues about time. Words like *hectic, whirlwind,* and *insane* are ubiquitous in every exchange. There is a perception that time is speeding up on us as we tally the number of days and weeks worked without time off, the number of hours we haven't slept, the holidays we haven't taken, or the mania of our kids' before and after school schedules. Some people even wear this "crazy busyness" as a badge of honour, as if it were a status symbol of success or a measure of capability; a personal branding that says they're *somebody,* going *somewhere,* and achieving *something.*

When you consider that we live in a world with washing machines, microwaves, the Internet, GPS enabled cars, supermarkets, email, and smart phones, it's hard to understand why we seem to have less time, not more, and that despite the wonders of this modern world, we're increasingly stressed. The American Psychological Association reports that a third of adults say their stress level has risen in the past year and their stress has a strong impact on their physical and mental health.[2] A 2015 report examined the health of the Australian workforce and found that 65.1 percent of employees had moderate to high stress levels.[3] It is a similar story in the UK where a 2015 report found there were 9.9 million lost work days because of stress, anxiety, or depression, and an estimated 234,000 new cases of work related stress that year.[4]

Apparently we're all stressed about pretty much the same stuff. Money, work, and family responsibilities constantly top the lists in stress surveys.[5] In the US, more than 120,000 deaths per year are associated with work-related stress such as long working hours, job insecurity, and work-family conflict.[6] And this isn't just a Western phenomenon; the Japanese even have a special name for death by overwork – *karoshi*, with an estimated 10,000 incidents each year. In China they call it *guolaosi*, with a staggering 600,000 incidents estimated each year.[7]

Stress is the reason many of us say we eat too much and sleep too little; it's the reason we're distracted, grumpy, impatient, and sick.[8] And if all that hasn't stressed you out, then this probably will: stress and disease are closely connected. Chronic stress is associated with a greater risk of depression, heart disease, diabetes, autoimmune diseases, upper respiratory infections, poorer wound healing, and increased susceptibility to infectious illnesses.[9] According to a study done by Emily Ansell from the Yale School of Medicine, stress shrinks key regions of our brain that are involved with emotion regulation and impulse control.[10] There is also an extensive body of work done by the pioneering husband and wife research team Ronald and Janice Kiecolt-Glaser from Ohio State University that irrefutably links high levels of stress to malfunction of the immune system.[11] There is even evidence from research done at the University of California, San Francisco that chronic stress can make cells age more quickly.[12]

With all this in mind, you might think my conclusions about stress are that it should be avoided at all costs. And given that this book is designed to offer practical ways to use the latest mind-body science to improve our health, you might expect me to now outline a step-by-step process on how to quit your stressful job, move to a low-cost beachside location, or run away to join a monastery. But although the science clearly shows that long-term stress can be bad for us, it also shows that some stress can be *good*. In fact, a robust and growing body of research shows that stress can have a positive effect on our health, wellbeing, and performance.[13]

Not All Stress is Bad

If you're anything like me and the 23 million others who have watched the YouTube video of surfer Mick "White Lightning" Fanning's shark encounter during the 2015 J-Bay Open surfing competition in South Africa, your heart started pounding right away.[14] The huge dorsal fin of what experts estimate to be a 3.5 metre (11.5 foot) great white shark rises up out of the ocean and takes Fanning by surprise.[15] By his own account given on live television moments after the encounter, the shark came from behind and Fanning instinctively lifted his leg out of the way before he started punching it. "I just sort of went into fight or flight, really," Fanning said later in an interview.[16]

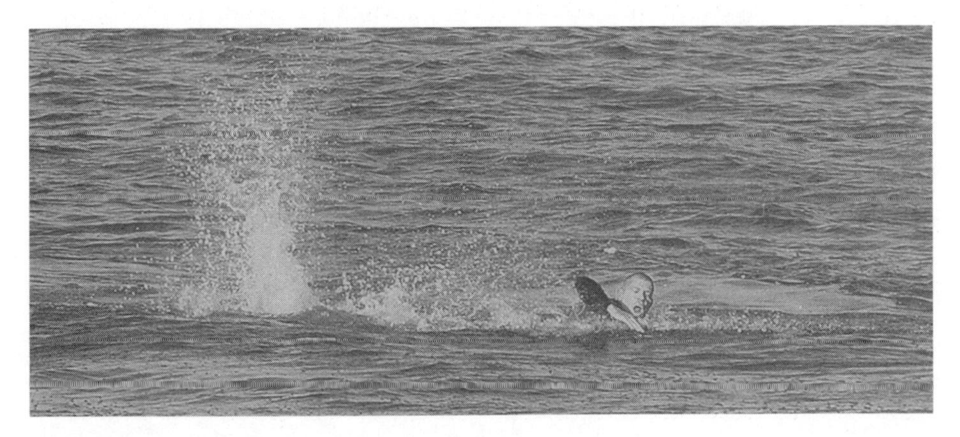

Mick Fanning moments after being knocked off his surfboard by a great white shark at the 2015 J-Bay Open. *Credit: Jimmy Wilson*

This "fight or flight" stress response to which Fanning referred is an evolutionary superpower designed to save your life. When the part of your brain called the amygdala detects a threat it sends a high-speed signal to another brain region called the hypothalamus – the stress response command centre – which immediately takes charge and sends urgent messages around your body to prepare for battle. As if you had hit the gas pedal of a car, your sympathetic nervous system, which operates without your having to think about it, instantaneously kicks in and sends a surge of powerful hormones, including adrenaline and cortisol, into your bloodstream. This amplifies your heart rate, muscle strength, and metabolism. Your body is flooded with glucose for energy and shuts down non-essential systems including your digestive system, sex drive, and complex thought processing. You begin to breathe faster, which boosts the amount of oxygen in your brain and sharpens your senses to put you on high alert. Your pupils dilate to let in more light and your hearing becomes more acute. Blood flow is diverted to your essential organs and muscles causing a clammy, sweaty feeling on your skin. Your immune cell troops muster in parts of your body at high risk of being wounded.[17] When the threat is over, your body's "rest and digest" parasympathetic nervous system takes over. Cortisol starts putting on the brakes. Your heart rate slows, your muscles relax, and your body returns to balance and calm.[18]

If you were facing a hungry sabre-toothed tiger on the savannah 11,000 years ago, or even a great white shark today, this vital physical response could be the difference between your life and death. But today, when you're in the helpless inferno of peak hour traffic, or impotently watching your favourite football team get trounced, a response like this is completely useless and can even be dangerous to your health.

If the fight or flight hormones that give you life-saving superpowers are released regularly, over a long period of time, they can have a devastating effect in your body. In what is called "immune dysregulation," your immune system can start malfunctioning, inducing low-grade chronic inflammation in your body, and suppressing the number, movement, and function of the good, protective immune cells. Chronic stress may also increase your susceptibility to some types of cancer by suppressing protective immune cells and increasing suppressor cells.[19] Your immune cells can also become insensitive to cortisol's regulatory effect on the stress response.[20] Essentially, the brakes on your stress response get worn through and a runaway train of inflammation can promote the development and progression of many diseases. Researchers call this effect "allostatic load."[21]

To explain the good stress/bad stress concept another way, consider this: when leading stress researcher Firdaus Dhabhar, an associate professor of psychiatry at Stanford University, takes his kids to be vaccinated, he first runs around with them in a park in order to trigger a mild stress response. He does this because his research shows that mild stress can enhance your immune system's response to a vaccine.[22]

Dhabhar's research also revealed that this healthy, useful, short-term stress can help you recover more quickly from surgery.[23] He's even found that when he induces cancer in mice by exposing them to ultraviolet light, the development of the cancer can be delayed by mildly stressing them before their UV sunlamp sessions. This has prompted him to speculate that giving cancer patients low-dose injections of stress hormones might one day be used to help prime their immune systems to better fight cancer. "It may not work out, but if it did, the benefits could be tremendous," he told *Stanford Magazine*.[24]

There is a crucially important distinction here between "good stress," which is an appropriate, short-term response and lasts for minutes or hours, and "bad stress," which is unnecessary, long-term, and lasts for months or years. Dhabhar uses a stress spectrum diagram to help explain what we should aim for.

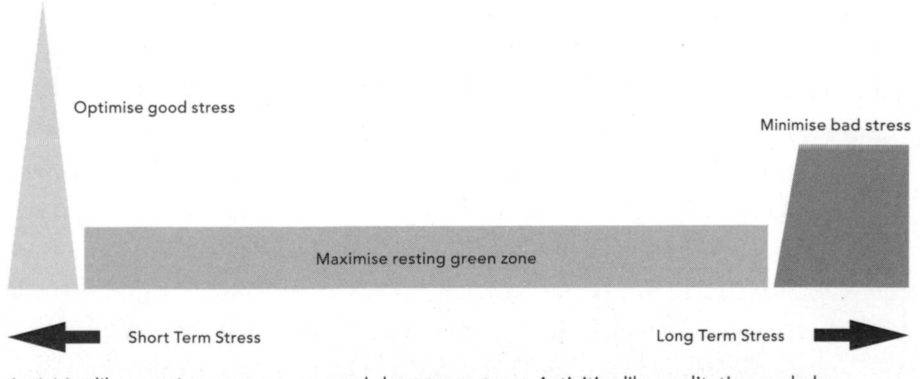

Activities like exercise can promote good short-term stress. Activities like meditation can help minimise bad long-term stress. Adapted from: Dhabhar, FS, 2014. Effects of stress on immune function: the good, the bad, and the beautiful. *Immunologic Research*, 58(2-3), 193-210, May.

At one end of the spectrum are brief episodes of stress where your body mounts a helpful, positive response to a threat. At the other end of the spectrum is long-term, dangerous stress. Right in the middle, taking up the ideal bulk of our time, is a "green zone" of low stress.

This doesn't mean you have to add base jumping, public speaking, or snake wrangling to your daily calendar. Instead, Dhabhar advises harnessing the everyday aggravations that life already throws at us. In essence, a hassle a day may keep the pathogens away.[25] He reminds us that getting regular exercise is helpful because it triggers a mild stress response. I'll have more about that for you in Chapter 5 (Exercise). I'll have more on how to nurture your low-stress green zone later in this chapter.

These new breakthroughs in stress research are forcing scientists to broaden the definition of stress beyond merely fight or flight. To explain this further, I want to take you back to the 2015 J-Bay Open and look at what else happened on that fateful day. Let's start with Fanning's good mate and competition rival, Julian Wilson, who, when the shark made its move, also happened to be in the water competing for world championship surfing points and the winner's purse. Instead of hastening away, Wilson plunged toward the danger. "I literally thought when I was paddling for him that I wasn't going to get there in time... I was like, I've got a board, if I can get there I can stab it or whatever, I've got a weapon," he said on television soon after they'd returned safely to shore.[26] Clearly Wilson was in full "fight" rather than "flight" mode, but what kind of biological insanity would compel him to paddle toward the threat?

Though adrenaline and cortisol are perhaps the best-known stress hormones, it turns out that an entire cocktail of chemicals may play as important a role in our stress response. For example, dopamine (a chemical associated with motivation, pleasure, and reward) and oxytocin (sometimes referred to as the "cuddle hormone") are both released during the stress response. Oxytocin is a hormone known for its role in intimacy and social bonding. It fine-tunes your brain to notice what others are thinking and feeling, and primes you to build and strengthen relationships. Scientists have called the oxytocin component of the stress response the "tend and befriend" response after observing that during stressful situations, people can engage in *tending* (as a parent would their vulnerable offspring during an attack) and *befriending* (handy for collaborating during times of peril).[27] So the effects of stress on our behaviour can not only be self-serving, but can also make us altruistic or even heroic in order to promote survival and wellbeing for the good of the tribe.

All that extra cuddle hormone that coursed through the bodies of the surf-riding gladiators at the J-Bay Open may also explain the numerous masculine embraces that followed soon after the immediate threat had passed. "We're all just trying to process more than anything, you kind of just want to hug him," said commentator Peter Mel moments after Fanning and Wilson were safely on board the rescue boat. Hearing his suggestion, the skipper left the helm to embrace Fanning. I lost count of the number of heartfelt hugs that followed. Given that hugging is known to lower levels of stress hormones such as cortisol, and that a recent study found hugging can reduce your susceptibility to fall ill during times of stress, all those manly moments may have given the guys just what they needed on what must have been a traumatic day for everyone concerned.[28]

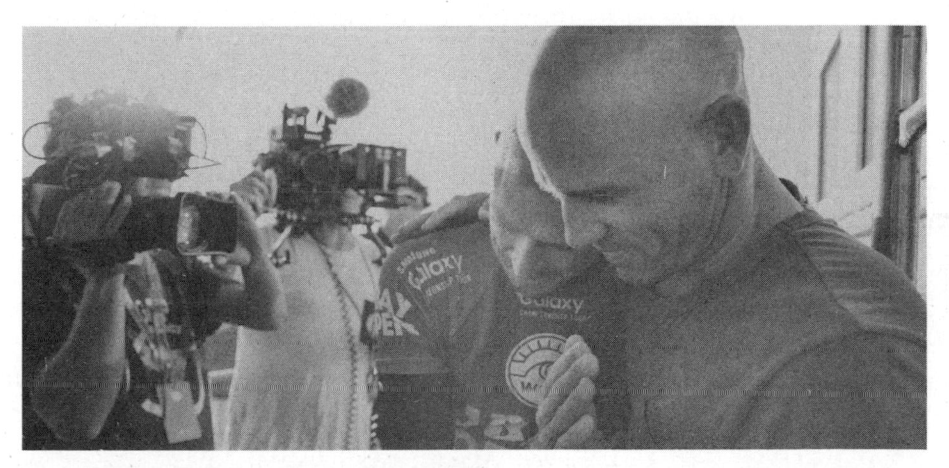

Mick Fanning and Kelly Slater hugging after Fanning's great white shark encounter at the 2015 J-Bay Open. *Credit: Jimmy Wilson*

The main point here is that although media headlines declaring "Stress May be the Worst Killer of the Modern Era" make us believe that all stress is bad, the latest research proves that this is far from the case. In fact, it's largely been forgotten that the father of our modern scientific understanding of stress, Hans Selye, actually distinguished between two kinds of stress – eustress (a word derived from the Greek root *eu* which means good, as in euphoria) and distress (stemming from the Latin root *dis,* meaning ill, or bad, as in disease or disabled).[29] We experience *eu*stress when we perceive a stressor as positive.[30] It warns and motivates us to rapidly adapt.[31] *Dis*tress, on the other hand, is negative, and we experience this when a demand is perceived to vastly exceed a person's capabilities.[32]

It was recently revealed that much of Selye's research was supported by Big Tobacco, which in the late 1960s and 1970s was searching for ways to dilute the emerging body of evidence against smoking and blame disease on anything other than cigarettes. Although his theories considered both the upside and downside of stress, Selye publicly emphasised the risks associated with stress in order to promote the benefits of smoking as a stress reliever. In light of the revelation about the tobacco industry's involvement, we start to see how the foundation was laid in the popular media for our modern perception of stress as a dangerous villain.[33]

Perception is the Key

These days, "stress" is a catch-all phrase we apply to a variety of negative mental states and circumstances. Exams are stressful. Our jobs are stressful. Moving house is stressful. So is being homeless. Years of infertility are stressful. And so is wrangling two children under the age of three in a supermarket. No matter where you sit on the continuum of life circumstances, when you say you're feeling stressed, you're probably referring to a negative, subjective feeling of being overwhelmed by the amount of responsibility you face – and which you might feel is too much to handle. And this feeling is different for everyone.

It was the less famous American physiologist John Wayne Mason, who in the 1960s and 1970s cohabited the Wild West of stress research frontiers with Hans Selye, who found that our perception of a stressful event was critical to how our body responded.[34] Mason discovered that the nature of our individual stress response depends on how we individually perceive each situation. Whereas one person may be consumed by terror at the thought of public speaking, another might see it as an exciting challenge. Research shows that each person's performance and biology responds accordingly.[35]

In a compelling study demonstrating that the same circumstances affect people in different ways, Firdaus Dhabhar teamed up with Nobel Prize winner Australian scientist Elizabeth Blackburn. They compared the cellular age of mothers of disabled children with mothers of healthy children. One surprising finding was that women who perceived themselves to have a great deal of stress in their lives had a greater rate of cellular ageing, regardless of whether they were carers of disabled children or not. In fact, women who perceived themselves to have high stress had aged the equivalent of 9-17 additional years, compared with the low-stress group.[36]

In another compelling study, researchers compared data from a national health survey of more than 28,000 people and data from national mortality records. They found that people who reported high levels of stress in their lives *and* who believed that stress was bad for them had a whopping 43 percent increased risk of dying prematurely.[37] To put this in perspective, the researchers say that if their posited causal relationship is valid, then 20,231 premature deaths each year in the US would be attributable to having a lot of stress *and* perceiving that stress negatively affects health.

Researchers are now turning their attention to working out what might be going on between our minds and bodies to help explain these stunning findings. If you'd like to read about one possible explanation, check out the section "When Your Body Believes Your Mind" in Chapter 3 (Belief).

If you're anything like me, it will take you a while to wrap your head around these ideas. When I first got sick, I definitely erred too much toward the chronic long-term stress end of the spectrum. I viewed all the stressors in my life (work, relationships, time, money) as monumental. I was chronically worried about my chronic stress. In a vicious cycle, I was stressed about my stress. I also knew that when I was stressed, my health suffered, and that I needed to do something about it. So I started researching proven, evidence-based ways to change my *perception* of stress so that I could spend more time in the low-stress green zone.

The Relaxation Response

In the late 1960s, a young cardiologist named Herbert Benson sneaked transcendental meditators through the side door of his lab at Harvard Medical School to study what happened to their bodies when they meditated. Benson was interested in the human stress response after becoming concerned that he was misdiagnosing people with high blood pressure. In what is now known as "white coat hypertension," he suspected that when his patients saw his white coat and measuring instruments they became worried and their heart rates rose in response.

Benson had studied the work of Harvard physiologist Walter B Cannon, who in 1915 was the first person to identify the fight or flight response, and he wanted to extend the research to investigate the relationship between our minds, our physiological stress responses, and our health.

Benson was approached by a group of devotees of Maharishi Mahesh Yogi, whose Transcendental Meditation teachings were gaining popularity in the counter-culture of the 1960s thanks to the admiration of celebrities like The Beatles. But studying meditation was considered career suicide by the scientific community, so Benson conducted his research after sundown, and by stealth. "If studying stress was in another world, studying meditation was in another universe with respect to science," Benson told me, as he described rigging up hippies with intravenous catheters, respiration masks, heart rate monitors, and electrodes on their heads in order to take physiological measurements while they meditated.

His work led to one of the major breakthroughs in modern mind-body medicine. Benson found dramatic physiological changes in his meditating subjects. He recorded decreased metabolism, heart rate, breathing rate, and slower brain waves. He called his discovery the "relaxation response" to suggest its role as a counter to the stress response. And although Benson never met his fight or flight predecessor, Walter B Cannon, the story comes full circle with the fact that Benson's secretive research took place in the same lab at Harvard that Cannon used 60 years before.[38]

But the enquiring mind of the young physician wasn't satisfied with just studying the meditators. He went on to determine that the relaxation response he had observed could be triggered using scores of different techniques embedded in different traditions around the world. Whether it was through the rituals of Judaism, Taoism, Buddhism, Hinduism, Christianity, Islam or various other religious or cultural practices, Benson realised there was a commonality among them all. Through different forms of prayer, contemplation, focused movement, or meditation, these different practices that have flourished over thousands of years all include the same two simple mental steps. "The two basic features of evoking the relaxation response are repetition and the disregard of other thoughts when they come to mind; and what those two things do is break the train of everyday thinking," Benson said, explaining that it's often this train of thought that causes stress in our lives.

Relaxation Response

1. Repetition (i.e., repeating a number, a nice word, or a musical phrase – out loud or in your head)
2. Disregard other thoughts when they come to mind (i.e., when you realise you forgot to bring the washing in, return to Step 1)

Benson took his theory back to the lab to see if untrained people could easily be taught to evoke the relaxation response using these two mental steps to stop the train of everyday thinking. He instructed medical school students to focus on counting from one to ten and back again, asking them to return to focus on counting when they got distracted. To his dismay, the experiments were a complete failure. "These bright students lost count, panicked, and that was the end of the experiment," recalls Benson. But he was determined to find the key that unlocked the relaxation response. He returned to the lab, this time asking the students simply to stay with the number one. To his delight, the physiological changes he observed in the aspiring doctors when they only counted to one were indistinguishable from those who practised transcendental meditation. Benson recalls some people telling him that it was wonderful that he'd chosen the number one, which they saw as the oneness of God and the oneness of The Universe. "Well, in truth it's because Harvard medical students couldn't count to 10," he told me with a glint in his eye. "This now was science. Here was something measurable, predictable, and reproducible."[39]

Benson, now in his 80s, is considered by many to be the founding father of modern mind-body medicine. He has dedicated his life's work to the study of the relaxation response and I was stunned when I learned that his groundbreaking research continues to this day. Recently, his team at the Benson Henry Institute for Mind-Body Medicine looked at how the relaxation response could affect the way genes function and learned that it can turn off genes that affect disease.[40] More remarkably, they discovered that these gene expression changes took place the *very first time* the response was elicited and that, as Benson explained, "The more times you do it daily, the more anchored the response will become."[41]

Learning about Benson's research was a breakthrough moment in my own health investigations. After I became ill, the first specialist doctor I saw told me that my autoimmune disease was likely caused by "bad" genes and that there wasn't much to be done beyond experimenting with different kinds and doses of medication. But here was a renowned professor of medicine from Harvard telling me it was possible to turn on and off the genes affecting my health. Moreover, it was simple and clear; there was no need to join a monastery or learn a dogmatic religious technique. It didn't even cost anything. This insight gave me hope and was a critical first step in my getting a handle on my stress and health. It inspired me to keep researching and to find help in developing a regular focused attention practice for myself. But where to start and which techniques would be best?

Meditation and Mindfulness

When Jon Kabat-Zinn walked into The Center for Mindfulness in Medicine and Healthcare at the University of Massachusetts, he was instantly mobbed. People around me gushed that he had arrived. One woman started shaking with nerves as she joined a line of people hoping to take his picture and get his autograph. He's a scientist and meditation teacher who counts among his friends fellow leading researchers, influential journalists, and His Holiness the Dalai Lama. In some settings, JKZ (as we like to call him in our office) is like a rock star. If you've looked into meditation or mindfulness in any small way, chances are you've come across his work. He's the founder of Mindfulness-Based Stress Reduction (MBSR), an eight-week program proven to improve stress, pain, depression, anxiety, and symptoms of chronic illness along with a number of other things.[42] More than 22,000 people around the world have completed the teacher training program, and the rate of scientific papers with MBSR at their core is increasing exponentially.

What got my attention was Kabat-Zinn's early research which showed that meditation, in conjunction with conventional medical treatment, could help people with the skin condition psoriasis heal more quickly. Kabat-Zinn, a microbiologist who studied under Nobel Laureate Salvador Luria, was having lunch with some dermatologists and listening to them describe how stress is linked to psoriatic flare-ups and how they treated the resulting skin lesions with a course of light therapy. In 1979 Kabat-Zinn set up the Stress Reduction Clinic to teach people with chronic illnesses non-religious meditative techniques in the hope of adding a new dimension to their health approach. Listening to the dermatologists gave him an idea. He convinced them to let him teach the patients to meditate while they were being treated under the ultra violet light. They set up a small, randomised trial to compare people who received only light therapy with people who also meditated during the treatments. It turned out that the meditators' skin cleared at four times the rate of the non-meditators.[43] "I didn't believe it. It was such a powerful finding," Kabat-Zinn told me. "So, we replicated it and tried to make a little bit more of a rigorous study design and, lo and behold again, the meditators were healing four times as fast as the non-meditators." For Kabat-Zinn, the study was an ideal scientific demonstration of the mind-body connection. The participants were doing something with their minds that appeared to affect what was happening in their skin. "It just doesn't get any better than that," he said, still amazed by the results decades later.[44]

The popularisation of meditation and mindfulness over the last decade must be mind-blowing for Kabat-Zinn who, along with Herbert Benson, was one of the first people to start bringing together traditionally Eastern practices with Western scientific enquiry. *TIME Magazine* recently hailed the "Mindful Revolution,"[45] Google has an in-house mindfulness program,[46] and lists of successful people who meditate make the rounds on social media memes,[47] including *Huffington Post* founder Arianna Huffington who champions its use in the workplace for boosting productivity and the corporate bottom line.[48]

What started as small, tentative steps toward evidence-based mind-body medicine a few decades ago has become a movement. Back then meditation was, at best, considered hippie juju and, at worst, heresy. These days it's considered self-evident and hundreds of researchers from top academic institutions all over the world are studying its usefulness, demonstrating that it can enhance your immune system,[49] help you cope with chronic illness,[50] and even change your brain structure to help with anxiety,[51] focus,[52] and attention.[53]

The great thing about meditation is that getting started doesn't require a major life upheaval. In fact, a recent breakthrough study by Harvard neuroscientist Sara Lazar on the effects of Kabat-Zinn's MBSR program showed that after just eight weeks, the amygdala (the stress centre) in the brain of the participants got smaller.[54] The effect occurred without their having to make major changes in their lives. These people went about their days as they normally would, adding only the techniques they'd learned in the program. As Lazar told me, "Their lives are exactly the same as they've always been. So they still have their stressful jobs and all the difficult people in their lives are still being difficult. But their amygdala has gotten smaller and they're reporting less stress."

Kabat-Zinn's MBSR course teaches different kinds of formal meditation such as the practical application of Herbert Benson's two mental steps through techniques such as progressively concentrating on relaxing muscles and other exercises that concentrate on focusing attention.

The program also introduces participants to an informal practice called mindfulness, which is simply paying attention, on purpose, in the present moment and without judgment. It involves taking time out of your day to observe the goings-on around you without judging them to be good or bad. For example, you might focus on your breath, the feel of sun on your skin, or the sound of the kettle boiling before you make a cup of tea.

When I started practising mindfulness and meditation I became far more aware of my own stress response. I realised that the alarm going off to wake me in the morning was stressful. Checking my emails on my phone before rising was stressful. Using my shower time to plan and prepare for the day was stressful. Even deciding what to wear was a source of stress as I contemplated the impression I wanted to make on the world. I must have had a dozen stressful thoughts before I even had my breakfast in the mornings.

The "without judgment" part of mindfulness and meditation has taught me the most. Rather than letting go of stressful things, it's often about letting them *be*. I am better able to accept many things that once weighed me down, and I feel less worried about things I cannot change. This acceptance is something I continue to work on every day. It is this fundamental shift in perspective that has brought about the greatest reduction of stress in my life and has helped me spend more time in Firdaus Dhabhar's green zone. This is not to say that I don't have daily stress, nor does it mean I ignore things that need to be addressed or tackled. But I try to notice my body's biological warning signs and use them to guide me, often reminding myself that a little bit of stress can be a good thing.

Does this mean that meditation and mindfulness are the only ways we can reduce chronic stress? Not at all. The good news for non-meditators is that science has validated the effectiveness of many other ways to reduce stress. Listening to music,[55] having a massage,[56] writing in a journal,[57] immersing yourself in art,[58] walking in nature,[59] taking a nap,[60] hugging it out,[61] or even drinking tea[62] and chewing gum[63] are all stress relievers. These activities may not have the exact same stress centre, amygdala-shrinking effects as mindfulness meditation, but they will all help.

Keep in mind that not everything we do for pleasure is an effective stress alleviator though. Alas, a survey done by the American Psychological Association found that gambling, smoking, shopping, playing video games, surfing the Internet, drinking alcohol, eating, and watching TV for more than two hours a day aren't particularly effective at relieving stress. So don't kid yourself that a marathon session watching your favourite TV series is an exercise in stress reduction.[64] All that intrigue and drama might also be enough to put your stress levels in the danger zone after a hard day.

The key – if you're anything like I used to be and need to reduce the chronic stress in your life – is to make healthy, relaxing activities a priority. Do something, at least one thing, every single day without compromise. For me, taking this time was the crucial first step in my whole-health evolution.

Meditation 101

In a world where we have bills to pay, bank balances to replenish and relationships to nurture, finding time for meditation can be tricky. Many of us struggle to carve out time to get even the recommended 30 minutes of exercise a day, let alone find enough time for mental stillness. It's also pretty confusing to determine what type of meditation is best. There are so many different "brands" that if you're new to the game, it's hard to know where to start. So when it comes to meditation, what does the research tell us about which kind is best and how long and how often we should practise it?

WHAT IS MEDITATION?

Meditation is a technique you use to train your mind. It can be used to enhance relaxation, prepare for a task, cultivate awareness, boost energy, or develop your awareness of emotions like compassion, love, or forgiveness. Some techniques, including mantra, mindfulness, and prayer involve focused thought (such as concentrating on an object, your breath, a word, a phrase, or simply paying attention to the present moment). You can meditate anywhere, any time. You can meditate with your eyes closed or open, when you are sitting, standing, walking, lying down, or when you are still. You can also use aids like music or prayer beads to help focus your attention.

WHAT TYPE OF MEDITATION IS BEST?

Despite there being thousands of studies about meditation, there is no clear evidence to suggest that one form of meditation is better than another. At the moment, the scientific community favours studying the health benefits of Transcendental Meditation (TM) and mindfulness meditation. TM is a mantra-style meditation taught by a TM teacher and is popular with celebrities. Mindfulness meditation is currently gaining favour in the corporate space. Mindfulness Based Stress Reduction (MBSR), the eight-week course developed by Jon Kabat-Zinn, combines mindfulness meditation with a simple style of yoga. That's not to say that TM or MBSR are the best. They just seem to be the buzz right now and research shows they both have benefits. What is also becoming clear is that various forms of meditation may affect our brains in subtle, yet different ways. For example, one study found that the effect of meditation on our ability to focus varies depending on whether the type of meditation encourages an inward or outward focus.[65] How you choose to get to a place where you can quiet your mind and stop the everyday chatter is entirely up to you.

HOW LONG AND HOW OFTEN SHOULD WE MEDITATE?

The good news is that we don't need to live in a cave or a monastery to derive benefits from meditation. The key is consistency. Sara Lazar from Harvard showed that the more experienced the meditator, the more the change in brain structure.[66] She looked at the brains of seasoned meditators who, on average, meditated once a day for 40 minutes over approximately eight years. They did this while living typical Western-style lives and working in traditional careers like healthcare and law. The main conclusion from the study was that meditating is like going to the gym. The more often you go, the stronger, fitter, and younger your brain. But 40 minutes a day can seem like a lot when we're busy dancing the work-life two-step. Unfortunately there is little agreement about the right "dosage" for meditation practice,[67] but studies show that 30 minutes a day for eight weeks can increase the density of grey matter in brain regions associated with memory, stress, and empathy.[68] Other studies show that meditating for only 20 minutes a day over four successive days improves cognitive skills[69] and that meditating for only 20 minutes a day over three days results in a significant decrease in sensitivity to pain.[70] The really good news is that one study found that just 10 minutes of meditation a day over 16 weeks significantly improved neural functioning associated with enhanced focused attention.[71]

If you think that finding even 10 minutes a day is impossible, then you might like to consider the advice of Associate Professor Craig Hassed, one of the world's leading experts in mind-body medical research, who is also the founding president of the Australian Teachers of Meditation Association. He says that mediating for just five minutes in the morning, and again in the evening, can serve as full stops, or moments of stillness, to punctuate your day. He also suggests trying a number of "commas" throughout the day as well. This might include a 30-second meditation before going into a meeting, or a one-minute session before lunch. I've found this to be particularly useful before public speaking. Taking 20 long, slow, focused breaths in the women's bathroom can quickly reset feelings of anxiousness and uncertainty.

Meditation is not a quick fix; rather, think of it as a lifelong practice. The idea is to develop a habit that becomes part of your daily routine. It's okay to start small. Don't expect to be able to meditate for 60 minutes or even 20 minutes straight away. As with any kind of exercise, start slowly and gradually build up. Finding a teacher and a meditation group is a fantastic way to make this part of your routine. You'll be held accountable and have other people to bounce off if you get stuck and need guidance.

If all this leaves you confused, you could always adhere to the ancient Zen proverb: You should sit in meditation for 20 minutes a day. Unless you're too busy, then you should sit for an hour.

Key Takeaways

1 Although the science clearly shows that inappropriate stress or long-term stress can be bad for us, research also shows that stress can be good for us too. The key is to minimise "bad" stress (such as flipping your lid in traffic, or enduring long-term negative stress) while encouraging short periods of "good stress" (such as exercising).

2 Our physical response to stressful events and situations is influenced by how we *perceive* each situation. Circumstances that might be detrimental for one person could be neutral or even beneficial for another. Learning to be more accepting of stressful situations can reduce its harmful effects.

3 Meditation is effective in reducing the harmful effects of an inappropriate stress response and chronic stress. Getting started doesn't require a major life upheaval such as running away to join an ashram. Whether you meditate for 10 or 40 minutes, there are benefits to be gained.

4 There are many other ways to reduce stress, such as walking or listening to music. The key is to do something every day and to prioritise spending time in your low-stress "green zone."

Getting Started

COMMIT to taking a "mindful moment" every day for a week during an activity you perform regularly. This means simply paying attention, on purpose, in the present moment and without judgment. You could do this while you're waiting for your bus, brushing your teeth, or making your morning coffee.

WRITE down three things you like to do that nurture your stress "green zone" and prioritise them into your weekly schedule. It could be anything from practising formal meditation to listening to music, getting a massage, writing in a journal, immersing yourself in art, or walking in nature.

LEARN mindfulness and meditation.

- *There are free guided meditations available for download on the resources page of my website. See the following Extra Resources section for details.*
- *Sometimes I use the help of a meditation app on my phone. I keep a list of recommended apps on my website that I update regularly.*
- *Find out about the Mindfulness-Based Stress Reduction program at The Center for Mindfulness in Medicine, Healthcare and Society at the University of Massachusetts Medical School at www.umassmed.edu/cfm*
- *Find out about Transcendental Meditation at www.tm.org*
- *Futurelearn.com offers a free, six-week online course that explores the science, practice, and philosophy of mindfulness. www.futurelearn.com/courses/mindfulness-wellbeing-performance*

Extra Resources

AVAILABLE AT
www.thewholehealthlife.com/resources

WATCH extended video interviews with the experts featured in this chapter including:

- *Craig Hassed (Associate Professor at Monash University and founding president of the Australian Teachers of Meditation Association)*
- *Jon Kabat-Zinn (Professor of Medicine Emeritus, University of Massachusetts Medical School and Founder of Mindfulness-Based Stress Reduction)*
- *Herbert Benson (Director Emeritus of the Benson-Henry Institute for Mind Body Medicine, Massachusetts General Hospital and Mind-Body Medicine Professor of Medicine, Harvard Medical School)*

DOWNLOAD the free first chapter of Craig Hassed's *Mindfulness Manual* which he wrote exclusively for The Whole Health Life website. This guide goes into more detail about how to make mindfulness part of your everyday life.

DOWNLOAD a free PDF outlining simple meditation exercises.

DOWNLOAD free guided audio meditations.

MY recommended reading list, which I update regularly, is available on my website. Books relevant to this chapter include:

- *Full Catastrophe Living: Using the Wisdom of Your Body and Mind to Face Stress, Pain, and Illness*, by Jon Kabat-Zinn
- *Mindfulness for Health: A practical guide to relieving pain, reducing stress and restoring wellbeing*, by Vidyamala Burch and Danny Penman
- *Mindfulness for Life*, by Stephen McKenzie and Craig Hassed
- *The Upside of Stress: Why Stress is Good for You and How to Get Good at it*, by Kelly McGonigal

Chapter 2

Emotions

Adrift

I'm not sure there is anything quite like the emotional turmoil that comes with being close to someone with an addiction. There is unpredictable drama, deception, and broken trust. There is hurt, pain, misunderstanding, and the heart-wrenching fear of losing them. There is terrible helplessness watching them try to escape their dark feelings and drown their sorrows in the oblivion of substance abuse. And there are few things in the world more emotionally fraught than having someone you love threaten to commit suicide when they're in the depths of despair.

In early 2006 I found myself walking into an unadorned room to attend my first group therapy session with about eight other people. Someone I was close to in my family was attempting to recover from a drug addiction and they were participating in a style of psychotherapy that encourages close friends, family members, and spouses to participate in their own support groups, even if they themselves don't express their troubles through substance abuse. The idea is to try to break dysfunctional relationship and behavioural patterns and in so doing, break the drug dependency.

I soon learned this circle was a sanctuary – a safe place where people could openly explore their darkest secrets. Over the weeks, months, and years I became a trusted member of the group, though I can't say I ever enjoyed the meetings. The therapy was confronting and called into question every behaviour, coping mechanism, and habit I had developed over my lifetime. It taught me to identify emotions lying under the surface and delve deep into past experiences I'd rather have forgotten. But in time, I also became more in tune with my feelings and I learned a new language for expressing them. I learned to notice the heat that rises in my skin with anger, the weight in my gut that comes with fear, the ache in my heart when I feel deep sadness, and the sickening nausea of regret. I learned to notice my feelings and to pause before acting on them. I had spent a lifetime trying to escape my dark emotions only to discover they could do me no harm.

I also began to realise that my emotions and health were connected. My autoimmune flare-ups ebbed and flowed with my inner emotional state, both because my symptoms always seemed worse during times of heightened emotion and because during these times I was more likely to engage in unhealthy behaviours. I began noticing that worrying led to sleeplessness, which led to days of fatigue and pain in my joints and muscles. Inner feelings of inadequacy were tied to my unhealthy drive to work harder and harder at the cost of my health. My need to feel needed had steered me into friendships that were all take and no give, leaving me depleted and reaching for unhealthy comfort foods I hoped would make me feel better.

Difficult as all this was, what emerged was self-honesty and a new freedom to make different choices moving forward. Although I had started on this path to help someone else, I soon realised that doing this hard emotional work was going to have health benefits for me.

When I first became ill in 2004, if I had asked my rheumatologist whether the emotional turbulence I was experiencing in my personal life was playing a role in my illness, he would have looked at me as though I were a delusional crazy hippie speaking the language of woo woo. Those were still early days for emotions research. And despite the credible and compelling evidence now emerging that proves a connection between emotions and health, there still remains a great divide between those in the healthcare system who treat the mind and those who treat the body. There are some outliers but, overall, neither side is much interested in working closely with the other.

There is a rich and fascinating history as to how this separation between the mind and body came about in the mainstream treatment of disease.[1] The short version is that thoughts and feelings are very difficult to put under a microscope and science is the foundation of modern medicine. What is an emotion anyway? What is a thought? Scientists still don't entirely agree on the answers to these two questions. And if we can't say what emotions and thoughts are, how on earth can we measure them? If we can't measure them, how can we even begin to fathom offering evidence-based advice? Despite these scientific obstacles, a brave troop of researchers working at respected academic institutions around the globe have put their careers on the line and, against the opinions of their peers, have persisted in studying this very topic.

Emotions Under the Microscope

It was a stroke of luck that gave rise to the seminal research that would lay the foundations for modern scientific enquiry into human emotions. In the mid 1960s, a US Department of Defense scandal prompted funds that were being used to cover up counter insurgency activity in South America to be redirected toward something international, but not controversial.[2] In his book *Emotions Revealed,* psychologist Paul Ekman tells how he just happened to walk into the right office on the right day to be offered those funds, and the idea for a cross-cultural study of emotions recognition was born.[3] Ekman was inspired by the work of Charles Darwin, who had outlined a theory for a universal language of human expression in his 1872 book *The Expression of the Emotions in Man and Animals* and he wanted to put the Darwinian theories of emotion to the test.[4]

In 1967, with his unexpected funding in place, Ekman trekked to the highlands of Papua New Guinea with the specific purpose of finding people who had never been exposed to a world outside their own. He was armed with a series of photographs showing people expressing six basic emotions: anger, disgust, fear, happiness, sadness, and surprise. The isolated villagers were able to identify each of the emotions expressed on the faces of the people in his photographs. In this way, he confirmed Darwin's theory of the universality of human emotions and began to develop a scientific methodology to measure emotions.

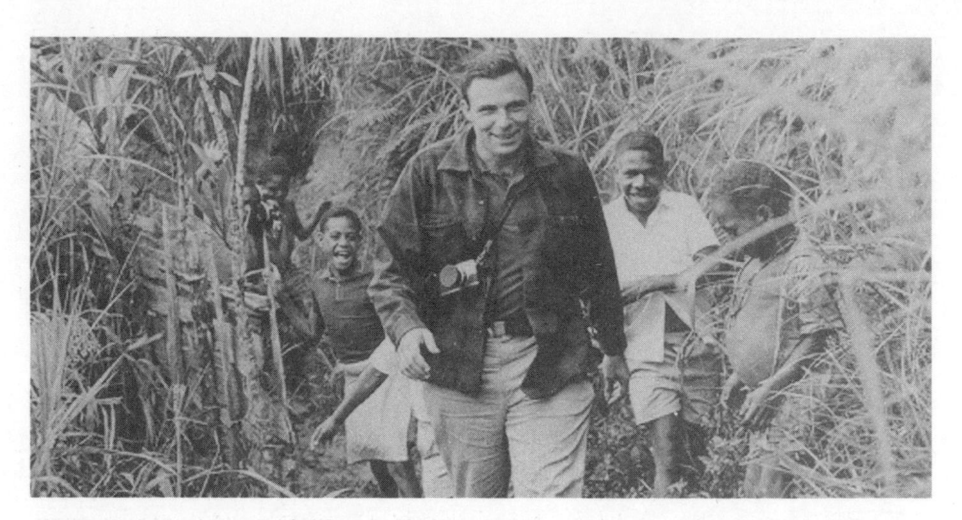

Paul Ekman in the highlands of Papua New Guinea, 1967. *Credit: Paul Ekman Group LLC*

Ekman went on to establish a detailed system for coding the muscle movements that constitute the facial expressions of specific emotions. He also discovered micro expressions – brief facial muscle movements that last only a fraction of a second and occur when a person either deliberately or unconsciously conceals a feeling. He became an expert in lie detection and is now famous for inspiring the character Carl Lightman in the US crime drama television series *Lie to Me* for which he served as a scientific consultant. But it was Ekman's groundbreaking work that gave researchers the ability to measure emotions and paved the way for thousands of modern studies.

In the late 1980s a young neuroscientist named Richard Davidson took Ekman's research to the next level and demonstrated not only a brain basis for emotions, but also a connection between emotions and immune function. When Davidson told his academic supervisors at Harvard University that he wanted to study the brain basis of emotions he was told it was a pipe dream, the scientific equivalent of wanting to hunt elephants in Alaska. Undaunted, Davidson and Ekman collaborated in a small study to measure emotional response. Their research subjects watched emotion-inducing video clips such as joyous puppies playing with flowers or a gruesome leg amputation procedure. Davidson used emerging technology called electroencephalography (EEG) to measure electrical activity in their brains, while Ekman measured their facial expressions. Their results showed that the expression of specific emotions was consistently correlated with activity in certain areas of the brain. They had clear evidence that the brain and body were connected in the expression of emotions.[5]

Soon after, Davidson found that women with extreme right frontal brain activation, which is associated with more negative emotional styles, also had lower levels of Natural Killer (NK) cell activity – a type of white blood cell that is a significant component of a working immune system.[6] In fact, as Davidson reported in his book, *The Emotional Life of Your Brain,* participants with high left frontal activation, which is associated with a more positive emotional style, had upward of 50 percent higher NK cell activity than those with high right frontal activation.[7] Just to be sure, Davidson repeated the study and again found that people with greater left frontal brain activity had higher levels of NK cell activity.[8] His remarkable findings clearly showed an emotion-brain-immunity connection.

Despite being seen as quacks when they first started out, both Ekman and Davidson went on to have long and distinguished careers that continue today. They were front-runners in a field of discovery called *psychoneuroendocrine immunology* – that is, the study of how our thoughts and emotions interact with our nervous, hormone, and immune systems. Their pioneering work has led to major breakthroughs in understanding the mind-body-health connection.

Positively Healthy

Whether you've got the flu, a broken arm, or a long-lasting chronic disease that is getting worse over time, if you're like me you've probably lost count of the number of times someone has told you to "look on the bright side" and "think positive thoughts" in order to overcome your ailment. A multitude of self-help books, magazine articles, and advertising campaigns have reinforced this idea, so it's little wonder that many of us believe that how positive our thinking is affects how well we are. But I wanted to delve into the scientific literature to see what the research says about the link between positive emotions and health, and to see if there were any specific hints about how I could use the science to approach my illness. Fortunately, a researcher who has dedicated her entire career to exploring this topic was happy to talk me through it all over a long conversation on Skype.

Associate professor Sarah Pressman has her own lab at the University of California, Irvine which is dedicated to investigating the interplay between emotions and health, with a focus on the physiological processes that underlie these associations. In 2005 she joined with a leading emotions researcher, Sheldon Cohen from Carnegie Mellon University, in order to explore whether good feelings like happiness, joy, excitement, enthusiasm, and contentment are actually linked to good health. Their review evaluated many research papers that together suggest that people who have a more positive outlook tend to feel healthier.[9] "So if you ask them, 'How do you feel?' they're going to say they feel healthier. They're going to feel that they are in less pain and report fewer symptoms. Even if you control for things like how severe their illness is, or how healthy they are objectively, you still see that kind of subjective difference," she told me.

So positive emotions might help you cope and feel better about your illness, but can they actually make you healthier? It's here that the scientific literature becomes a little murky. Certainly there is vast recent research linking positive emotions such as joy, love, hope, wonder, and awe to good health. For example, a study that followed more than 6000 university students for more than 40 years found that pessimistic students tended to die younger than their optimistic peers.[10] A 2011 review of more than 160 studies found "clear and compelling evidence" that people who have positive dispositions tend to live longer and experience better health than negatively-inclined people. The reviewers estimated that when all was said and done, having higher levels of positive emotions may add 4-10 years to your life.[11]

But why exactly do people with a positive outlook seem to have better health? Is it because they're better at looking after themselves? Perhaps they eat healthier foods and exercise more? Is it because cheerful people have more friends, get more support, and might experience less chronic stress? Perhaps these sunny-side-uppers are more likeable and therefore attract more attention from their doctors? One likely explanation found in an extensive body of research is that optimists are more likely to take proactive steps to protect their health, whereas pessimists are more likely to engage in health-damaging behaviours.[12] Optimistic people set goals and persist longer in working to achieve those goals despite challenges and setbacks.[13]

But there's also some fascinating preliminary research showing that positive emotions may also have direct biological benefits. Positive emotions may actually be able to "get under the skin" and to interact with our immune and other biological systems to influence our health.

In one fascinating study, Pressman gave willing volunteers a minor skin wound by putting adhesive tape on their arms and then ripping it off about 50 times. She reported that people with higher levels of positivity healed more quickly than those with less positive outlooks.[14] This ability to influence rapid healing is very important, Pressman explained to me. "If you're seriously injured or have had surgery, you want to heal quickly because the amount of time it takes you to heal can influence whether or not you get secondary infections or whether you get injured again," she said.

Pressman's fellow health-emotions researcher colleague, Sheldon Cohen, also showed that when he quarantined people in a hotel room for five days and exposed them to the rhinovirus (also known as the common cold), positive people were less likely to develop a cold.[15]

At this point you might be thinking, well that's not revelatory, positive-minded people are probably more likely to look after themselves and therefore be healthier. But what's interesting is that Cohen and his team found that positivity correlated with a lower risk of getting a cold *independently* of healthy behaviours and other factors such as age, weight, gender, and whether a person was already immune to the virus. His conclusion was simple – a tendency to experience positive emotions is associated with greater resistance to developing a common cold. He has even replicated the findings.[16]

The Upside of Negativity

It's easy to understand how positivity has become so much more popular than its darker sibling, negativity, and why it forms the nucleus of many bestselling self-help books. Positive emotions feel great. They lift us up and promise the holy grail of happiness, life satisfaction, and contentment. On the flip side, we think negative emotions feel terrible. Many of us spend a lifetime trying to escape their grip. We fear the pain of losing those we love, suppress anger that rises in order to keep the peace, or try to escape our guilt and regret by pushing them to the backs of our minds, even to the point of turning to self-destructive behaviours to do so.

But it may surprise you that so called "bad" feelings are an essential element in our emotional repertoire. Anger, fear, sadness, grief, guilt, and even anxiety can not only be useful, they can be a force for good. For example, one study found that anxious people were more alert to sensing a threat when researchers put them in a room that slowly filled with smoke.[17] If you're like me, watching the video of smoke filling the room will make you want to shout a warning to these poor test subjects, even though you know the whole thing is a set-up. (The link to watch this video is at the end of this chapter.) The researchers theorised that having people in our community with an anxious disposition may be an important part of humanity's evolution and that as humans evolved, it was to our benefit to have a diverse range of emotional types in a community, including anxiety.[18] After all, we all benefit from being in the company of someone with danger-detecting super-powers.

There is also a compelling body of research by Joseph Forgas, a professor of psychology at the University of New South Wales, who suggests that a temporary, slightly negative mood can make us less prone to judgmental errors,[19] better at remembering details,[20] more polite,[21] and more persuasive, regardless of whether we are advocating popular or unpopular positions.[22] Howard Friedman, Distinguished Professor of Psychology at the University of California in Riverside, who has spent three decades studying the personality predictors of longevity, believes that even a "healthy neuroticism" can be a good thing if it makes us more vigilant about our health.[23]

Think about it this way – you need a touch of anxiety if you're facing rush-hour traffic, otherwise you'd be blind to the potential dangers lurking in the behaviour of your fellow drivers. If your kids are being threatened by a schoolyard bully, a swelling of anger will motivate you to take (hopefully appropriate) action. Feeling frustrated or inadequate at work may be exactly what you need to get motivated to step up. When you feel the guilt that comes with failing to recognise a friend in need, bingeing on unhealthy food, or doing anything that goes against your own moral code, that's a signal that something is wrong and needs your attention. When it comes to good health, a touch of worry may well be the push you need to go for regular checkups or take your medication.

Another consideration is that while thinking on the bright side is correlated with a better chance of staying healthy if you are well, other studies show that positive emotions make no difference to outcomes for people who are already seriously sick. In fact, there's evidence to suggest that people with end-stage disease and diseases from which they are likely to die quickly may be harmed by high levels of positivity.[24] In 2007, researcher James Coyne who was then from the University of Pennsylvania, studied 1,093 people with head and neck cancer and found that a patient's emotional state did not predict whether they lived or died, even after controlling for several other factors such as gender, tumour site, or disease stage.[25] While the methodology and findings of Coyne's head and neck cancer study have been queried by other leading researchers,[26] in 2010, Coyne also published a systematic review that found when it came to cancer progression and survival, having a "fighting spirit" had no benefit.[27]

The reason for these slightly confusing findings is that emotions research is highly complex. Sarah Pressman explained to me that the current line of thinking among researchers is that sick people with a highly positive outlook might make a conscious choice to live out the rest of their lives without the pain and invasiveness of medical treatments and therefore die sooner. It may also be that ill people who are highly positive underreport their symptoms, or are overoptimistic and don't follow recommended medical advice. Another consideration is that the physiological health benefits that may be gained by boosting positive emotions like love, joy, and inspiration may simply not be powerful enough for people who are gravely ill.[28]

When Negativity Goes Too Far

In a similar way that being overly positive might be harmful for our health, too much negativity can also swing us too far to the wrong end of the emotional pendulum and become problematic. Estimates are that more than 350 million people around the world suffer from depression.[29] The 2012 World Mental Health Survey conducted in 17 countries found that on average about one in 20 people reported an episode of depression in the previous year.[30] In the US, 15 percent of people will become clinically depressed at some point in their lives.[31] At its worst, depression can lead to suicide. Almost one million people commit suicide every year – this translates to 3,000 lives lost every single day. For every person who completes a suicide, it's estimated that 20 or more attempt to end their lives.[32]

If you've suffered from depression or know someone who has, you'll know that the experience is like thinking and moving in slow motion. Everything is difficult. Getting out of bed. Planning a meal. Committing to a future event. You're forgetful and never truly present. It's lonely and seems to have no end and no beginning. And despite the well-meaning words of those around you, it's not something you can just snap out of. It's hard on you, and it's hard on those who love you.

People with depression not only have unhealthy thoughts like persistent sadness, worthlessness, and helplessness, they also have unhealthy habits and behaviours like insomnia, and over- or under-eating.[33] So it's no surprise that people with depression have a greater risk of becoming sick, and people who are sick have a greater risk of becoming depressed.[34] For example, if you have type 2 diabetes or heart disease, you're two to three times more likely to have major depression than a healthy person.[35] A large study of more than 100,000 Canadians showed that having one or more long-term medical conditions was associated with having major depression.[36] Twenty-three percent of depressed patients report health difficulties severe enough to keep them bedridden.[37] The World Health Organization predicts that by the year 2020 depression will be the second leading cause of mortality in the world, affecting 30 percent of adults.[38]

Feeling sick is awful and can affect your mental state. You may be experiencing high levels of pain, insomnia, or worry. Over time this mental state can become your new "normal" and develop into full-blown depression. The reverse can also happen; if you're depressed you might stop exercising or getting enough good sleep. You might self-medicate with cigarettes, mood-altering drugs, or alcohol. These unhealthy behaviours can contribute to the escalation or worsening of an illness.

Although scientists don't yet know the exact physiological pathways to explain the depression-health correlation (it may be genetic, it may be circumstantial or, most likely, it may be a combination of many factors), the correlation between depression and illness is too conspicuous to ignore. The tragedy is that those people who are most vulnerable are also the least likely to look after themselves. Less than 25 percent of those affected by depression receive treatment.[39] A systematic review found that compared with non-depressed people, people with depression are three times more likely to be noncompliant with medical recommendations.[40]

If you're suffering from depression, or suspect that someone you know might be, the good news is that a variety of treatments, including cognitive behavioural therapy,[41] mindfulness based cognitive behavioural therapy,[42] positive psychology interventions,[43] and other therapies, as well as antidepressant medications that can be prescribed by experienced doctors,[44] have been shown to be effective. It is essential to consult professionals and get help. Research shows that most people don't get help until 10 years after their first depressive episode.[45] With a myriad of proven techniques at your disposal, don't let another 10 years slip by – or even another day.

Emotional Wholeness

Often when researchers tackle the question of the relationship of emotions and health, they tend to view it from one end of the emotional spectrum or the other. That is, they ask whether or not positive emotions are good for us, or whether or not negative emotions are bad for us. Indeed when their messages are translated into book titles and headlines, they often drill down to a single argument such as: "Positivity: Top-Notch Research Reveals the Upwards Spiral that Will Change Your Life"[46] or "Bright Sided: How Positive Thinking is Undermining America."[47] There is, however, an emerging line of enquiry pondering what the interplay might be between health and having a varied range of emotions. That is to say, taking the good *with* the bad may in fact be the key to good health.[48] For example, when suffering the loss of a loved one, allowing positive memories to be experienced alongside sadness could lead to a healthier bereavement process.[49]

This *mixed emotions* research is coming from a surprising place. Hal Hershfield is an expert in behavioural economics at the University of California, Los Angeles. When he's not studying topics like how to make discretionary money last,[50] he's delving into the link between varied emotions and health. He told me that the thread running through his work is studying how people can simultaneously hold two opposing positions. "My interest in mixed emotions stems from asking how can we hold positive and negative emotions in mind at the same time, and how can doing so affect behaviour and decisions?" he said.

In one study, Hershfield observed 47 adults undergoing psychotherapy to help them with difficult life events such as divorce or the transition to parenthood. They were given questionnaires and asked to write personal narratives reflecting on their thoughts and feelings. The results showed that people's wellbeing wasn't improved simply by increasing levels of happiness. It was the people who experienced a mixture of happiness and sadness who saw improvements in their wellbeing.[51] Here are two examples of personal reflections from people in the study who expressed a mixed emotional experience. You'll note that they highlight both their sadness and their happiness:

1 "I am committed to trying to make every day better than the day before. So far, it's been tough going at times, with frequent setbacks involving much sadness and feelings of helplessness at times. But the fact that I'm working on improving in and of itself makes me feel better about my future and makes me happy and hopeful despite my slow progress and often listless feeling."

2 "This has been a difficult couple of weeks. My wife and I celebrated the good news of a healthy pregnancy report at nine weeks (the time when we lost our pregnancy last January). But I also feel the sadness of still looking for a job and for my wife and my pending loss of my wife's grandmother. It feels as if "what more can I take." But, in reality I also feel reasonably confident and happy. Not that I don't feel down, but I also feel happy with my marriage."

Adapted from: Adler, JM, & Hershfield, HE, 2012. Mixed emotional experience is associated with and precedes improvements in psychological well-being. *PLoS ONE*, 7(4), e35633

Hershfield's case for the role of mixed emotions in health is strengthened by another study in which he and his colleagues gave electronic pagers to 184 people, then buzzed them five times a day for a week to remind them to fill out an emotions questionnaire. This data-gathering process allowed them to get a well-rounded picture of their subjects' emotional states over a period of time, rather than relying on one-time reports that may have skewed assessments of their subjects' moods one way or another. Over the 10 years of the study, they found that not only were frequent experiences of mixed emotions (both positive and negative) strongly associated with relatively good physical health, but that when people experienced an increase of mixed emotions over many years, this counter-balanced typical age-related health declines.[52]

This research is still very much in its infancy. The physiological mechanisms that might explain how a mix of positive and negative emotions can have health benefits are still unknown, but there is a clear takeaway from what we do know. Rather than only searching for the next thing we think will make us happier, or trying to escape pain and suffering, this research indicates the answer may instead lie in seeking balance in our lives. In their book *The Upside of Your Dark Side: Why Being Your Whole Self – Not Just Your "Good" Self – Drives Success and Fulfillment,* psychologists Tod Kashdan and Robert Biswas-Diener call this concept *wholeness*.[53] They believe the key lies in mental agility – that is, the ability to access our full range of emotions in order to respond appropriately in any situation.

Learn to Let it Out

When we suppress our emotions we avoid distressing feelings by distracting ourselves or holding things in. We may even repress our negative emotions to the point of not being consciously aware of them.[54] Some of us go to enormous lengths to run from our negative feelings, yet research shows that our efforts may be to no avail, and in fact may do more harm than good.

Suppression affects our health by making it more likely we will engage in harmful coping behaviours such as overeating. A 2012 study on emotional eating found that suppressing feelings led to increased consumption of comfort foods like chocolate, crisps, and cookies. Interestingly the researchers found that it wasn't the emotions themselves that drove people to their unhealthy treats, but rather their attempts to suppress their emotions.[55]

All that hard work trying to repress or inhibit the expression of our emotions may also have a direct impact on our health. An analysis of 22 studies on repression, which in total included 6775 participants, found that people who repress their emotions are more likely to suffer from chronic disease, especially cancer and hypertension.[56] People who suppress their emotions have more physical signs of stress, such as elevated blood pressure.[57] Separate studies in the US, Holland, and Germany link suppression of anger to death from all causes over a number of years.[58]

All this is not to say that we should go around blowing up in a raging fit every time we feel the burn of anger, or spend our days planning revenge on people we think have wronged us, nor does it mean that crying is the only appropriate action during times of grief. There are a number of healthy ways to handle our difficult emotions.

Of particular note is the power of expressive writing. The process of expressing information, thoughts, and feelings about personal and meaningful topics can have various health and psychological consequences.[59] In a series of studies, James Pennebaker and his colleagues from the University of Texas found that expressive writing about negative experiences can improve health problems and bolster coping and wellbeing. Compared to groups assigned to write about trivial or non-traumatic events, people who engage in expressive writing exercises experience reduced medical visits,[60] improvements in immune function,[61] increases in antibody production,[62] increases in psychological wellbeing,[63] reduced anxiety,[64] and reduced depressive symptoms.[65]

Pennebaker believes that writing forces us to stop and reevaluate our life circumstance and further speculates that the act of writing encourages us to acknowledge and label our emotions. When we translate our emotions into words, we can start to see things differently and can therefore behave differently in ways that may be better for us.[66]

Can We Change?

You've probably heard that people who win the lottery ultimately end up no happier than if they hadn't been blessed by their financial stroke of luck. It's a well-known anecdote based on a study done in 1978, and it's often used to demonstrate that the emotional disposition we're born with cannot be changed.[67] The argument is that, despite the highs and lows we may experience in our lives, we all have a wellbeing baseline to which we are destined to return. Research published since that 1978 paper continues to support this viewpoint. For example, an Australian study that tracked people for six years found that over time, despite fluctuations in subjective wellbeing that coincided with the ups and downs of life, people tended to return to a predictable emotional range.[68] Richard Davidson (whom you'll remember is the neuroscientist studying the brain basis of emotions) can scan your brain to determine whether you're inclined to be positive or negative, how focused you can be, how socially sensitive and self-aware you are, and even how resilient you might be after a setback.[69] In fact, a growing body of research done with identical and fraternal twins suggests that how happy you'll be is likely to be 35 to 50 percent due to your genetic make-up.[70] Two researchers think this factor may even be as high as 80 percent.[71] So regardless of where you live, how much money you have, whom you marry, how good looking you are, or any of the windfalls and challenges that come your way, it seems your genes are largely responsible for your emotional wellbeing.

With all this in mind, it would be easy to take the fatalistic view that you're stuck with a particular genetic blueprint that will forever form the foundations of your emotional architecture and that all your tendencies toward positivity or negativity, toward optimism or pessimism, toward resilience or rumination, are set in stone for the rest of your life. But before you fall into a pit of despair and curse the money you've spent on happiness books, ask yourself this: if 50 percent of our emotional life is governed by genetics, what governs the rest? And if even some of our emotional disposition is within our power to change, what is the best way to go about it?

Two of the world's leading happiness scientists, Sonja Lyubomirsky, a professor in the department of psychology at the University of California, Riverside and Ken Sheldon, a professor of psychological sciences at the University of Missouri have teamed up over the last two decades to answer these questions. The good news is they have demonstrated it is possible to become happier.[72]

In a 2012 study, they found that when a participant sowed the seeds for a happiness boost by making a positive life change, such as getting a new job or starting a new relationship, they were able to maintain the uplift if they made an effort to cultivate those seeds. The study demonstrated that appreciation and gratitude preserved the boost in wellbeing by encouraging people not to take the good stuff for granted. It also demonstrated that people who continued to derive varying experiences from the life change were more likely to experience a sustained boost in happiness, indicating that variety and surprise spice up life in ways that can help sustain wellbeing. Sheldon and Lyubomirsky ultimately concluded that increased happiness "is an attainable goal, realizable when people make efforts to be grateful for what they have and to continue to interact with it in diverse, surprising, and creative ways."[73] In an email sent from his office in Missouri, Sheldon told me, "So, yes, it is possible to become happier, but it takes effort and awareness."

I thoroughly enjoyed my email exchanges with Sheldon because although he's a world leader in the study of happiness, he confesses to not buying in to the smiley face, cuddly-kittens, "think happy thoughts, count your blessings" side of an ever growing movement called *positive psychology*. "Actually, I find contemporary positive psychology to be a little bit gross. People selling out the science to get famous, that kind of thing," he said.

When it is not selling self-help books, the positive psychology research movement is making headway in discerning what the best ways are to go about boosting positive emotions. So far, things such as deliberately practicing gratitude, savouring positive experiences, and being kind are proving to be promising ways to become happier.[74] A 2009 analysis that combined results from 51 randomised controlled interventions found that people who were prompted to engage in positive intentional activities, such as thinking gratefully, optimistically, or mindfully were able to become significantly happier[75] and a 2013 follow-up analysis also found that positive psychology interventions can be effective in boosting psychological wellbeing and may help to reduce depressive symptoms.[76]

I've summarised some of the key positivity techniques being tested and how you can use them in your everyday life in a free download you can access on my website. But it's important to remember that, because each of us is unique, we don't all need positive psychology interventions and not all positive psychology interventions will work for everyone. "I'm not big on disciplined exercises," Sheldon told me. "I guess I don't believe in setting out to make myself happy, or buying books on happiness. Instead I set out to do something fun and interesting, which will lead to new discoveries and realisations."

It's interesting that these positive interventions have been shown to be less effective over time, probably because of our innate tendency to adapt.[77] People who use positivity-boosting exercises get used to them, just like lottery winners get used to being millionaires. To date, the evidence suggests that interventions are most successful when participants know about them, endorse them, and commit to them.[78] In other words, you have to want to make a change and fully engage in deliberate and ongoing action to make it happen.

Swimming Back to Shore

I've lost count of the number of conversations I've had with people about whether our emotions can affect our health. Inevitably, anecdotal stories are evoked to make one argument or the other – "My uncle was the angriest, meanest man on the planet and he lived to the age of 94" or "My auntie was told she had six months to live, but she's the happiest, most positive person I know and is still alive and kicking five years later." When we hear these stories it's easy to become confused and wonder what to believe. Should we strive for ultra positivity at the risk of glossing over important details? Or should we harness the power of pessimism to motivate us to cover all possible bases?

The current science of emotions suggests that the answer is highly complex. It's not as simple as saying "do whatever makes you happy" in hopes it will boost your immunity. After all, people can feel happier by eating junk food, taking drugs, and partying all night. Emotions are also highly subjective. For some people, there is nothing better than a fiery argument to get the blood pumping or having a good cry during a sad movie. Emotional advice, unfortunately, is not black and white and there is no one-size-fits-all diagnosis or prescription.

We can, however, draw on the latest scientific research to make a road map and determine the right path to travel. Perhaps you have a tendency to drift too far toward the positive side of life where you may be blinded to reality, or perhaps your pessimism stops you from taking healthier action. If you'd like to gauge where you sit on the positivity-negativity scale, a good starting point could be two quizzes often used by researchers in their studies: The Subjective Happiness Scale and a depression questionnaire. Both are available for download from my website.

Even the most critical of sceptics must acknowledge that there is evidence to strongly suggest that the functions of our mind do influence the health of our body, and that disease in the body can affect our moods and emotions. While there is no evidence that suggests emotions *cause* illness, or that disease arises from some kind of innate personality defect, or even that psychotherapy can stop the progression of cancer or heart disease,[79] we do know that actively working to change our emotional outlook can motivate us to eat better, get out of bed, attend medical appointments, and connect with other people.[80] Whether through positivity exercises, meditation, psychotherapy or just having a good old natter with a close friend, attending to our emotions is a fundamental necessity when we want to get healthy or stay healthy.

As I write these words, the person in my life who initially sparked my emotional deep dive is still weighed down heavily with their problems, but I am not. I have learned a great deal about letting things be and taking the good with the bad. I am no longer afraid of my difficult thoughts and feelings, and I now see them as an effective gauge on my emotional barometer. I've stopped asking questions about whether I somehow caused my illness by thinking negatively or whether if I just somehow thought happier thoughts I could cure my disease. If I fall into a funk for more than a day I try to catch myself before plummeting deeper into a rumination trap. At these times I make a conscious effort to practice loving kindness, forgiveness, gratitude, and generosity. Doing this boosts my mood and brings me back to reality. I use meditation and journal writing to regulate my emotions, and rely on a close network of trusted friends with whom I can share my burdens openly. While I haven't yet gotten all this right (after all I've spent a lifetime of laying down particular neural circuitry and the rebuilding is an ongoing renovation project) my emotions are far more balanced and my recovery from setbacks is far swifter.

I am also eternally grateful for the time I spent in group therapy. It changed the course of my life. But there came a point when reflecting on my past had served its purpose and it was time to move on. It took me years to fully take in the central adage held by those who successfully bear the burden of loving an addict – that the only person who can motivate recovery is the person with the addiction. I had viewed myself as the heroic rescue worker swimming out to save my drowning loved one, only to have them swim into deeper waters as I approached. I followed them farther and farther out to sea until we found ourselves too far from shore to make it back. I was exhausted and drowning. For my own sake, I had to let go and swim back alone. While they are still adrift, I am now stronger and better able to protect myself in times of heightened emotion. If they ever need me, I'll be waiting on the shore to support them as they catch their breath.

Key Takeaways

1 Having more positive emotions is linked to better health and living longer. This may not only be because positive people are more likely to take proactive steps to protect their health, but also because there are physiological benefits to be gained from positive emotions, such as having a stronger immune system.

2 People who are already sick and people with end-stage disease may be harmed by high levels of positivity because they may underreport their symptoms, or be overoptimistic and not follow recommended medical advice.

3 So called "bad" feelings are an essential element in our emotional repertoire. Anger, fear, sadness, grief, guilt, and even anxiety can be not only useful, they can be used as a force for good. For example, a touch of anxiety can make us more vigilant about our health.

4 Negative emotions can swing too far in the wrong direction. Depression is a serious illness linked to poor health, but there are a now a variety of effective treatments for depression.

5 The key to balancing emotional and physical health may lie in practicing emotional wholeness, taking the good with the bad, and learning to access our full range of emotions in order to respond appropriately in any situation.

6 Despite the influence of our genetic predispositions and the world around us, a large proportion our happiness is within our control. By practicing proven positivity-boosting techniques we can shift our disposition towards positivity, but it takes commitment to do so and we may need to keep mixing things up in diverse, surprising, and creative ways.

Getting Started

LEARN to identify your emotions by keeping track of how you're feeling throughout your day. You can do this by setting a reminder on your phone to buzz every few hours and manually noting down what you are doing in that moment, along with your mood and any associated physical sensations. There's a template for this emotions tracking diary available for download on my website. There are also mobile apps available to help you do this. I keep a list of recommended apps on my website that I update regularly.

IF you'd like to gauge where you sit on the positivity-negativity scale, there are two quizzes often used by researchers available for download on my website that you can use as a starting point. See the following Extra Resources section for details.

CHOOSE one of the ten happiness-boosting activities to work on each month from the positivity boosting techniques summary available on my website. See the following Extra Resources section of this book for details.

SEEK professional help. If you're sitting too far to one extreme on the emotions scale, don't hesitate one more day before getting help from a qualified professional. Different experts offer different types of services and treatments. A good starting place is your local doctor who will be able to provide an initial assessment and then point you in the right direction as to who you should see next.

HERE are some key organisations that provide information and support for people seeking help for mental health.

- **AUSTRALIA**
  www.beyondblue.org.au
- **US**
  www.mentalhealthamerica.net
- **UK**
  www.mind.org.uk

Extra Resources

AVAILABLE AT
www.thewholehealthlife.com/resources

LISTEN to extended audio interviews with the experts including:

- *Sarah Pressman (Associate Professor of Psychology & Social Behavior at the University of California, Irvine)*

DOWNLOAD a free summary of the key positivity-boosting techniques being tested by scientists and how you can use them in your everyday life (including practicing gratitude exercises, learning expressive writing techniques, practicing optimism, practicing kindness, learning to use strengths in new ways, affirming important values, practicing loving-kindness, meditation, and savouring).

DOWNLOAD a template for an emotions tracking diary to help you keep track of how you're feeling throughout the day.

DOWNLOAD the Subjective Happiness Scale quiz and a depression questionnaire to see where you sit on the emotional spectrum.

WATCH the video filmed during the study that found that anxious people are more alert to sensing a threat. Just try to stop yourself from shouting a warning to them, even though you know the whole thing is a set-up.

MY recommended reading list, which I update regularly, is available on my website. Books relevant to this chapter include:

- *Emotions Revealed: Recognizing Faces and Feelings to Improve Communication and Emotional Life*, by Paul Ekman
- *The Emotional Life of Your Brain*, by Richard Davidson and Sharon Begley
- *The Upside of Your Dark Side, Why Being Your Whole Self - Not Just Your "Good" Self - Drives Success and Fullfillment*, by Todd Hasdan and Robert Biswas-Diener
- *The How of Happiness, A New Approach to Getting the Life You Want*, by Sonja Lyubomirsky

Chapter 3

Belief

Merry Christmas?

Shortly after Christmas I was sitting in a doctor's waiting room surrounded by torn magazines, an indifferent receptionist, and a clock ticking away reminding me how late my appointment was running; it was a scenario that was by now all too familiar. I had spent the holiday feeling fragile and sore following surgery two days before and I was there for a post-surgical check-up. Several weeks earlier I had begun feeling pain in the right side of my pelvis. It started as a dull ache, which I tried to ignore. At work I was juggling various productions at a time when everyone seemed to want everything wrapped up before the end of the year, as if the 31st of December was a mystical date after which no work could take place. I spent my days bouncing between meetings and edit suites. And although I had been working on reducing my stress and balancing my emotions, I still had a long way to go. I had disregarded and pushed through the uncomfortable ache, but in the quiet of the night it demanded my attention and was keeping me awake. My insomnia gave way to rumination about the pain's origin. The more I thought about it, the more I noticed it. The more I noticed it, the more anxious I felt. I thought of all the stories I'd heard of people ignoring their symptoms only to discover the cause was something serious. I cleared my schedule so I could see a doctor.

I was referred to a specialist who wanted to perform a laparoscopic surgical procedure to determine whether I had endometriosis, an often painful disorder that affects about 10 percent of women.[1] I was newly wed to Jules and we hoped to start having children sometime in the next few years. With my history of autoimmune disease (which by now had been labeled by different doctors as everything from lupus to Sjögren's syndrome to fibromyalgia), and given that endometriosis can cause fertility problems, the doctor wanted to check things out.

He had good news. The surgery showed no sign of active endometriosis and the biopsy was clear. My nervous wait to hear the results was over and there would be no need for further treatment. But my initial relief soon passed and I asked the doctor what he thought was causing the pain. I explained that since recovering from the surgical tenderness I had noticed the original ache I'd seen him for was still there, less severe, but still there nonetheless.

His response was frustratingly vague as he explained that pelvic pain was one of the great mysteries of his profession. He was a kind man and a good doctor who meant well, but I left the consultation feeling confused and uncertain. Despite the drama of medical appointments, surgery, and a miserable Christmas Day recuperating, the whole thing was still unresolved. Part of me felt as if I had wasted everyone's valuable time and resources. Had I imagined the pain? Was it all in my head? Had I somehow manifested this brouhaha?

There was no path to follow. What could I do? Where should I turn? I was determined to avoid the Dr. Google trap, knowing that the hours I'd spent in online forums reading anecdotal stories about autoimmune disease, catastrophising about this or that, had brought little relief in the past. But the research I had delved into about the stress-health connection and the emotions-health connection had me intrigued and I wanted to see what science had to say when it came to chronic pelvic pain. So rather than typing things like "pelvic pain cure" into the search engine, I used terms like "research on pelvic pain treatment."

My investigations led me to a small but interesting study on the effect of laparoscopic surgery on pain and quality of life for women with endometriosis. In the study, 39 women were divided into two groups. The first group underwent surgical treatment for their endometriosis. The second group had exploratory surgery, but (unbeknownst to them) did not receive surgical treatment for their condition. In other words, they underwent fake surgery. While the study found that being given the real treatment was effective for just over half the women in the group, what was fascinating was that in the fake surgery group, 6 out of 19 women reported a reduction in their pain levels and an improvement in their quality of life. In other words, 30 percent of women in the placebo group felt better without their condition having actually been treated.[2] I should highlight that in the interest of ethical considerations, the women who were given the fake surgery were given real surgery at a later date. But the study piqued my curiosity. What was it about the fake surgery that caused women who had been experiencing severe pelvic pain to suddenly feel better? Had they been imagining their illness? Had their belief in a treatment made their pain evaporate?

In another pelvic pain study I came across, the researchers noted that the placebo response – in which patients improve just because they expect that a treatment will work – is recognised as a contributing factor in recovery from illness, and the authors cited other research scrutinising the effect.[3] I was stunned that this information wasn't more widely known. If what the study's authors were suggesting was true, the implication for my own health and the health of others was profound. Was it possible that I could somehow harness the power of belief to change my health?

The Powerful Placebo

During World War II, in a field hospital at Anzio beachhead in Italy, an American anaesthetist named Henry Beecher was attempting to treat a husky 19-year-old soldier wounded by a mortar shell. The young man was wild with pain from a meat cleaver-like wound through his chest and it took the strength of three men to hold him down. The patient had lost so much blood that his skin had turned purple. His condition was rapidly deteriorating and he complained bitterly of pain. Beecher administered an injection and the soldier calmed down at once, allowing the medical team to examine his wounds. Eight of his ribs had been cut in two by a shell fragment and one rib had penetrated his diaphragm and a kidney. But Beecher had not given the distressed man a shot of the powerful pain relieving drug morphine, which was commonly being used to treat severely wounded soldiers. Instead, he had administered a sedative, in a dose too low to have any kind of pain-relieving effects.[4]

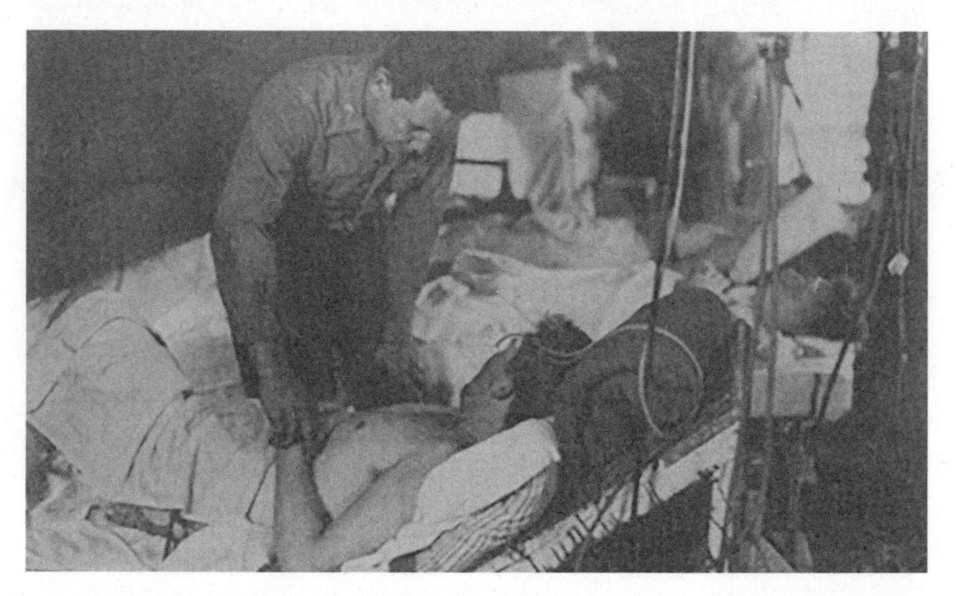

Postoperative ward in 1st Platoon, 33d Field Hospital, Italy, 1944. *Credit: U.S. Government*

Beecher was acting on well informed instinct. The Harvard-trained doctor was concerned that wounded soldiers were being poisoned from too much morphine, so he started closely observing their pain levels before offering them the potent opiate. Rather than automatically giving soldiers pain relief, he paused to ask them how they felt. In his 1946 paper based on his observations of more than 200 gravely wounded soldiers in Africa and Europe, Beecher challenged the commonly held belief that the more extensive the wound, the worse the pain. He was surprised when three quarters of the wounded soldiers had so little pain they declined morphine.[5] Injured though they were, these men had a one-way ticket home and their spirits were high. In the case of the distressed young solider with the chest wound, Beecher suspected that his pain was worsened more by his anxiety than by his wound. It was a story he used throughout his career to passionately argue that our state of mind can have a significant impact on how we feel pain, and how we heal.

It's unlikely that during the war Beecher knew his experiences marked the beginning of a career that would change the course of medical research and inspire the development of new treatments for disease. Ten years after his paper on pain in men wounded in battle was published, he published a seminal review paper in which he analysed 15 studies where "dummy" pills or placebos were used, concluding that in about 35 percent of cases, placebos relieved "a fairly wide variety of conditions, including pain, nausea, and mood changes." In other words, about one third of people recovered directly because of their belief in a drug or treatment rather than because of the treatment itself.[6]

Although we now know there were methodological errors in his analysis,[7] the paper established the template for the process by which all new drugs are tested for the pharmaceutical industry today and is considered one of the most influential scientific papers of all time. Beecher became the trailblazer for the Randomized Clinical Trial or RCT – the double blind, placebo-controlled method accepted as the gold standard for scientific research. His work has since inspired thousands of doctors and scientists to study what we have come to know as the "placebo effect," in which a fake treatment such as sham surgery or an inactive substance like sugar, water, or saline solution improves a patient's condition simply because they have an expectation that it will be helpful.

We've all heard stories about gifted healers producing miracle cures and tales of witch doctors in far-off places putting curses on people that result in their untimely deaths. These stories are often dismissed as fantasy or the result of a person's psychosis or gullibility rather than acknowledged as a physiological phenomenon. But in recent decades there's been an uprising of independent researchers around the world who are extending Beecher's work and taking it to a whole new level. Instead of asking *whether* the placebo effect works, they're now studying *how* the placebo effect works.

Overall, studies suggest that the effects of our expectations and beliefs may account for good-to-excellent health improvement for almost 70 percent of us.[8] Here are some fascinating findings that might make you reconsider the seemingly innocuous placebo effect:

TAKING a placebo four times a day can make an ulcer heal more quickly than taking a placebo twice a day.[9]

PATIENTS who adhere to taking their prescribed fake pills do significantly better than those who take only some of them.[10]

FOR people being treated for severe nausea and vomiting, placebo tablets can be just as effective as taking drugs.[11]

THIRTY percent of people with a moderate to severe migraine can recover with a placebo, and the effect is enhanced if the placebo is administered via an injection rather than in a tablet.[12]

MIGRAINE patients who were given an active drug deceptively labeled as "placebo" reported the same degree of pain relief as patients who were given a placebo labeled with the correct drug's name.[13]

THE more expensive the placebo, the better it is at reducing pain.[14]

THE colour of a pill makes a difference depending on where you're from. In many parts of the world, red and orange placebo pills act as uppers; blue and green placebo pills act as downers,[15] except in Italy where men are fans of their beloved Forza Azzuri (Blue Force) national soccer team and blue pills have the opposite effect.[16]

ONE stunning finding from a 2015 review of 21 minor surgical procedures, such as arthroscopic knee surgery, found that they were, on average, no more effective than sham surgeries.[17]

The Physiology of Belief

More than 40 years ago at the University of Rochester, a researcher named Robert Ader was studying taste aversion in rats when he began to form a theory that the mind could significantly affect the ability of the immune system to fight disease. His colleagues greeted the idea with scepticism, but nevertheless, in the mid-1970s he conducted a game-changing experiment that proved he could suppress the immune systems of rats by making them "believe" they had been given a drug.[18] He did this by giving the rats sweetened water and at the same time injecting them with a drug that induced a stomach upset and suppressed their immune systems. The rats soon started associating the water with feeling sick and learned to avoid drinking it. Ader then stopped giving the rats the drug but continued to force feed them the sugar solution by dropping it in their eyes. He was stunned to find that the rats began to die and realised that, in addition to training the rats to avoid the sugar water, he had been training their immune systems to become suppressed merely through exposure to the taste of sugar water. With suppressed immune systems, the rats succumbed to infections and died. This effect is an example of "classical conditioning," and Ader's research was one of the first scientific clues to suggest that the brain and the immune system are connected. This research launched the field of psychoneuroimmunology (mind-brain-immune science) and inspired a large body of research that suggests our mind can unconsciously have profound effects on our body's functions.

Ader's work was the foundation for many later research papers, including a 2002 study in which researchers showed they could reproduce the effect in humans.[19] A 2007 study found that athletes given a performance-enhancing drug during pre-competition training could be given a placebo on the day of competition and still experience an increase in pain endurance and physical performance. (This opens up a whole can of worms for anti-doping authorities in sports.[20])

Ader also continued the research and in 2009, two years before his death at aged 79, he published a paper in which he and his fellow researchers at the University of Rochester Medical Center used classical conditioning to successfully treat people with psoriasis using a quarter to a half of the usual dose of a widely used steroid medication.[21] "Our study provides evidence that the placebo effect can make possible the treatment of psoriasis with an amount of drug that should be too small to work.... While these results are preliminary, we believe the medical establishment needs to recognise the mind's reaction to medication as a powerful part of many drug effects, and start taking advantage of it," Ader said at the time.[22]

Ader's call to the medical community to take the role of the mind seriously when considering the best treatment path for patients is one echoed today by a pioneering group of placebo researchers in locations dotted around the world.[23] Fabrizio Benedetti, a leading neurophysiologist from the University of Turin in Italy, is at the forefront. Recently he demonstrated it is possible to reduce medication given to people suffering from Parkinson's disease by first treating them with the anti-Parkinson's medication apomorphine and then, on a subsequent administration – and unbeknownst to the patient – giving them a fake. After first training subjects' bodies to respond to the real drug, Benedetti was able to give them a placebo and elicit the same response as if they'd been given the real drug. In fact, the greater the number of previous apomorphine administrations, the larger the magnitude and the longer the duration of the placebo responses.[24] During our chat from his office in Turin, Benedetti explained that "If you give an anti-Parkinson agent on Monday, on Tuesday, on Wednesday, on Thursday, and on Friday, and then on Saturday you replace the real drug with a fake drug, virtually all patients will respond."

This is not to say that you can be given any fake pill to heal any ailment. Benedetti is careful to highlight that drinking a glass of water to cure a bacterial infection is not likely to work, no matter how much you believe in its power. "I don't think that a glass of fresh water can kill bacteria or viruses, and I don't think that fresh water or a sugar pill can produce general anaesthesia. There are some conditions in which a placebo response is not present at all. It's completely absent. There are other conditions in which the placebo response is very important, like depression, pain, movement disorders, and the general neuropsychiatric disorders."

Working out exactly when, where, and how our beliefs and expectations can induce a physical response is precisely the focus of the work being done by researchers like Benedetti. Remarkably, the latest evidence reveals that classical conditioning isn't the only way the placebo effect works in your body.[25] For example, we now know that placebos can work in a way similar to morphine by using the endogenous opioid system, the body's innate pain-relieving system.[26] Another way placebos can work is by triggering dopamine, the chemical in your brain that makes you anticipate pleasure and reward. In a study of Parkinson's disease patients who were told they would be given either an active drug or a placebo, researchers witnessed a 200 percent increase in dopamine in their subjects' brains. That is the same increase of dopamine observed in healthy people given the powerful stimulant amphetamine.[27] It's interesting that the people with Parkinson's who experienced the highest levels of dopamine also reported greater relief from the stiffness and inflexibility in their muscles that comes with having the disease.[28]

The main point here is that although there is still much to discover, we now know there exists not one single placebo effect, but many placebo effects that work in different ways.[29] If you respond to a placebo it may be because you've been conditioned to respond (like Ader's rats), it may be that pain-relieving chemicals are triggered in your brain, or that your doctor has reassured you enough to make you feel less anxious, which improves your mood and makes you feel better. Scientists are really just starting to uncover the mysterious underpinnings of placebo and I won't be surprised if before this book goes to print more biological mechanisms of belief are revealed.

Worried Sick

In 2007, a 27-year old man was rushed to hospital after taking a drug overdose. When he arrived at the emergency department he collapsed, dropping a prescription bottle for an experimental antidepressant medication on the floor. His blood pressure was crashing and he was hyperventilating and shaking. Nurses sprang into action and inserted an intravenous line into his arm to try to maintain his blood pressure and save his life.

This man had been enrolled in an antidepressant drug trial. In the first month he reported that his loneliness and depression had improved significantly, but in the second month he had an argument with his ex-girlfriend and became suicidal. He took the remaining 29 pills all at once but immediately regretted his action and was rushed to the hospital by his neighbour.

The case was written up in the medical journal *General Hospital Psychiatry,* because four hours after he collapsed it was revealed that "Mr. A" had been in the placebo arm of the clinical trial. He had taken an overdose of *sugar pills.* When he discovered the news, the man was surprised and tearful with relief, and within a short time he recovered completely.

This phenomenon is called the "nocebo effect" – when you have a negative response to a harmless substance that you believe is harmful. In 2014 Fabrizio Benedetti wanted to test just how easy it would be to trigger a nocebo effect. Before taking 121 students to a medical research facility located 3,500 metres (11,500 feet) above sea level in the Italian Alps, he deliberately started a rumour about the risk of altitude sickness and the possible occurrence of severe headache. He instructed only one student to bring a specific dose of aspirin in case he succumbed. Benedetti gave the young man a brochure depicting a headache sufferer at 3,500 metres lying on a bed, grimacing, and taking pills.

It took just one week for Benedetti's "social infection" to spread, during which time another 36 students contacted the university asking for more details about high altitude headache and the doses of aspirin needed for their trip. Unbeknown to these students, they would become Benedetti's nocebo experimental group. On the day of the trip, 86 percent of those in the nocebo group got a headache versus only 52 percent in the control group. Those who had heard the rumour were also the ones who suffered the worst headaches.

While it is largely thought that the nocebo response works by directing our attention toward symptoms that would have been there anyway, it is interesting that in Benedetti's study, analysis of the students' salvia revealed a genuine biological response to the low oxygen conditions including a proliferation of the enzymes associated with altitude headache. It's also interesting that the students in the nocebo group showed an increase of the stress hormone cortisol, though the students in the control group did not, indicating that the stress hormone rise was due to the anxiety primed by the rumour.[30]

The study raises interesting questions about the idea of a *social* nocebo, where negative expectations can be communicated by our friends, colleagues, family members, and doctors, especially in the age of smart technology and social media when information can be shared very quickly. "The propagation of negative and positive expectation could be very important in illness in general and in the generation of pathology or disease," Benedetti told me. "It shows there is what we call 'social learning.' Social learning could be really very important in everyday life because expectations about something like pain can be communicated across different individuals, across colleagues, across friends, across relatives. Chronic pain is a major problem today and I would say that the social communication about chronic pain could play a very important role in the propagation of pain between different individuals."

When Your Body Believes Your Mind

Wendy Berry Mendes first became fascinated by mind-body interactions when she was an undergraduate student applying for an internship with the Federal Bureau of Investigation (FBI). As part of her application, she had to undergo a lie-detection test in order prove her trustworthiness for working in a position that gave her exposure to high-level security information.[31] Rigged to a number of sensors to measure her respiration, heart rate, skin conductance, and skin temperature, Mendes recalls feeling her entire body go on edge. She had cold, sweaty palms, a dry mouth, and her heart raced when she was asked the questions, "In the past seven years, have you been 100 percent honest all the time?" and "In the past seven years, have you ever said something negative about a friend?" Thinking she wouldn't have a chance at getting the job if she answered yes to these questions, which spoke to her character and integrity, Mendes fibbed. Her deception was immediately recorded by the machine. "My body betrayed me and exposed me for my white lies and gossipy ways," Mendes said.

The experience planted the idea for her that our mental states and bodily responses are inextricably linked. "For me, this experience was foundational. I was fascinated that my body could betray me, and that no matter how much I tried to control my internal responses, I was a slave to them in many respects," she said. Despite her deceit, Mendes got the internship and it was to be the beginning of her highly awarded research career. She is now a professor in the School of Medicine at the University of California, San Francisco and an expert in using physiological markers to study how our mind influences our body, and how our body can influence our thoughts and emotions.

In what I can only describe as comfortable society's most severe form of torture, Mendes joined with Jeremy Jamieson and Matthew Nock from Harvard University for a study that involved the two tasks many of us fear most – public speaking and mental arithmetic. Participants had to perform an impromptu five minute speech about their personal strengths and weaknesses. The speech was delivered in front of a camera and a panel of hostile evaluators who gave negative feedback by furrowing their brows, crossing their arms, and frowning at the participants. If the participant ran out of things to say, they were told to keep going until their five minutes was up. Following their speech, they had to complete a mathematics task, counting backwards by seven from 996, all the while being interrupted and told things like "You're not very good are you?" and "Other people seem to be able to do this."

This task is called the *Trier Social Stress Test,* and in the last 15 years it's been shown to raise the stress hormone cortisol by up to 300 percent in test subjects.[32] "I think imagining the absolute worst job interview you have ever been on and then multiplying that experience by two or three and that gets you to a TSST," Mendes told me.

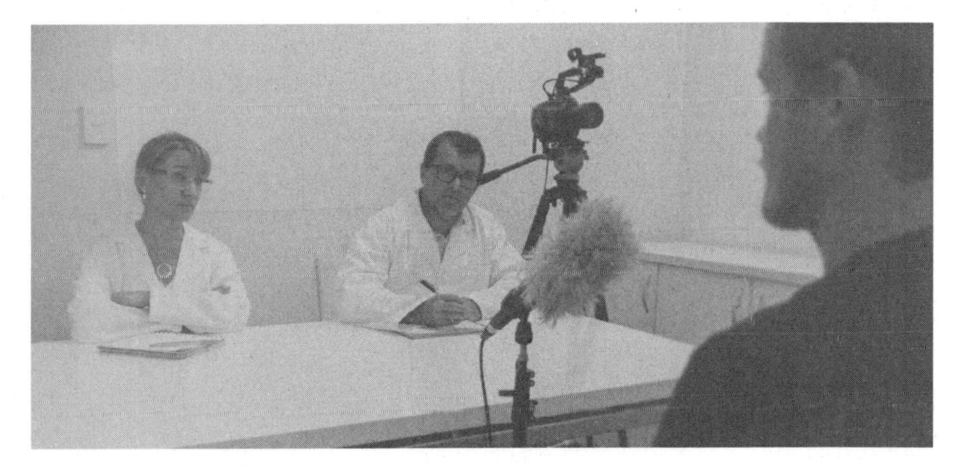

The Trier Social Stress Test.

In a torturous version of the Trier test, Mendes and her colleagues assigned participants to one of three conditions. One group was told the best way to deal with stress is to try to ignore it. Another group was told about the human challenge response and instructed to see their stress as positive, functional, and adaptive, and that the response would give their heart and brain more blood which would help them perform better.[33] A control group was given no specific instructions.

Taking advantage of Mendes's specialty in using biological markers, the researchers measured the participants' stress responses during the experiment, including their cardiovascular reactivity and cognitive functioning. The results were astounding. The people in the *stress is good* reappraisal group not only reported feeling they were better-equipped to handle the task, but also responded on a physiological level. They still had high levels of stress hormones and increased heart rates, but their physiology was more efficient. Their hearts pumped out more blood with each beat and their blood vessels were less constricted.[34] In other words, reframing how they thought about stress shifted their physiological responses in positive ways.

Those in the control group and in the group instructed to ignore their stress unfortunately had a different physiological experience. They had the usual stress response hormones, along with less efficient hearts and more constricted blood vessels. "Think of the diameter of a fire hose getting smaller so less water can move through the hose; this is what happens in the arteries. Less oxygenated blood can move freely through the system and the extreme periphery, like hands, fingers, feet, and toes, receive the least amount of blood," says Mendes, who explained that if you had felt the hands of the people in the "ignore stress" group, they would likely have been stone cold.

Although Mendes is careful to highlight that this is not about "thinking our way to a better life" and that we don't yet know whether these changes can persist in the long run, the study showed it is possible to immediately change our biology simply by changing the way we perceive life events such as the nerve-racking task of having to give an impromptu speech and by reappraising our beliefs about a situation.

Mendes's work is further strengthened by another study done by Yale researchers during the 2008 Global Financial Crisis (GFC). You may recall this was a very difficult time for people; unemployment rates were in double digits, widespread dismissals took place, and employees faced unknown futures alongside increased pressure to perform.[35] Amid this turmoil and uncertainty, researchers Alia Crum, Peter Salovey, and Shawn Achor set out to test if by changing people's mindsets, they could change the way people were responding to the crisis psychologically, behaviourally, and physiologically.[36]

Nearly 400 men and women from the financial firm UBS took part in the experimental mindset intervention and were divided into three groups. Over the course of a week, one group was emailed links to videos designed to reinforce the common belief that stress is bad for you and should be ignored or avoided where possible. These videos contained information about stress being America's number one health issue as well as examples of people being unable to perform under stress. A second group – the control group – was not given any stress related materials. A third group was given a stress-is-enhancing mindset intervention. The employees in this group were shown videos about the benefits of stress. They were taught how stress can make people stronger, more creative, and strengthen relationships. They were given examples of companies that performed well in the face of adversity and told stories of leaders who took remarkable actions while under great stress.

At the end of the study the stress-is-enhancing group reported higher levels of engagement and performance at work and fewer negative health symptoms including fewer back aches, less muscle tension, and less insomnia.[37] The researchers also demonstrated in a follow-up study that having a stress-is-enhancing mindset lowered levels of the stress hormone cortisol in people who tended to have high levels of stress reactivity.[38] Overall, they concluded that having a stress-is-enhancing mindset can engender positive effects in both health and performance, and having a stress-is-debilitating mindset is more likely to engender debilitating effects.

It's common sense that the mindset we take with us when we face the challenges of everyday life can have an effect on the choices we make and the behaviours we adopt.[39] But this new research demonstrates that what we think and believe can also influence physiological outcomes that affect our health.

Turning Back the Clock

In 1979, Ellen Langer piled two groups of men in their seventies and eighties into vans and drove them to an old monastery in New Hampshire. When the men arrived, they discovered they had time-traveled 20 years into the past. For the next week their environment was a complete replication of what life was like in the 1950s. They were surrounded by old issues of *Life* magazine and the *Saturday Evening Post*; a black-and-white television and a vintage radio broadcast "live" programs from 1959.

Langer was a researcher from Harvard who wanted to test what effect turning back the clock psychologically would have on participants' physiological states. She wanted to see if by immersing them in an environment 20 years in the past she could make them biologically younger. One group of men was asked to act as though they were living in the 1950s and were instructed only to talk as though 1959 were the present day. As they watched old movies like *The Diary of Anne Frank* and *Ben-Hur*, discussed pressing issues of the day such as communism and the need for bomb shelters, and listened to Nat "King" Cole on the radio, they were instructed to "let themselves be who they were 20 years earlier." The second group of men was the control group. They also spent a week in the 1950s environment, but they were instructed only to reminisce about that era.

In her book *Counterclockwise; Mindful Health and the Power of Possibility*, Langer reported remarkable transformations in the men. "At the end, one of them had begun to walk without using his cane," she wrote. Both groups of men showed improvements in measures of their physical strength, manual dexterity, gait, posture, perception, memory, cognition, taste sensitivity, hearing, and vision. The group for whom Langer had turned back the clock, who were experiencing their surroundings as if it were 1959, showed even greater improvements on most of the measures. When independent observers looked at "before" and "after" photos of the men who had been living as though the past were the present, they rated the subjects' appearances as being more than two years younger at the end of the study than they had been at the start.

Captivating as this experiment was, it was never submitted to peer-reviewed scientific journals. There were only nine men in the experimental cohort of the study, and eight in the control group, and the intervention lasted only five days. There were just too many variables and possible explanations for the men's transformation. Despite Langer's being a professor at Harvard Medical School, her work is regularly called into question by sceptics.[40] Nevertheless, the Counterclockwise experiment has generated significant buzz. Actress Jennifer Aniston has reportedly signed on to play Langer in a Hollywood film about the experiment.[41] A replication of the study by the BBC that used ageing celebrities as the test subjects made for compelling television viewing, especially with memory, mood, flexibility, stamina, and even eyesight improvements being recorded in almost all the participants. Studies were also conducted by other researchers demonstrating that if people felt older than their actual age, they were more likely to die earlier.[42] As Langer writes in her book "These improvements were the result of one week spent with a group of strangers. Imagine the possibilities if our culture afforded us a different set of mindsets than we have about old age."[43]

Placebos in Action

Whichever way we look at it, more research must be done before we can fully understand when and where the power of belief might be necessary, called for, and effective. It's likely that in the future, targeted placebo responses will be effective for treating some diseases but not others, or to alleviate some aspects of disease but not others. For example, at this stage there's no evidence that placebos can make cancer tumours shrink. In fact, a review of 37 "gold standard" double-blind clinical studies found that tumours rarely respond to placebos.[44] On the other hand, a review of treatments for osteoarthritis concluded that there is a significant placebo effect on pain, stiffness, and function.[45]

It's interesting, however, that the tumour analysis also found that placebos could help relieve symptoms; this is an especially important point for people in pain looking for improved quality of life, and should not be disregarded as meaningless. It's also interesting that the osteoarthritis review found that trials using injections, acupuncture, and placebo surgery (with lots of flashy theatrics and interaction with medical experts) had the largest placebo effects. This finding illustrates one of the key directions in which placebo science is heading. It seems that the "ritual of medicine," with its impressive instrumentation and fancy language, can enhance a patient's expectations of recovery and can therefore enhance placebo effects. Increasingly, research indicates that the medical settings in which we receive our treatments, and the words used by medical professionals, may have a significant effect on our health outcomes. This important subject warrants an entire discussion of its own, which you'll find in Chapter 8 (Healthcare).

Also at the very frontier of this placebo research is fascinating evidence that our genetics play a role in determining who may respond well to placebo treatments. This potential was first identified in 2008[46] and taken to a whole new level in 2012 when Kathryn Hall and her team at Harvard Medical School, who were studying people with irritable bowel syndrome, discovered that people with variations of the gene COMT (which affects levels of dopamine in the brain) responded more strongly to placebos.[47] In 2015, Hall and her team wrote a headline-grabbing review paper that identified specific genetic pathways implicated in the placebo response.[48] The idea of genetic signatures of placebo – the placebome is very new and the science is in its "proof of concept stage," but the implications are wide-reaching. A day may come when drug companies can speed up their research processes by genetically testing potential participants and culling out placebo responders in their trials. There may also be a time in the not too distant future when your doctor tests your placebo response before determining your treatment path.

The common misunderstanding of many people, especially medical professionals, is that the placebo response is only a subjective phenomenon (that is, that it exists only in their patient's mind). I hope the information here helps convince you that there is more to it than that, and that your beliefs, expectations and mindsets are an important part of your health. But compelling as the new science of placebo is, it should not be thought of in any way as a replacement for the active treatments of modern medicine. When compared to proven therapies, placebo responses are often smaller, less reliable, and less predictable. There is still a long way to go in understanding how placebos can be used effectively in medicine. "I think the future challenge will be to answer these four questions: where, when, how, and why placebos work," Fabrizio Benedetti told me. He stressed this is not something you can do at home yourself, explaining that "Before a decision of whether or not to take a placebo is made, there should be a very good diagnosis by a doctor. A headache could be only a headache. A headache could also be the expression of a brain cancer. It's very important that the physician, that the doctor, that a good health professional, makes a good diagnosis before deciding whether or not to give a placebo."

As for my own experience with chronic pain, I now see that my beliefs, expectations, and mindset can trigger a significant biochemical effect in my body that I can use to improve my mental and physical wellbeing. Having explored all the available medical options for my pelvic pain, in the months following the surgery I made significant lifestyle changes. I used meditation to relieve my worry and stop my ruminating thoughts. I developed a level of acceptance around my condition and, rather than perceiving it as *pain*, began thinking about it as a *sensation*.

Having read papers published in academic journals demonstrating that acupuncture had been effective in helping people who experience chronic pain, I turned to a Japanese acupuncturist who also practiced shiatsu massage, which I thought would also be helpful for my arthritis.[49] Although I couldn't really understand his accented English, his needles and massages brought great relief. It didn't matter to me whether this was because of an unseen energy force he called *chi*, or because his massages helped my muscles relax, or because the attention he gave me stimulated the pain relief pathways in my brain. To me, as a sick person experiencing chronic pain, it only mattered that I *felt* a little better.

Key Takeaways

1 It's now well-established that your beliefs and expectations can have a profound effect on your perception of pain, your quality of life, your physiology, and your health. The "placebo response" – in which patients improve just because they *expect* that a treatment will work – accounts for good-to-excellent health improvement for a majority of people.

2 There exists not one single placebo effect, but many placebo effects that work in different ways – for example, classical conditioning (where your immune system becomes programmed to respond by expectation of the treatment), pain relief (where your expectation activates your brain's pain relieving pathways), stress relief (where a treatment brings a reduction in anxiety), and the promise of reward (where your expectation activates your brain's feel-good, reward pathways).

3 We can literally worry ourselves sick. Negative expectations can trigger a physiological effect called "nocebo"– that is, when you have a negative response to something that is actually harmless. These negative expectations can be propagated by your friends, colleagues, family members, and doctors, as well as by the media.

4 Your mindset influences not only your choices and behaviour, but also your physiology and health. By changing the way you view something like the nerve-racking task of having to give an impromptu speech, and by rethinking your beliefs about a situation, you can trigger positive physiological changes in your body.

5 Researchers are still in the very early stages of determining where, when, how, and why placebos work. It is likely that placebos will be found effective for treating some diseases but not others, or some aspects of disease but not others. Do not rely entirely on belief and expectation in place of conventional medicine.

Getting Started

NEXT time you find yourself in a challenging situation, consider a mindset reset. Thinking things like "This task is exciting" rather than "This task is scary" can help you to change the way you view a situation. There's a video on my website to help you change the way you view stress, based on the Yale mindset reset study. See the following Extra Resources section for details.

PAY attention to the influence of negative expectations that might be created by the people around you including your friends, colleagues, family members, doctors, and the media. Once you notice them, you can then actively realign them with helpful beliefs and expectations.

USE meditation and mindfulness to reduce your health-related worry and rumination. For more information, refer to Chapter 1 (Stress).

MAKE a ritual around your treatment to enhance the possibility that classical conditioning can take place. For example, if you take medicine every day, rather than swallowing your pill absentmindedly as you're racing out the door, follow a repetitious routine such as always taking it in the same location and eating a jelly bean afterwards.

BE thorough and attentive to instructions from healthcare providers and medicine labels to enhance the expectation effect. For example, if your doctor says to take one tablet three times a day after meals for two weeks, be sure to follow the exact prescription. Adherence to a treatment can boost the expectation effect and help program your body's response.

Extra Resources

AVAILABLE AT
www.thewholehealthlife.com/resources

ACCESS extended audio and video interviews with the experts including:

- *Fabrizio Benedetti (Professor of Physiology and Neuroscience at the University of Turin Medical School and at the National Institute of Neuroscience, Turin, Italy)*
- *Damien Finnis (Associate Professor at the University of Sydney Pain Management Research Institute, Royal North Shore Hospital and the School of Rehabilitation Sciences, Griffith University)*

WATCH a video I've created based on the Yale mindset reset study, designed to encourage a "stress-is-enhancing" mindset.

MY recommended reading list, which I update regularly, is available on my website. Books relevant to this chapter include:

- *Placebo Effects: Understanding the mechanisms in health and disease*, by Fabrizio Benedetti
- *Meaning, Medicine and the 'Placebo Effect,'* by Daniel E Moerman
- *Counterclockwise: A Proven Way to Think Yourself Younger and Healthier*, by Ellen J Langer

Chapter 4

Food

What to Eat?

With a renewed sense of determination after my inexplicable pelvic pain episode, I was intent on finding answers to my ongoing health questions. Overall, I was feeling a little better with more energy and the odd symptom-free day or week, but I was still pushing myself too much at work and convalescing on the weekends as my body demanded time to catch up on sleep and rest. There were still flare-ups, with lethargy and soreness. I was also experiencing a good deal of stomach upset and found myself waking in the middle of the night with crippling cramping. On some sleepless nights, the pain was unbearable.

I'd long been experimenting with my diet hoping to find a solution to the stomach upsets that had plagued me for as long as I could remember. But working in the fast-paced burn and churn of television often meant that my experiments were compromised. I was forced to eat on the run, often having to choose from the best of a range of bad options. There never seemed time for me to research for myself what I should be eating, so I relied on the opinions of others and followed the advice of "experts" who promised they could cure my ills if I simply cut out this or that type of food or bought this or that type of supplement.

One "medical nutritionist" I saw asked all manner of important-sounding questions, charged me $200, and promised to email me a report with her recommendations. She never sent the report, despite my numerous follow-up phone calls and emails. Another time I visited a place with the scientific sounding name *Advanced Allergy Elimination* that promised to identify and cure my food allergies. They diagnosed me using a "non-invasive muscle strength indicator test" and told me that I had a vast number of allergies that would need to be treated in a certain sequence, one session at a time, by using a technique based on "acupressure and positive conditioning." Each time I sat in that waiting room alongside mothers with their asthmatic kids and people who had suffered from hay fever all their lives, I was full of hope. Was this finally the answer? In 2009 the Federal Court in Australia declared that the company had violated Australian law by making "false, misleading and deceptive" representations. The company no longer operates.[1] You probably won't be surprised that the treatments did not resolve my issues.

While there are, of course, many scrupulous and highly-qualified practitioners working in the nutrition field, my experience was by then thoroughly tainted, leaving me feeling used, abused, and confused. Nevertheless, I continued with various diet experiments, including, most recently, juicing. A popular documentary in which people were featured recovering from illnesses just by drinking freshly squeezed fruit and vegetable juice had inspired some of my friends to take up "cleansing." I kept hearing about the huge hit of micro-nutrients I would get by squeezing fruit and veggies through a machine to extract their juices. I bought two top of the line juicers, one for home and the other for the office, and the fridges at both locations were soon bursting with fresh produce ready for me to extract all the health benefits they had to offer.

To be really honest, the fact that what effectively became juice-fasting coincided with my wedding preparations was no coincidence. My desire to look good in my strapless wedding dress when I walked down the aisle to marry Jules was a strong motivator in my swapping out one or two meals a day with veggie juices – and I did lose a few kilograms in a relatively short stretch of time. But once the wedding was over, my main source of motivation passed and my appetite started winning out over my willpower. Although I was still drinking a freshly squeezed juice every day, my old eating habits returned, resplendent with a weakness for chocolate and anything involving caramel. Once more, I was choosing convenience and availability over nutritional integrity. The weight crept back on and my stomach issues continued throughout.

There's little doubt that diet is one of the most important influencers of our health.[2] Insufficient fruit and vegetable intake is among the top ten risk factors contributing to mortality worldwide[3] and it's estimated that in 2013, 5.2 million people died worldwide because of inadequate fruit and vegetable consumption.[4] In fact, worldwide, insufficient intake of fruit and vegetables is estimated to cause around 14 percent of gastrointestinal cancer deaths, about 11 percent of ischaemic heart disease deaths, and about nine percent of stroke deaths.[5] It is also estimated that factors related to nutrition could account for more than one third of cancer deaths.[6]

I knew that my constant gut issues were likely linked to my autoimmune illness, and I knew it was time to use my journalistic and investigative skills to find out for myself what I should or should not be eating. But the more I dove into nutrition science, the more I realised just how muddy the waters are. One major problem is that the leading diet researchers are still divided about what exactly a healthy diet looks like. The subject of what to eat is an absolute minefield if you're looking for credible, unquestionable, absolute, and conclusive advice. There are vegans and vegetarians, omnivores, carnivores, flexi-tarians and veg-aquarians; low carb vs low fat, high carb vs high protein, slow cooked vs raw, organic vs conventionally grown, preservative-free, gluten-free, dairy-free, sugar-free... whatever diet people advocate, there is a wealth of scientific reasoning and an abundance of anecdotal stories that can spark fiery debate. So where should we turn and whom should we believe?

The Right Diet

If you're like me and feel confused and overwhelmed by the latest diet information, you're not alone. According to one US report, three out of every four people claim that today's ever-changing dietary guidelines make it hard to know what to believe. In fact, over half of Americans say it is easier to figure out their income taxes than to figure out what they should and shouldn't eat to be healthier.[7] Fortunately, there is the nonprofit publisher *Annual Reviews,* which is dedicated to helping scientists cope with ever-increasing volumes of research and data by providing robust and systematic reviews of important topics in the scientific and medical literature. In 2014, the publication shone the spotlight on diet.

To perform the analysis, the editors selected two researchers from Yale University who had no agenda regarding any one particular diet, but were both experts on nutrition science. David Katz and Stephanie Meller spent a year poring over studies of the most popular mainstream diets, including low carb, low glycemic, low fat, Mediterranean, paleo, vegan, and diets that conform to various authoritative dietary guidelines.

I interviewed Katz in a series of emails. In addition to being the founding director of the Prevention Research Center at Yale University, he is also an associate professor of public health practice at the Yale University School of Medicine and has authored or coauthored over 200 scientific papers. He explained that he was likely invited to conduct the review not just because he had written three editions of a leading nutrition textbook for healthcare professionals, but because he was not tethered to any particular diet. "Most leading nutrition experts have spent their careers studying some particular diet: vegan, paleo, Mediterranean, etc.," he wrote. "I have spent my career focused on helping people actually apply the best dietary advice we have. So it is probably easier for me, than for many, to see the big picture, and follow the evidence wherever it leads."

He and Meller published their findings in a paper titled, "Can We Say What Diet Is Best for Health?"[8] Their conclusions are fascinating:

"There have been no rigorous, long-term studies comparing contenders for best diet laurels using methodology that precludes bias and confounding, and for many reasons such studies are unlikely. In the absence of such direct comparisons, claims for the established superiority of any one specific diet over others are exaggerated."

Translation – there is no one diet to rule them all, nor will there likely be one in the future.

This is disappointing news for those of us who want to know what to eat. But it makes sense because nutrition science is fraught with difficulties including the fact that it's impossible to lock 20,000 people of a variety of ages, body types, ethnicities, and genders into a lab for 50 years and feed them specific diets, while keeping every other variable the same. This is further complicated by emerging evidence indicating that the dietary advice of the future may need to be different for different people depending on their individual genes.[9]

Considering all this, it would be easy to give up on the search for the right diet and just eat whatever you want. After all, for every study showing [insert ingredient here regardless of whether it's a fruit, vegetable, sweet treat, caffeinated or alcoholic beverage] is bad for you, you'll surely find a study to show that [that same ingredient] is good for you. What's the point? Life's short. We may as well eat whatever we want. Right? Well... let's not be so hasty. When you take a second look at Katz and Meller's paper, there are actually some very concrete and heartening findings. While they did conclude that no one diet is best, they also found a very clear and compelling universal thread across them all:

"A diet of minimally processed foods close to nature, predominantly plants, is decisively associated with health promotion and disease prevention."

In a table from the article, shown below, Katz and Meller demonstrate that all these seemingly-conflicting diets actually have many things in common. They limit refined starches, added sugars, and processed foods. They also emphasise whole plant foods (with or without lean meats, fish, poultry, and seafood). In all the noise about what we should *not* eat, the fundamental message about what we *should* eat is being lost. Katz and Meller finally conclude:

"The case that we should, indeed, eat true food, mostly plants, is all but incontrovertible."

	Low-carbohydrate	Low-fat/ Vegetarian/ Vegan	Low-glycemic	Mediterranean	Mixed/ Balanced	Paleolithic
Health benefits relate to:	Emphasis on restriction of refined starches and added sugars in particular.	Emphasis on plant foods direct from nature; avoidance of harmful fats.	Restriction of starches, added sugars; high fiber intake.	Foods direct from nature; mostly plants; emphasis on healthful oils, notably mono-unsaturates	Minimization of highly processed energy-dense foods; emphasis on wholesome foods in moderate quantities.	Minimization of processed foods. Emphasis on natural plant foods and lean meats.
Compatible elements:	Limited refined starches, added sugars, processed foods; limited intake of certain fats; emphasis on whole plant foods with or without lean meats, fish, poultry, seafood.					
And all potentially consistent with:	Food, not too much, mostly plants[a,b].					

a) Portion control maybe facilitated by choosing better quality foods which have the tendency to promote satiety with fewer calories.
b) While neither the low-carbohydrate nor Paleolithic diet need be "mostly plants", both can be.

Diverse diets making competing claims actually emphasise key elements that are generally compatible, complementary, or even duplicative. *Credit: Katz, DL, & Meller, S, 2014. Can we say what diet is best for health? Annual Review of Public Health, 35, 83-103.*

"Actually, I think it's pretty simple," Katz wrote during our email exchange. "The evidence indicating that all the best diets emphasize vegetables, fruits, whole grains, beans, lentils, nuts, seeds, and water for thirst is rather overwhelming. But whole industries run on pseudo-confusion: big food, big pharma, big media, big publishing. As for scientists, we tend to emphasize the thing we work on all the time. So, naturally, someone who studies vegan diets will talk about the benefits of those diets; and someone who studies Mediterranean diets will talk about those. It may sound as if they are disagreeing, because they are making different choices, but they would actually agree about the fundamentals that make good diets good in general."

I'm very aware that a take-home message to eat less processed food and more plants is not particularly sexy or groundbreaking. I certainly won't be inspiring a whole new health movement and I'm not the first person to come to this conclusion. But despite how seemingly obvious this message is, it's just not getting through. For example, most people eat well below the World Health Organization's recommendation of a *minimum* of 400 grams of fruit and vegetables (approximately five portions) per day.[10] Specifically, illnesses that are highly diet-related, like heart disease, could be reduced by 31 percent if people ate just 600 grams of fruit and vegetables every day. A more recent analysis published in the highly-regarded journal *PNAS* demonstrated the significant benefits for not only health, but also to the environment and the global economy, if we were to eat more plants. A global change to more plant-based diets could, in 2050, save up to 1 trillion US dollars annually by reducing health care costs and lost productivity. That figure balloons to as much as $30 trillion annually in 2050 when we also consider the economic value of lost life.[11]

Although experts will continue to debate what a healthy diet looks like for the next century and beyond, it would be hard to find a credible authority who would argue that a diet high in sweets, refined and processed grains, French fries and potato chips, sugary drinks, and low quality, processed meat (also known as the typical Western diet) is healthier than a diet high in unprocessed, nutritious whole foods and fresh fruits and vegetables. As Katz wrote to me, "There just isn't as much sex appeal or profit potential in conveying that message! But it does have the potential to add years to lives, and life to years – which really ought to matter more."

My foray into nutrition science continues even as this book goes to print, but if there's anything I've learned so far in my investigations it's that the topic is complex and multi-dimensional. At one point when I started looking into the detailed science of Omega-3 fatty acids, I spoke to two different academics at the same university who fundamentally disagreed with each other. I'm not the first journalist to come up against this problem. As New York University nutritionist Marion Nestle told food journalist Michael Pollan in a famous 2007 essay, "Unhappy Meals," published in the *New York Times Magazine,* "The problem with nutrient-by-nutrient nutrition science is that it takes the nutrient out of the context of food, the food out of the context of diet, and the diet out of the context of lifestyle."[12]

The more I read, the more I realised that while the reductionist scientific approach to nutrition has brought us tremendous insights into the function of food by breaking down complex processes into smaller basic parts, it has led us to lose sight of the fact that, as Aristotle said, the whole is indeed more than the sum of its parts.[13] I realised that instead of getting caught up in epic debates about which macro- or micro-nutrient of the moment was villainous or virtuous, I needed to zoom out and look at the whole picture. I was already coming to an understanding that the two-way interactions between my mind and my body were playing a significant role in my health, and I wanted to investigate how this could also be playing out when it came to my diet. Was there any evidence to suggest my gut, my mind, and my health were all connected, and more important, that this interconnectedness could somehow be used to improve my health?

In the meantime, I decided that my whole-health, whole-life approach to food would be to eat a whole-food, plant-focused diet. In essence, I came to the exact same conclusion as Michael Pollan did in that influential *New York Times Magazine* essay in which he attempted to answer the incredibly complicated and confusing question of what we should eat in order to be maximally healthy. He said, simply: "Eat food. Not too much. Mostly plants."

The Second Brain in Your Gut

In 1899, British physiologists William Bayliss and Ernest Starling were studying the gut of an anaesthetised dog when they made an intriguing observation. They were trying to understand the movements and contractions by which food was moved through the digestive tract when they realised that when they cut communication between the gut and the central nervous system, the motion of the gut was not interrupted. Specifically, they observed that the motion of the gut was stimulated by the presence of food itself within the tract. They theorised that nerves in and around the gut were responsible for coordinating this autonomic function, an effect they called the "law of the intestine." In other words, Bayliss and Starling had discovered that the gut can still perform its duties even if it's not talking to the brain.[14]

Unfortunately, for a hundred years or so, the world more or less forgot about the discovery of this autonomic response and we continued along as though the brain were an almighty dictator of bodily function, as well as the single determinate of all things emotional. But in 1998 Michael Gershon, a professor at Columbia University, published a landmark book called *The Second Brain: Your Gut Has a Mind of Its Own* and the game changed. The book was part memoir and part detailed explanation of Gershon's discovery of the neurochemistry of what he called the "second brain." The book's publication and Gershon's subsequent appearances on television talk shows and in mainstream magazine feature articles finally gave the remarkable second brain the limelight it deserved.

Gershon is regarded as the pioneer of the field now known as neurogastroenterology. Through his work and the work of others we have come to understand that the lining of the gut wall contains the enteric nervous system, a semi-autonomous network of neurons (or second brain) that can not only talk to the brain, but can also function independently and influence our mood and modulate our emotions.[15] In fact, based on research in rats, about 73 percent of the signals passing along the vagus nerve that connects the brain to the gut come not from above, but from the second brain below.[16]

As scientists inch toward greater understanding of the gut-brain conversation, they're beginning to investigate whether the relationship can be harnessed for the treatment of a number of illnesses. For example, researchers are experimenting with inserting a pace-maker-like device to stimulate the vagus nerve of severely-depressed people who have failed to respond to any kind of drug treatment. In one study, 44 percent of the participants who had run out of all other treatment options for their severe depression responded positively to the treatment. Two years later, 42 percent were still responding.[17] In the US, vagus nerve stimulation in conjunction with other therapies is now approved for treatment of depressive disorders.[18]

Although we are not conscious of this second brain, and it is unlikely to ever write a sonnet or invent a rocket ship, emerging research suggests that the second brain has a good deal of influence on our everyday lives, an idea that gives us a whole new appreciation for the notion of having a "gut feeling." But the two-way conversation between the brain in our head and the brain in our gut is not the only frontier being explored in the new science of gut-mood interconnectedness. Scientists have realised that these "conversations" are actually more like a teleconference that includes not only the brain and the gut, but also the bugs living in our gut, which can also receive and send signals that are passed to and from our brains.[19]

Meet Your Microbes

When Rob Knight's first child was delivered via an emergency Caesarean section in 2011 he was worried, not because his wife wasn't in the hands of medical experts, but rather because his newborn daughter had been delivered in the sterile surgical theatre of a modern hospital and thus hadn't been exposed to his wife's intestinal and vaginal microbes by coming out the old-fashioned way. As a professor at the University of California San Diego Medical School and a leading researcher of the human microbiome, Knight had in mind a paper he had co-authored just one year earlier that demonstrated that the microbial populations living in the guts of babies born via C-section looked very different from the populations living in the guts of babies born by vaginal delivery.[20] He was also aware of a growing body of research demonstrating that disrupting the mother-to-newborn transmission of these good bacteria by C-section delivery may increase the newborn's lifetime risk of allergy, asthma, type 1 diabetes, and obesity.[21]

With all this in mind, Knight did what any scientist who believed passionately in his own research findings would do. He used cotton swabs to take samples from his wife's vagina and dab them in his newborn daughter's ears, skin, and mouth. Essentially, he was coating or "inoculating" his daughter with what the latest research indicates may be nature's way of providing us with our first protective layer against the world.*

The human microbiome is a bacterial world that exists in and on humans. It is a world consisting of complex communities of single-celled organisms. They're found on your skin and hands, in your belly button and nose, and throughout your body. It is thought that up to 100 trillion microbes call the human gut home.[22] Scientists have made recent breakthroughs in studying these minuscule organisms because of the development of new technology that allows them to analyse their DNA. In Medline (PubMed),

---

*The procedure done by Knight and his wife, which is being called "vaginal seeding" by those who advocate its use might, in theory, restore the microbiota of infants born by Caesarean section to a more natural state,[1] but large clinical trials with many years of follow-up are still a long way from publication. A 2016 editorial in the Journal of the British Medical Association encouraged medical professionals not to recommend the practice due to risk of infecting the newborns with harmful bacteria and viruses like genital herpes.[2] "Although that article represents one view in the obstetrics community, I have also seen many positive messages of support," says Knight. "I think at this point it's a biologically plausible idea that remains to be clinically proven. Of course, prospective users of the technique should get tested for group B strep and other transmissible pathogens." At the moment hospitals do not routinely screen a mother's vaginal fluid for potentially harmful bacteria and viruses, so until the evidence of the health benefits of vaginal seeding builds in more clinical trials and those benefits can be proven to outweigh the risks, the practice is unlikely to go mainstream any time soon.

1. Dominguez-Bello, MG, De Jesus-Laboy, KM, Shen, N, Cox, LM, Amir, A, Gonzalez A, Bokulich, NA, Song SJ, Hoashi, M, Rivera-Vinas, JI, Mendez, K, Knight, R, & Clemente, JC, 2016. Partial restoration of the microbiota of cesarean-born infants via vaginal microbial transfer. *Nature Medicine*, 22(3), 250–253, March
2. Cunnington, AJ, Sim, K, Deierl, A, Kroll, JS, Brannigan, E, & Darby, J, 2016. "Vaginal seeding" of infants born by caesarean section. *BMJ*, 352, i227–i228, 23 February.

the vast medical database produced by the U.S. National Library of Medicine, the number of articles that include the word "microbiome" has increased from just two in 2002 to more than 7,000 in early 2016.

In the past, Western thinking viewed these bugs as foreign disease-causing invaders that must be eradicated with everything from antibiotics to antibacterial wipes and hand sanitisers. But that idea is now under serious review as scientists begin to understand the degree to which humans and their microbes share a mutually beneficial relationship. "The three pounds of microbes that you carry around with you might be more important than every single gene you carry around in your genome," Knight told me in an email.

Estimates are that in the average human gut, approximately 500 to 1,000 different species of bugs are battling it out for survival.[23] But rather than being parasites or passengers hitching a ride, these microscopic creatures are more like co-pilots, playing a crucial role in harvesting energy from our diet, protecting us against infections, training our immune system, providing nutrition to cells, influencing the size of our waistline, affecting our resilience to stress, and even influencing our mood and behaviour.[24] Disruptions to the balance of this gut "wildlife" are associated with obesity, diabetes, colon cancer, various inflammatory bowel conditions, and autoimmune diseases, including multiple sclerosis.[25] There is also emerging evidence that suggests the microbiome may be, beginning at birth,[26] a key player in the development of food allergies, which is one reason Rob Knight was so keen to inoculate his C-section delivered daughter. In fact, these highly-diverse, highly-prolific living creatures have such a broad influence on our bodies' physiological regulation that they are recognised by some as a separate organ within the human body.[27] "Gut bacteria could play as powerful a role as genetics, lifestyle, and environment in determining health," Knight told me. The day when it is mainstream practice to analyse a patient's gut bacteria in order to treat their chronic illness may not be far off.

Cut the Crap

In their endeavour to learn more, the passionate scientists at the forefront of gut health research are known for constantly sampling their own microbial make-up and that of their children. My favourite story came from an Australian microbe researcher, Phil Hugenholtz, who bumped into Rob Knight in an airport in the US. Knight was holding a thermos flask of his own faeces. "I asked, 'What's in there?' And he said, 'Diarrhoea – I got a bad case of the squirts in Mexico, so I've been tracking it,'" Hugenholtz told the magazine *The Monthly*.[28]

Studying their children seems to be a trend too. While Knight swabbed his newborn daughter after her emergency C-section delivery and has been tracking her gut bugs ever since, Tim Spector, a professor of genetic epidemiology at King's College London, convinced his son to take part in an experiment to serve his quest for microbial knowledge.

Spector has an important role as the gatekeeper of the Twins UK Registry. For more than two decades he's been tracking 12,000 identical and fraternal (non-identical) twins, examining information about their health, lifestyles, and diet habits in an effort to discover the role of environmental and genetic factors in disease. He also leads the British Gut Project and is currently using DNA sequencing to study the microbiomes of 5,000 twins.

Inspired by the filmmaker Morgan Spurlock (who made the documentary *Supersize Me*), and in the name of science, Spector convinced his 22-year-old son Tom to eat nothing but junk food including Chicken McNuggets, Big Macs, McFlurry ice-cream, crisps, Coke, and beer, for 10 days. In that short time, Tom gained two kilograms (four and a half pounds), started to feel bloated and sluggish, had difficulty sleeping and, needless to say, was relieved when the experiment ended. Tom, a young genetics student wrote up the experiment for his final year dissertation and Spector used it as research for his book *The Diet Myth*.[29] Their findings were fascinating. In just 10 days on the junk food diet the diversity of Tom's community of microbes was devastated. He'd lost an estimated 40 percent of the total detectable species in his gut.[30] While the father-son experiment was not published in an academic journal, a similarly interesting experiment led by Harvard researchers demonstrated that a microbial population shift occurred within five days of eating either a plant-based diet (rich in grains, legumes, fruits, and vegetables) or an animal-based diet (composed of meats, eggs, and cheeses).[31]

In another landmark study, researchers swapped the diets of US-based African-Americans with South Africans living in a rural area of South Africa. The 20 American volunteers were asked to eat an African-style diet while the 20 Africans were asked to eat a typical American-style diet. Instead of their traditional plant-rich, high-fibre meals, the rural South Africans ate a high-fat, high-protein diet of sausages, hash browns, burgers, and fries. Meanwhile, the Americans switched to a low-fat, high-fibre diet that included corn fritters, mango slices, bean soup, and fish tacos. While you might think that the US diet sounds delicious, it was the South Africans who had the raw end of the deal in this experiment. In just two weeks, their gut microbes began producing more secondary bile acids, which have been linked to increased cancer risk.[32] The microbes of the Americans eating the rural South African plant-heavy high-fibre diet produced more butyrate, a chemical with anti-cancer properties. The study demonstrated just how rapidly our gut microbe populations can shift and how quickly those shifts may begin to affect our health.

It is ironic that scientists are beginning to understand the importance of the microbiome just as modern diets and lifestyles are ravaging it.[33] It turns out that our friendly microbes don't like substances like the emulsifiers, preservatives, and artificial sweeteners found in processed foods.[34] These artificial substances can kill off the friendly bugs.[35] When researchers at Université Catholique de Louvain in Brussels fed a junk-food diet to mice, they observed not only that the community of microbes in the mouse guts changed, but that the diet made the animals' gut barriers notably more permeable, allowing endotoxins to leak into the bloodstream. This constant leakage caused a low-grade inflammation that eventually led to metabolic syndrome, a collection of symptoms that increases the risk of diabetes, stroke, and heart disease.[36]

If you look at a typically Western diet, many of us are eating excessive amounts of cheap, nutritionally-deficient, low-quality food.[37] Just over one third of American children and adolescents eat fast food every day,[38] which is alarming when you consider that 2016 research, done on mice by researchers at the University of New South Wales, demonstrated that eating a poor diet that includes things like meat pies, cakes, and cookies even three days a week can change the balance of bacteria and lead to weight gain and ill health.[39]

If you visualise your body as a high-performance sports car that you saved your hard-earned money to buy, you wouldn't want to power it with cheap, low-quality fuel and oil. Your car would be a wreck within months. When I began thinking about my food as my fuel, I made a decision to stop limping along, powered by inferior products. I now focus on eating whole foods that pack the most powerful nutritional punch available rather than eating food that has been stripped back in the manufacturing process, even if it carries a health halo of "added vitamins," is organic, or preservative-free. I also started trading up – eating the whole fruit, rather than drinking its juice, whole wheat pasta instead of white pasta, and brown rice instead of white rice. Though I'm not yet completely junk-free, I've stopped walking down the cookie and sweets aisles in the supermarket entirely.

Gut Napalm

The use of antibiotics is known to have long-term effects on the compositions of gut microbiota.[40] For example, a single course of commonly prescribed antibiotics has enough strength to disrupt your gut ecosystem for as long as a year.[41] In fact, the rapid increase in allergies coincides with a rise in the use of antibiotics, and recent research shows that the two may be connected.[42] Researchers found that babies exposed to antibiotics in the first 4-6 months of their lives have a 1.3- to 5-fold higher risk of developing an allergy.[43] Babies with reduced bacterial diversity in their guts, which can occur with antibiotic use, have increased risk of developing eczema.[44]

This is not to say that antibiotics must be avoided at all costs. Antibiotics have been used effectively to treat bacterial infections for over half a century. They save lives and have played a pivotal role in achieving major advances in medicine and surgery.[45] But we need to be highly aware of the potential for their overuse and their unnecessary use. For example, 89-95 percent of cases of acute bronchitis are viral, passing after a few weeks, so the use of antibiotics to treat these cases is superfluous.[46] Studies show that antibiotics are used incorrectly in 30-50 percent of instances,[47] and the antibiotic resistance crisis currently spreading around the globe is attributed in part to the overuse and misuse of these medications.[48]

Unfortunately, it's not as simple as saying that we need only take probiotic (good bacteria) supplements along with our antibiotics and a healthy gut ecosystem will be restored. A comprehensive review of research published between 1985 and 2013 found that more studies are required to determine which probiotic strains have a beneficial impact after microbiota have been disrupted, and that many probiotic products overstate the strength of their claims to restore normal microbiota.[49] So, if you do need to take a course of antibiotics, be sure to maintain a high-fibre, microbe-friendly diet, rich in diverse whole foods with lots of fresh fruit and vegetables and low in junk and processed food. Also keep in mind that other factors affecting our gut bacteria include illness, stress, ageing, and lifestyle.[50]

The Good, the Bad, and the Ugly

In 2014 Tim Spector contributed to a study that identified a family of microbes that seemed to help people stay thin. Analysis of more than 1,000 stool samples from 416 sets of twins registered in Twins UK revealed that a relatively newly described family of bacteria called *Christensenellaceae* were far more abundant in healthy or underweight people than in people who were overweight or obese. When researchers transplanted the microbes into skinny germ-free mice, they found the mice did not get fat, even though they were on high-fat diets.[51]

Already microbiologists can predict with up to 90 percent accuracy whether someone is lean or obese from their gut bugs alone, which is more accurate than using human genetic testing,[52] and the race is now on to determine how other specific species in our gut might influence our health and whether altering our gut microbes through diet, tablets, or even microbial faecal transplants (commonly called poo transfusions) might be the silver bullet for ailments that medicine has so far found difficult to treat. To date most of the research has been done on mice, so it's still early days, but let me tell you some of what we do know of who's who in the gut zoo...

- *Lactobacillus helveticus* can decrease anxiety-like symptoms in mice if it is given in conjunction with a healthy diet. [53]
- *Lactobacillus reuteri* can reduce the likelihood that mice will get infections when they're stressed.[54]
- *Lactobacillus kefiri* CIDCA 8348 reduced gut inflammation in mice.[55]
- *Lactobacillus casei rhamnosus* can improve symptoms for irritable bowel syndrome patients complaining of diarrhoea.[56]
- Drinking a probiotic mixture containing *Lactobacillus helveticus and B. longum* for 30-days has beneficial effects on anxiety and depressive measures, as well as reduced levels of the stress hormone, cortisol, in healthy volunteers.[57]
- People with rheumatoid arthritis are much more likely to have a bug called *Prevotella copri* in their intestines than people who do not *have the disease.*[58]
- Patients with psoriatic arthritis have significantly lower levels of other types of species such as *Akkermansia, Ruminococcus,* and *Pseudobutyrivibrio.*[59]
- Healthy women who drank a fermented milk product containing *Bifidobacterium animalis* subsp *lactis, Streptococcus thermophilus, Lactobacillus bulgaricus* and *Lactococcus lactis* subsp *lactis* for four weeks were shown to have robust alterations in brain regions that control emotion and pain sensation.[60]

There's no doubt that the microbiome is an exciting new frontier of research and that the potential for human health seems immense. Stanford University microbiologist Justin Sonnenburg, a leading gut bug researcher, predicted in 2015 that, "In the not too distant future each of us will be able to colonise our gut with genetically modified 'smart' bacteria that detect and stamp out disease at the earliest possible moment."[61] The day when probiotics, or "good bacteria," are tailored for us to compensate for our personal microbial deficits may not be far off. But I must stick a red flag on all this, lest we get carried away in our enthusiasm for the next big thing. We're still very much only beginning to understand the application of all this research in the real world. We actually know very little about how our gut bugs interact with each other, how they interact with us, or how they interact with their environment. Our microbial make-up is complex, varied, and ever-changing. Scientists don't even yet know what exactly constitutes a "normal" or "healthy" microbiome.

Taking advantage of the speed with which personal anecdotes of cures and instantaneous improvements spread by word of mouth, you can find on supermarket and pharmacy shelves all manner of products promoting the health benefits of different microbial species. In fact, this lucrative probiotic marketplace is predicted to be worth 96 billion US dollars by 2020.[62] But it's unlikely that the probiotics used in scientific trials are the same probiotics you're buying at your local shops. In some ways it's like saying "I'm going to take a drug to cure my headache" without considering what specific drug to take. "Probiotics are not all the same, just like drugs are not all the same, and as always, studies in mice are far ahead of what we can do clinically in humans," professor Rob Knight told me. Furthermore, specific probiotics will have different effects in different people; a probiotic that works for one person for a certain set of symptoms will not necessarily work for another person with different symptoms.[63] More research is needed to determine which probiotics and which dosages are associated with the greatest efficacy and for which patients.[64]

Another drawback to using probiotics is that the minuscule microbes have to be alive when you take them in order to get the full benefits they offer.[65] They're rather fussy and need specific conditions to survive. It's unclear whether the preparations you buy contain any living organisms after being manufactured, packaged, shipped, unpacked, and stored on shop shelves. And because they are not subject to regulatory review, manufacturers can be lax with ingredients and labelling. One review of 14 commercially available probiotic products found that only one actually contained the ingredients listed on the label.[66] Another review of probiotics for pets found that out of 25 products analysed, only two actually contained the microorganisms listed on the label. More than one actually misspelled their names.[67]

So if not probiotics, where can we turn if we want to take advantage of the latest evidence on gut bacteria for good health?

Operating alongside the flourishing probiotic industry is another, rather less conventional marketplace. Taking advantage of the evidence showing that poo transfusions have been effective in helping people infected with clostridium difficile (C-diff, a difficult-to-treat bacteria that causes diarrhoea and serious intestinal conditions such as colitis), companies have sprung up with the express purpose of collecting poo samples from healthy donors to be used in clinical treatments. The commercial response hasn't been fast enough to meet consumer demand though, and there's now a burgeoning do-it-yourself internet market that helps people perform their own poo transfusions in the comfort of their homes. Yes, you read that right. People are finding donors to provide them with poo and then giving themselves poo enemas. Given that these treatments are still very much in the experimental phase, the danger of a DIY approach cannot be over emphasised. Even in the relative safety of a clinical setting, there have been reports of negative consequences. In one case, reported in a medical journal in order to spark discussion about the risks and benefits of poo transfusions, a healthy weight woman (62 kilograms, or 136 pounds) with a C-diff infection elected to try a faecal microbial transplant donated by her 16-year-old daughter who was healthy but gained weight soon after the sample was taken from her. Within 16 months, the mother receiving the transplant had become obese, gaining 15 kilograms (34 pounds), despite her attempts to lose weight via a medically-supervised liquid protein diet and exercise program. Her weight gain continued and three years later she weighed 80 kilograms (177 pounds) and had developed constipation and unexplained indigestion.[68]

The good news is that the prevailing winds of current research are pointing us toward an understanding of how we might be able to cultivate a healthy gut, and researchers are beginning to think that it's not about trying to somehow take or insert more specific species of good bacteria into your gut, but rather about maintaining a healthy balance of the species.[69] Think of your microbiome as being an ecosystem or food web. You may have a gut ecosystem that looks like the Great Barrier Reef, teeming with corals and fish life, or you might have a microbial community that looks more like a rainforest in Borneo bursting with thousands of plant species, birds, and mammals. Either one may be vibrantly healthy. It's the people who lack diversity in their microbiomes who seem to be vulnerable to disease such as C diff.[70] The same is true for obesity, inflammatory bowel disease, and rheumatoid arthritis.[71]

So for the everyday person, rather than recommending and espousing the benefits of particular supplements or clinical procedures, experts recommend working on cultivating gut diversity. And the accumulating evidence suggests the way to do this is by eating a long-term, highly diverse, high fibre diet.[72] By eating a wide variety of fibrous plants, we are essentially feeding and encouraging a thriving, diverse population of good bugs. Rob Knight follows this advice and adds foods containing living bacteria (such as yoghurt and fermented foods) to his list as well. "I had already largely cut out junk food before the recent microbial evidence on artificial sweeteners and on sugar-rich diets came out," he told me, "but on the basis of recent work, I try to eat more whole foods containing fermentable fibre, a greater variety of fruits and vegetables rather than just more of a few kinds, and more yogurt and nuts."

With this "eat a variety of plants" and "cut the crap" message coming out loud and clear from the gut microbe experts, I started thinking about my food as not only feeding me, but also feeding my gut bugs. I upped my game on eating more diverse and fibrous whole foods – vegetables and fruit, whole grains (like brown rice, oats, rye, and whole-wheat), beans and legumes (like chickpeas and kidney beans), nuts, and seeds. Once again all this seems to boil down to Michael Pollan's simple message: "Eat food. Not too much. Mostly plants."[73] But when I started factoring in the idea of nourishing a healthy gut bug community, I decided to slightly tweak the famous expression and add four additional words to my food mantra –

"Eat *real* food. Not too much. Mostly *a variety of* plants."

The Big MAC Diet

HOW TO FEED YOUR BUGS

We know that microbiome diversity is linked to human health[74] and we know that while several factors influence our microbiota, what we eat seems to be one of the key influencers.[75] So what should we eat to promote healthy gut microbiota diversity?

Our gut bugs eat what we eat. Specifically, they eat "Microbiota-accessible carbohydrates" or MACs, a term coined by Erica and Justin Sonnenburg, a husband and wife duo who lead a team of microbiota researchers at Stanford University. MACs are carbohydrates we can't easily digest ourselves but that our gut bugs can ferment or metabolise into beneficial compounds such as short-chain fatty acids.[76] Essentially, MACs are the components within dietary fibre on which gut microbes feed. So eating more MACS can provide more nourishment to the microbiota, help gut microbes thrive, and improve the diversity of this community.

The most common source of MACs is fibre – both soluble and insoluble – which includes fruits, vegetables, starchy plants, unrefined whole grains, nuts, seeds, legumes, and other foods that are poorly absorbed by us, but can be utilised by our gut bugs as a food source.[77]

Unfortunately you can't read a food label or ingredient list to get an idea of the MACs contained in different foods. But it is clear that when we're eating a typical Western diet high in bad fat and simple carbohydrates, many of us are not getting enough dietary fibre. The average American consumes a measly 16 grams of dietary fibre per day.[78] This falls far short of the 25-38 grams recommended by the FDA, and is even farther still from the 100-150 grams of fibre consumed by modern day hunter-gatherers such as the Hadza of Tanzania.[79]

In practice, a "Big MAC diet" means that each meal should include a healthy portion of plant foods so that you are consuming at least 29-38 grams of dietary fibre per day. For example, the Sonnenburgs recommend that your day could start with a bowl of steel cut oatmeal topped with berries, then a leafy green salad sprinkled with nuts and seeds for lunch, and finally a dinner comprised of a veggie-filled Mediterranean bean soup. This type of diet ensures that our microbes have plenty to eat so they can maintain a robust and thriving community within your gut. Although research on the gut microbiome is still in its early days, I think you'd be hard-pressed to find a doctor who would argue that eating more fresh fruit, vegetables, whole grains, nuts, seeds, and legumes is fundamentally unhealthy.

Key Takeaways

1 Despite the wealth of conflicting and confusing information about what you should eat, the answer is actually very simple – Eat *real* food. Not too much. Mostly a *variety of* plants.

2 In recent years, our understanding of the mind-body-health connection has been taken to a whole new level with the knowledge that a three-way teleconference is taking place between the brain in your head, the brain in your gut, and your gut microbes.

3 The microbiome has become one of the most important areas of nutrition research. Gut bacteria could play as powerful a role as genetics, lifestyle, and environment in determining health. Rather than espousing the benefits of particular supplements or clinical procedures, experts recommend working on cultivating gut diversity.

4 Eating a junk food or low-fibre diet, or taking antibiotics is likely to be detrimental to your microbial diversity. You can boost your gut bug diversity by eating a high fibre diet containing a wide variety of fresh fruits and vegetables, whole grains, beans, lentils, nuts, and seeds.

Getting Started

CLEAR your house of junk foods and remove temptation. Instead, fill your pantry and fridge with fresh, whole, plant foods.

TRADE up your foods so they pack the most powerful nutritional punch available – e.g, choose the whole fruit, rather than drinking its juice, choose whole wheat pasta instead of white pasta, and brown rice instead of white rice.

KEEP a food diary for a month to get a clear picture of what you're actually putting into your body with each meal. You can do this by writing in a physical diary (a template download is available on my website), or use an app (I keep a list of recommended apps on my website that I update regularly). See the following Extra Resources page for details.

FIND a healthy eating buddy or food coach with whom you can swap ideas, tips, and tricks, and get the people in your household on board with your plan so they won't be a source of temptation.

ENROLL in a vegan or vegetarian cooking class to learn how to plan and prepare delicious whole-food, plant-based meals.

HAVE your gut bugs tested. You can send in samples to the American Gut Project or the British Gut Project. An Australian Gut Project is also in the planning stages, and there are several commercial companies that offer microbial testing. Keep in mind scientists can't yet tell precisely what your results mean for your health and they are still trying to find ways to standardise their tests. Nevertheless, having your microbiome tested by one of the organisations listed below is a great way to participate in citizen science and help fund research into the microbiome.

- *http://americangut.org/*
- *http://britishgut.org/*

Extra Resources

AVAILABLE AT
www.thewholehealthlife.com/resources

DOWNLOAD a template food diary.

DOWNLOAD some of my favourite Big MAC recipes that I make for my family each week.

MY recommended reading list, which I update regularly, is available on my website. Books relevant to this chapter include:

- *What to Eat*, by Marion Nestle
- *Secrets From the Eating Lab: The Science of Weight Loss, the Myth of Willpower, and Why You Should Never Diet Again*, by Traci Mann
- *The Diet Myth: The Real Science Behind What We Eat*, by Tim Spector
- *The Good Gut: Taking Control of Your Weight, Your Mood and Your Long-Term Health*, by Justin and Erica Sonnenberg
- *Follow Your Gut: The Enormous Impact of Tiny Microbes*, by Rob Knight with Brendan Bugler
- *The Second Brain: A Groundbreaking New Understanding of Nervous Disorders of the Stomach and Intestine*, by Michael D. Gershon
- *Nutrition in Clinical Practice*, by David L. Katz, Rachel S.C.Friedman and Sean C. Lucan

Chapter 5

Movement

India

The sun was setting over the ocean as I breathed in the humid air, arms above my head – stretching, reaching, extending. I was midway through an Ayurvedic health retreat near Goa in the south west of India. Each morning and afternoon I'd been moving my body in this way. I was practising a yoga sequence called *Surya Namaskar* or the Sun Salutation, a series of postures coordinated with breathing, performed one after the other in flowing motion – *inhale as you extend and stretch, and exhale as you fold and contract.* I felt strong. I felt relaxed. I felt good.

Before I got sick, I stayed fit by running and weight training a few times a week, but the arthritic joint and muscle pain, alongside the heavy fatigue that arrived with the onset of my autoimmune disease, had been too much of a barrier to motivate me to keep moving my body regularly. Pretty soon lethargy set in and my health declined even further. The medication I was taking contributed to weight gain, and my aching muscles would seize and spasm. Some days, just getting out of bed was too much.

I first gave yoga a try after years of living with the chronic pain that came with arthritis. I was looking for something that would help loosen my stiff muscles and go easy on my inflamed joints. At first I wondered what on earth I was doing. I'd compare myself to the strong, fit, lean people beside me who gracefully moved through each motion while I wobbled and wavered and could barely hold a pose. The instructor would encourage us to co-ordinate our breath with the movement, and I'd end up confused and out of sync. During some classes I just felt stupid, chanting meaningless *oms* and mantras in a language I didn't understand. I shopped around at a number of studios before I found a style and teachers that I liked. With regular practice, I noticed a difference in my sore and tired body and I was encouraged. My balance improved and I became stronger. I began to challenge myself further, participating in "40 Day Revolutions" and other programs designed to lead to "personal transformation." These were great, but to be honest the "transformation" never lasted and within a few months I'd find myself back in my old habits. Urgent work deadlines would take priority and my mental fatigue only motivated me to collapse on the couch in front of the television after a hard day at work.

That is how I came to be in India, a country that first captivated me when I studied it for a research topic during my final year of high school. There was something about the blend of ancient wisdom, the scintillating history, the diversity of people and culture, and the rise of modern India making its mark on the world that enchanted and called to me. In the 14 years that followed high school, I visited a travel agent three times with the intention of organising a trip, but I never actually made it onto the plane. For one reason or another my plans were always thwarted. Now, when I was in my early 30s and still looking for answers to my chronic health problems, India took on new significance for me. I wanted to extricate myself from the everyday of my busy life at home, get some perspective, and dedicate time to my health. Although by that time my arthritic flare-ups were less debilitating and my energy levels were improving, the good days were still being tempered by bad days, and at times I was still utterly wiped out and barely able to function. Whether it was a looming deadline, a social pressure, or my own choices, things just kept getting in the way of putting my health at the top of the priority list. Going to India was my way of saying enough is enough, I'm putting health number one.

Ayurveda is a "science of life" – *Ayur* being the Sanskrit word for life and *Veda* being science or knowledge. It is an ancient system based on the belief that there is an interconnectedness among people, their health, and the universe.[1] Ayurvedic physicians prescribe individualised treatments, including compounds of herbs, diet, exercise, and lifestyle recommendations. I was hoping that by dedicating time to attend the retreat, despite all the frenetic shenanigans going on back home, I would learn ways to make healthy changes that would be lasting and sustainable in my life (preferably without the need to quit my job, shave my head, and give up all my worldly possessions).

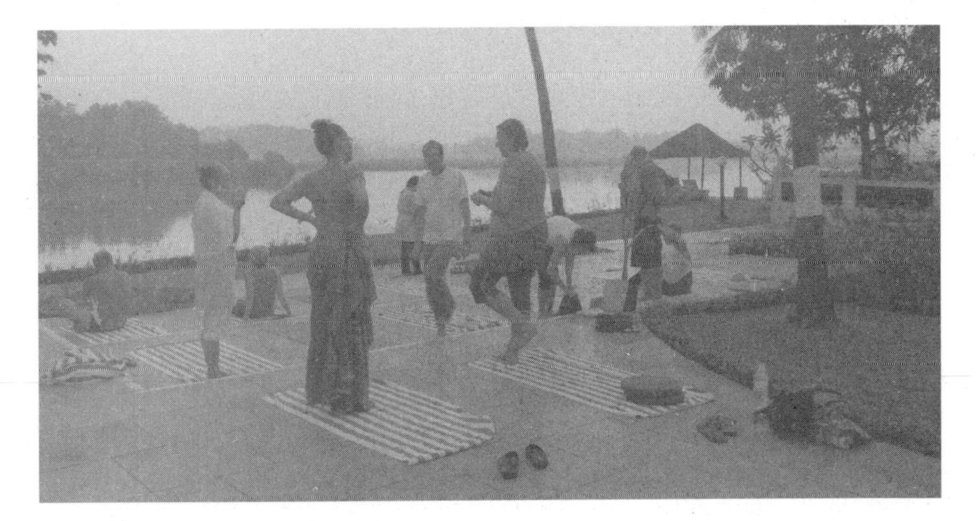

Sunrise yoga in Goa, 2013.

I confess that my Western thinking made some of the concepts in Ayurvedic medicine difficult for me – for example, that my health could be influenced by "life forces" or energies called *doshas,* and that we become sick when the balance of these *doshas* is disrupted. I'd recently developed a habit of taking scientific papers with me to bed as nighttime reading so I struggled to connect the more esoteric ideas in Ayurvedic principles with the answers I was finding in modern science. Nevertheless, the actual practical application of the Ayurvedic concepts fit in well with what I had been learning. The retreat involved twice daily yoga and meditation, an organic, plant-based diet, and twice daily treatments that were mostly vigorous, oil-infused massages. I also took the time to do a lot of personal reflection, writing in my diary and chatting with others at the retreat who were on health journeys similar to mine.

What I hadn't foreseen was that it wouldn't be the retreat itself that brought me the answers I sought. In fact, I found what I was looking for after a day trip outside the retreat. I spent a Wednesday morning wandering through the famous market at Anjuna beach, which my travel guide book had told me was an essential part of the Goan experience. The market was established in 1975 by Yertward Mazamanian, an American man of Armenian descent, known as the "Godfather of Hippies." He set up the market so that he and his fellow free-thinking nomads could sell their unwanted possessions and handmade jewelry to help fund the rest of their stay in India. But in early 2012 when I arrived, I didn't find a quaint bohemian market. I found a sprawling hectic centre of commerce where I could buy anything from cheap clothes and tacky jewelry to pirated DVDs and plastic statuettes of any spiritual luminary I desired. One statuette even had a Made in China sticker on the bottom. The stalls offered few things for sale that I couldn't get back home at my local mall.

Back at the retreat, I discovered that my outside excursion meant I'd missed an afternoon yoga class, and I returned to my room feeling disappointed. I had an hour before dinner would be served and I was tempted to pull out my computer and check in with my work emails. But I did not want to feel as if my entire day had been wasted, so I decided I would practice yoga anyway, even without a teacher. I walked out onto my balcony, which overlooked a peaceful river, rolled out my mat, and began working through a sequence of poses, concentrating on coordinating my breath with my movement. Pretty soon I found myself lost in the flow. After my day at the frantic market, my tired and stressed-out muscles began to relax and release. I felt my mind and body reconnect. I felt a deep sense of calm, balance and restoration.

There had been a time not too long before when doing a sequence of simple postures like that was a near impossibility for me. After my practice, as I was reflecting on my experience at the souvenir market and eating a tasty but uncomplicated vegetarian curry in a setting that was beautiful – but no more extraordinary than the beaches back home in Sydney – I was hit by a blinding flash of the obvious: the answer to my health questions were not to be found in the ancient wisdom of a far-off country. I didn't need to come all the way to India to find what I was looking for. I had actually already laid the foundations for my whole-health life. I already had a path to follow. It was just a matter of continuing my research and committing to putting into practice what I was learning.

The New Science of Exercise

The researchers standing around looking at the brain scan images of one of the world's greatest athletes were impressed. This particular athlete held over 30 world records and had won over 750 gold medals. Her fitness scores were streaks ahead of her peers and, based on the scans that had just been done, it was clear that her brain was also in great shape. The white-matter tracts associated with reasoning, planning, and self-control were in particularly good condition. It was also especially impressive that there were relatively few signs of ageing-related damage to the white-matter tracts in the region of the brain called the *corpus callosum,* which connects the right and left hemispheres at the very front of the brain and allows one side of the brain to talk to the other. But the really interesting thing about this brain is that it belonged to a 93-year-old woman named Olga Kotelko. Overall, Kotelko's brain was comparable in some ways to those of women decades younger.[2]

The encounter with Kotelko continues to be a source of inspiration for the researchers at the Beckman Institute for Advanced Science and Technology at the University of Illinois who specialise in studying the effect of exercise on the brain. Kotelko hadn't taken up the sport in which she had excelled - track and field - until she was 77 years old. While we can't say for sure that the youthful condition of Kotelko's brain was a result of her athletic training (researchers hadn't been tracking her over time), it certainly looks that way when you consider other research results coming out of the Beckman Institute.

In 2010, the Institute Director at the time, Arthur Kramer, and his team studied 120 men and women aged between 55 and 80 who were not doing any exercise and put half of them through an aerobic training program. After one year they measured changes in their subjects' brains and discovered increases in the size of the *anterior hippocampus* and related improvements in spatial memory, which helps us find our way around our environment and remember where things are within it. This part of the brain typically shrinks in late adulthood, causing impaired memory and increased risk for dementia. Kramer found that the simple exercise training program increased hippocampal volume by two percent, "effectively reversing age-related loss in volume by one to two years."[3]

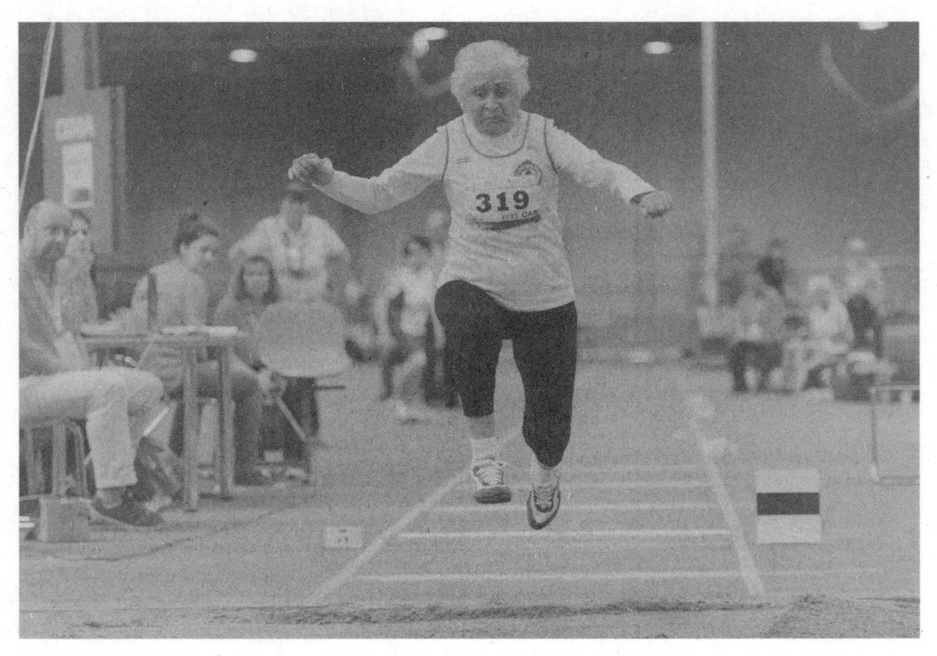

Olga Kotelko at the 2014 World Masters Track and Field Championships in Budapest. *Credit: Rob Jerome*

Exercise is also associated with greater levels of brain-derived neurotrophic factor (BDNF) in the blood. Often described as "brain fertiliser," BDNF is an essential substance that nurtures the development of new brain cells and the growth of existing ones.[4] (If you sprinkle BDNF on neurons in a Petri dish, they literally sprout branches.[5]) The movement-related increases were seen after the participants did only moderate levels of exercise, highlighting that we don't need to be world champion athletes to get the brain benefits of moving more. In a Skype interview I did with

Kramer he explained that people can ease into an exercise routine. "A lot of older folks will say to me, 'I'm too old. I can't do vigorous exercise,' but it was pretty modest exercise," he said, adding, "we would start off on day one having them walk about 15 minutes and gradually over the first two months build up to 45 minutes to an hour a day, three days a week. I can tell you, nobody in our groups was winning any medals."

We've long known that it's good for us to regularly move our bodies. Movement helps maintain blood pressure, reduces inflammation, and boosts lung function.[6] It can make us stronger, fitter, and slimmer.[7] But the more I looked into the new science of exercise, the more I realised that the benefits of moving my body went far beyond building muscles and staying thin. Studies like those coming out of the Beckman Institute and other research centres around the world are increasingly demonstrating the benefits of exercise for our *whole* body, including our mind and brain. We now know that exercise improves blood flow to our brain and in doing so gives it an oxygen boost, which feeds neural tissues and enhances memory.[8] Even briefly exercising for 20 minutes facilitates information processing and memory functions.[9] We all have an exercise-enthusiast in our lives who tells us they "have to" work out every day because it makes them feel good. Today the anecdotal mood-boosting benefits of exercise are increasingly being proven in studies that demonstrate exercise's effectiveness in helping people with mild to moderate depression, anxiety, and other mental health issues.[10]

We also now have compelling evidence about the effectiveness of regular physical activity in the prevention of several chronic conditions (such as heart disease, diabetes, cancer, hypertension, obesity, depression, and osteoporosis), as well as premature death.[11] Research done in the US estimates that inactive people who become active from age 50 will live between 1.3 to 3.7 years longer than they would have if they did not exercise.[12] No wonder doctors call exercise "The Miracle Drug."[13] The message is loud and clear. The research is unequivocal. For whole health, from top to toe, exercise is a fundamental human need. We should all move regularly... and yet, we don't.

What We Should Do and What We Do Do

In the same way that navigating nutritional advice can be a hazardous walk through a minefield, the subject of what exercise is best, and how much we should do, can be conflicting and confusing – even explosive. The various tribes advocating one form of movement or another will passionately argue their case as to why you should join them, espousing health benefits that range from having boundless energy and superhuman strength to everlasting good looks. Given that it's hard enough finding time in our busy day for exercise, we also want to make sure we're getting the best return on our time investment. From Zumba to CrossFit, marathons to martial arts, yoga and Pilates, sprints to squats, and weights to treadmills, the choices seem endless and it can be bewildering to try to figure out what is best.

The World Health Organization recommends that people between 18 and 64 years of age should aim for at least 150 minutes of moderate aerobic exercise throughout the week, or at least 75 minutes of vigorous aerobic activity, or some combination of the two. (In case you are wondering, if you are doing a moderate intensity activity, you will have enough breath to talk during the activity, but not to sing. If you are doing a vigorous intensity activity, you won't be able to say more than a few words without needing to take a breath.) WHO makes a few other recommendations too (such as doing strength training at least two days a week), but on the whole it's all pretty straightforward.[14] In fact, many experts and health organisations simplify this even further by recommending that we should exercise for 30 minutes a day, five days a week.[15] The American College of Sport Medicine, the largest sports medicine and exercise science organisation in the world, adds another element to its guidelines, advising that:

> "A program of regular exercise that includes cardiorespiratory, resistance, flexibility, and neuromotor exercise training beyond activities of daily living to improve and maintain physical fitness and health is essential for most adults."[16]

In other words, if you thought that exercise was just about choosing to either pound the pavement, hit the gym, or pump weights, think again. The advice from medical experts is that we need to be getting a variety of movement types into our week.

One reason Arthur Kramer thinks 93-year-old Olga Kotelko's brain was in such great shape was because her track and field training involved a variety of activities including high jump, long jump, triple jump, shot put, javelin, hammer and discus throws, and sprints. Kotelko passed away at age 95, but was still competing the weekend before her death. "She was a field athlete doing you name it. Usually, the impression is the big men throw the hammer. Olga was probably about five foot tall, weighed about 90 pounds and threw the hammer. Although she might have been small, she sure as hell was tough," Kramer told me.

Now in his early 60s, Kramer has recently moved to Boston for a new role at Northeastern University. When he's not setting up and conducting new studies, he takes a leaf out of Kotelko's book and focuses on variety in his activities. "I always recommend a variety of exercise because I certainly want to be fit in the cardiorespiratory sense, be able to walk up stairs, be able to take hikes, and enjoy life. You also need sufficient strength to do various things. During my move to Boston I lifted several 100-pound dressers. It's good to have the ability to do that at my age. You also want to have the balance. Nobody wants to fall over and break a hip or break their arm or worse, damage their brain. I most certainly recommend all forms of exercise for people at any age," he said.

Unless you're the only person on the planet who has nothing to do but focus on your health, by now you're likely reading all this information and thinking that the new science of exercise is asking the impossible - cardio, strength, stretching *and* neuromotor exercise (whatever that means!) - there's no way you can possibly fit in all the exercise recommendations on top of your other commitments. But don't feel overwhelmed. There are many activities you can do that combine all the recommended categories of exercise. For example, a vinyasa yoga class can get your heart pumping, your muscles stretching and strengthening, and your mind-body connected (that's neuromotor exercise). A salsa dancing class ticks many of the boxes, as does rock climbing or a martial art like Wing Chun. Swimming can also get your heart going and strengthen your muscles at the same time. The important thing is to make sure you *move*. Remember, doing some exercise is better than doing none. "I think there are a number of things we can do to ensure that we get some exercise, even when we're not in the gym. Even when we're just living our life. If you have the opportunity, instead of taking an elevator, walk up a few flights of stairs several times a day – that's a plus," Kramer said.

This clear message from the new science of movement – that we need to be regularly doing a variety of different things – is all well and good, except that despite the recommendations, most people aren't getting anywhere close to moving enough *at all*, let alone moving in a variety of different ways. In Canada, for example, 75 percent of adults don't meet national physical activity recommendations. In the US and UK, nearly 80 percent of adults are falling short.[17] And this is not a problem attributed to a few lazy countries, it's global. At least 31 percent of the world's population does not get enough exercise. This is true for both children and adults in almost all developed and developing countries.[18]

One reason for the gap between what we *should* do and what we *actually* do has a lot to do with the changing nature of the world.[19] We now get around in cars, buses, and trains instead of cycling and walking. Modern luxuries like washing machines and supermarkets have taken much of the physical demand out of basic living activities in our homes. The advent of digital devices and screens usually means we're spending our down time sitting down. Having a physically demanding job is now the exception, not the rule, and some researchers directly attribute the weight gain epidemic that is crippling healthcare systems to the change in the nature of our work.[20] Since the 1960s, the number of jobs requiring physical activity has plummeted. Once these jobs accounted for 50 percent of the labor market, but today it's estimated that 80 percent of jobs are sedentary or require only light physical movement. The great shame about the current crisis is that we should have seen it coming. It was forewarned by a pioneering doctor and scientist whose work laid the foundation for what we now know about physical activity, but his early discoveries were largely ignored in our push toward ever-sedentary modernity.

You May Not Want to Sit Down to Read This

Scottish physician and epidemiologist Jeremy Morris was one of those researchers who acted whole-heartedly on his own discoveries. Well into his mid-90s, Morris swam, pedalled his exercise bike, or walked for at least half an hour every day. In 1949, Morris, known as "The Man Who Invented Exercise,"[21] laid the scientific foundation of our modern understanding of the importance of movement when he began tracking the heart attack rates of 15,500 drivers and 9,500 conductors working on buses, trams, and trolleybuses in London. His data showed that drivers who sat for most of their shifts were more than twice as likely to suffer heart attacks as the more active conductors who were up and down the stairs of their double-deckers many times a day. Morris's data was the first clue to understanding that exercise helps us stay healthy. But this was completely out-of-the-box thinking at a time when the medical community firmly believed that heart disease was caused by high blood pressure, high cholesterol, and obesity. Morris kept silent and waited to publish until he had more proof. He did a follow-up study in which he compared British postmen who walked or bicycled all day to their postal colleagues who worked at desks and telephones in the office. Again he found that the posties who were moving all day were much less likely to die from heart attacks than their sedentary peers.[22]

There are few better advertisements for his discovery of the link between moving more and good health than Morris himself; he lived to be 99 ½. "He always insisted on adding the ½," said his daughter, Julie Zalewska, in a *New York Times* tribute published after his death.[23] Morris was well-known for encouraging more exercise among his friends and in society as a whole and these days you'd be hard-pressed to find a credible expert who would argue that physical exercise is fundamentally not linked to good health. But almost seven decades on, another critical warning that was coded into Morris's bus driver data is only now starting to become apparent as the vast majority of us start emulating the lifestyles of the sedentary transport workers of the 1950s. It's not just that the drivers weren't getting enough exercise; it may also have been that they were sitting down too much.

In 2012, researchers conducted a major analysis of the results of 18 studies that, when combined, involved almost 800,000 people. They found that compared with those who sat the least, people who sat the longest had a:

112% increase in risk of diabetes
147% increase in cardiovascular events
90% increase in death caused by cardiovascular events
49% increase in death from any cause[24]

While you might think this doesn't affect you because you're not sitting all day as Morris's bus drivers were, you might want to think again. Researchers found that the average American adult spends the majority of the day sitting.[25] Findings from the Australian Health Survey 2011-12 indicate that, on average, adults spent 39 hours per week sitting or lying down for various activities.[26] Meanwhile, evidence is accumulating that links activities like watching TV, computer use, driving in a car, and working at a desk with an increased risk for developing obesity, type 2 diabetes, hypertension, metabolic syndrome, cancer, osteoporosis, and heart disease.[27] In other words, the more you sit, the greater your risk of developing chronic illnesses.

If all this is still a little bit too much to fully absorb and apply directly to your own life, let me put it a different way. An Australian study performed by researchers from the University of Queensland found that people who watch six hours of television a day can expect to live about five fewer years than people who do not watch television. So every hour of television viewed after the age of 25 could reduce your life by nearly 22 minutes.[28] When you compare this with research showing that smokers shorten their lives by about 11 minutes per cigarette,[29] it's easy to see why experts are starting to call sitting "the new smoking."[30] It's estimated we can prevent five million premature deaths each year by getting people to quit smoking.[31] By getting people who sit too much to move more, we could prevent 5.3 million deaths each year.[32]

With all this research buzzing around in my head, I became acutely aware of how much sitting I was doing during my average day. I started my mornings by sitting at my kitchen bench to eat breakfast. Then I spent up to an hour and half sitting in traffic during my commute to work. When I arrived, I spent the next 8-10 hours sitting at my desk or in an edit suite. After my seated commute home, I sat down for dinner before settling on the couch for an hour or two of TV time, and then finally heading to bed.

It turns out that even the yoga that I was practising a few times a week and the walks I took after work or on my weekends may not have been undoing the harmful effects of sitting all day. Emerging research shows that too much sitting may be bad for our health in itself, despite other time spent moving. For example, one large meta-analysis of studies that examined almost 70,000 cancer cases found that sitting is associated with an increased risk of certain cancers *even when people were getting the daily recommended levels of exercise.*[33] Another study, which looked at the sitting habits of 11,000 adults, found that the more time people spent watching television, the more likely they were to have abnormal glucose metabolism (where your body converts glucose into energy to fuel your cells) and metabolic syndrome (which is a fancy way of saying you have a number of risk factors that raise your chances of heart disease and other health problems like diabetes and stroke). This was true even if they were exercising regularly.[34] In other words, we may not be able to exercise away the harmful effects of sitting.

Researchers are starting to turn their attention to the underlying physiological mechanisms that might explain these findings. We now know that sitting for long periods changes our biochemistry. For example, when we sit, our body stops producing lipoprotein lipase, an enzyme crucial in helping us absorb fat. In a study where rats were inactive for 24 hours, the activity of this enzyme became virtually nonexistent.[35] Without this vacuum cleaner in the blood stream, fat is left to deposit itself in the body. Researchers also found that just a few hours of sitting suppresses a gene that helps keep your circulatory system healthy by controlling inflammation and blood clotting.[36] While the complexities of this new science of movement are still being explored, and new papers continue to be published at rapid pace, the takeaway message from the current evidence boils down to one very simple message: *We need to move more and sit less.*

What if You're Sick?

When most of us think of the 26th President of the United States, Theodore Roosevelt, we usually call to mind an intrepid explorer, nature conservationist, and war hero. What we may not recall is that he was also a sickly child who suffered from debilitating asthma. In fact the small, thin, pale boy with poor eyesight and skinny legs repeatedly experienced sudden nighttime asthma attacks and had to sleep propped up in bed or slouching in a chair. He was not expected to survive childhood.

His father, Theodore Senior, was determined to create an alternative destiny for the boy. When his son was 10-years-old he began encouraging him to build strength through systematic exercise, saying "You have the mind but you have not the body.... You must make your body."[37] He installed a gymnasium in the family home and the future president trained every day, lifting weights, doing pull-ups on the rings, and working out on the parallel bars. In time, the sickly youth transformed himself into a muscular, broad-shouldered man.[38] As an adult, Roosevelt exercised regularly and took up boxing, tennis, hiking, rowing, polo, hunting, and horseback riding. Despite being plagued by constant health issues (partial blindness, tropical fevers, rheumatism, partial deafness, and a gunshot wound in the chest, just to name a few) during his 60-year life, Roosevelt climbed mountains, became a cattle rancher, led a cavalry into battle, and explored the Amazon rainforest.

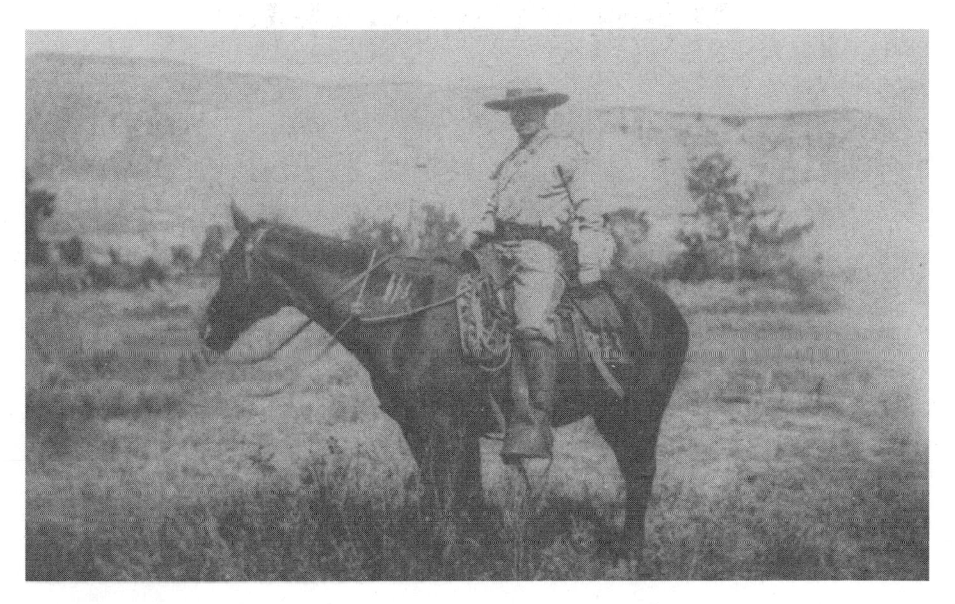

Theodore Roosevelt, 1903. *Credit: T.W. Ingersoll*

In the past, doctors would have recommended rest and relaxation for those of us coping with chronic illnesses. But with evidence increasingly pointing to the benefits of being active, medical advice is starting to shift in that direction and we're now being encouraged to exercise despite obstacles. A 2015 review highlighted that considerable knowledge has accumulated over the last two decades concerning the significance of exercise as the first-line of treatment of several chronic diseases.[39] While the authors acknowledged that exercise should be attempted only when a patient is medically stable and their symptoms are under control, they demonstrated that exercise can have many benefits for people with several chronic conditions including mental illness, Parkinson's disease and dementia, diabetes, heart disease, asthma, osteoarthritis, back pain, rheumatoid arthritis, and even cancer.

Arthur Kramer, the researcher specialising in the brain benefits of exercise, has demonstrated that exercising regularly may help mitigate the damaging effects that some treatments for breast cancer can have on the brain.[40] "Usually 'chemo brain' is associated with fogginess, difficulty remembering information, and so forth," Kramer told me. "What we found is that those women who worked out on a fairly regular basis tended to have higher levels of memory and decision-making than women who didn't. We can think of it as less chemo brain." Research like this helps build the case that exercise in and of itself can now be considered medicine.

If you're new to physical activity and are concerned about the safety of being active, speak with your doctor or health professional about the most suitable activities for you. Don't force yourself to run a mile if you're aching all over or feel flat with fatigue. Take a slow and steady approach. I started by simply circling my joints or doing gentle hatha yoga. These days I'm highly active and I don't feel as if there's anything my illness prevents me from doing. But my attitude on both good days and bad days is to follow the lead of Theodore Roosevelt who in his autobiography quoted his friend William "Squire Bill" Widener's advice: "Do what you can, with what you've got, where you are."[41]

Closing the Gap

Starting an exercise program is consistently near the top of the list for New Year's resolutions. For example, a study of almost 4,000 people in the UK found that 36 percent of people *intend* to exercise.[42] But unfortunately, 48 percent of people who intend to exercise don't actually follow through.[43] Having an intention to be active is not always enough to change behaviour,[44] a concept that researchers call the "intention-behaviour gap."[45] For me, the real world translation of this concept is that despite all the research I'd gathered, all the knowledge I now possessed, and all my good intentions to move more and sit less, it still didn't mean that I actually would.

I spoke with Professor Stuart Biddle who dedicates his time to understanding the fundamentals of exercise psychology – from theories of motivation, to adherence, to the design of successful interventions for increasing participation. Biddle has not only been instrumental in shaping UK Government recommendations for exercise and sedentary behaviour, he's also published over 250 research papers, 14 books, 70 book chapters, and presented over 750 papers at conferences. If anyone could explain the best way to go about actually implementing my intention to move more and sit less in my everyday life, it was him.

Formerly at Loughborough University in the UK, Biddle has recently moved to Australia and is leading a research team at Victoria University's Institute of Sport, Exercise and Active Living. When his video image came up on my computer screen for our interview, I couldn't help noticing that, like Jeremy Morris who lived and breathed his discoveries, Biddle was putting his own research into practice and was broadcasting to me from his stand-up desk.

At first you might think a stand-up desk rather peculiar, but Biddle's method of working is based on his evidence. In 2016, he and his colleagues published a review paper that looked at all the available research on how to get people to sit less. Although it is early days, one of their key conclusions was simple – *Environmental structuring has been shown to effectively reduce sitting time.*[46] "The simple notion of a standing desk is an environmental restructuring intervention," Biddle explained. "You've restructured the environment of a sitting desk into a standing desk and therefore you sit less. It's relatively straightforward." While their review of the evidence to date found that active workstations like standing desks promote decreased sitting time, have a positive effect on several health markers, and have no detrimental effect on work performance,[47] Biddle is careful to emphasise that this isn't about saying we need to stand all day long. "Of course we need to sit down and we have the absolute right to sometimes just relax and switch off and sit in front of a good film and so on. That's absolutely fine. What we're trying to avoid here are excessively long periods of sitting, or just too much sitting overall," he said.

It took me a little while to get used to it, but I wrote this book at a work station that I can raise and lower throughout the day. I stand up after I've been sitting for a while, and then sit when I get tired. I also look for other opportunities to stand throughout my day; for example I now stand when I'm eating at my breakfast bench rather than slouching on a stool.

Biddle's review paper also found that self-monitoring is an effective method of getting people to sit less, so I wore a fitness tracker on my wrist for a few months. It vibrated every hour and was really helpful in training me to get up and move with more regularity. "Self-monitoring is quite important. You need to know what you're doing in order to change it because some people probably think they're not sitting very much when in fact they are, and that awareness is definitely very helpful," Biddle said.

It's surprising and encouraging that breaking up sitting time every 20 minutes with just two minutes of light walking significantly improves glucose and insulin regulation.[48] So something as easy as making a cup of tea and walking around while the kettle boils could very well make a big difference to your health. I've noticed that these small changes have made a real difference for me, especially in providing relief for my general aches and pains.

By tweaking our environment and monitoring our behaviour, we can easily and inexpensively address the issue of too much sitting in our lives. But what about the bigger, more complex problem that most of us don't get enough exercise? Fortunately, this is a problem that Biddle has dedicated most of his career to solving. He has literally written *the* textbook on the psychology of physical activity, now in its third edition.[49]

Exercise Motivation 101

(With Professor Stuart Biddle)

ENJOY IT

In the moment-to-moment pace of everyday life when we need to constantly reaffirm our commitment to move, it can be hard to find the motivation to do something if you don't actually like doing it.[50] Unsurprisingly, when we feel good as a result of exercising, we are more likely to be regularly physically active, and as important, to maintain physical activity over the long term.[51] For example, one study found that sedentary people who felt good after a single session of moderate exercise reported doing more physical activity 6 and 12 months later.[52] Another study found that women with low levels of self-motivation were more likely to stick to their exercise activities if it made them feel revitalised.[53] Researchers also found that asking 150 students to recall a positive memory about exercise inspired the students to exercise more the following week.[54] "Certainly any behaviour that is unpleasant or produces a lack of reward, or even a negative punishment if you like, is really not going to be pursued unless you absolutely have to do it. Not many people will stick to an activity that's really unpleasant," Biddle says.

IT'S YOUR CHOICE

When you feel as though you're being forced to exercise, it has a negative impact on your motivation. In a study by researchers at the University of Alberta, women enrolled at a health club were asked to list their preferred exercise activities and then assigned to either a "choice" group and told their exercise programme was based on the choices they had made, or to a "no choice" group and told their programme was based on a standard format, not their preferences. In reality, both groups received the activities they had originally chosen, but the "choice" group had a significantly better attendance record after six weeks.[55] "I think we've probably gone about this the wrong way on many occasions in the past; the way we've used our language, where we use the term *should*. You *should* be physically active, you *must* be physically active. Really it should ultimately come down to individuals making the choice. I want individuals to use the phrase I *want* to be physically active, I *choose* to be physically active," Biddle says.

BELIEVE IN YOURSELF

When it comes to exercise, your belief in your ability can predict whether or not you'll go through with your intention to exercise and this is particularly true in the early stages of a new program.[56] Aim for small, achievable and gradual improvements, especially if you're just starting out in establishing a regular exercise routine. Overcoming self-doubt can be a challenge if you've tried to start a program before and failed. You may believe that exercise won't work for you, that your life is too hectic to add another thing to your To Do list, or that there are too many obstacles to overcome. When you're starting out, set goals you believe you can achieve.

PLANNING

Planning when and where you'll exercise, and planning how you'll cope with setbacks and obstacles, are keys to changing your behaviour.[57] A Polish study of people who had suffered heart attacks and had very compelling reasons to stick to a regular exercise program found that only patients who participated in a special planning intervention, which taught them to specify when and where they exercised each week and to plan for how they would overcome obstacles, actually stuck to the recommended three or more sessions of moderate physical activity per week eight months later.[58] A meta-analysis of 94 studies examining the effect of forming "if-then" plans (i.e., "If it's 5:30pm on a weekday, then I will go for a 30 minute walk, and if it's raining, I'll wear my new rain jacket and go anyway.") showed a significant impact on people following through with their intentions.[59] More on this in Chapter 10 (Lasting Change).

FEELING LIKE YOU BELONG

Belongingness is the human need to form and maintain positive, stable relationships.[60] Whether it's being part of a family group, a circle of friends, or a sports or work team, the "belongingness hypothesis" states that a major part of innate human behaviour is to seek intimate, coherent, and meaningful relationships. This fundamental need to belong has also been shown to be a key driver in motivation.[61] One study showed that while the majority of a group of 34 inactive and overweight women who went through a 24-week exercise program were initially motivated to train because they wanted to get into "a structured exercise programme," social contact with other participants was cited by 60 percent of the women as the primary reason for their adherence to the program.[62] Feeling as if you don't belong somewhere, or feeling nervous can undermine your motivation. "Some people are quite happy being the lone exerciser, a bit of running time, think time on their own, and that's all fine. Generally speaking though, if there's a social element to it, it helps. We're social beings and normally that's a helpful way to go about things," Biddle says. More about this in Chapter 9 (Relationships).

Unexpected, Surprising, Joyful News

I went home from the retreat in India feeling inspired, energised and, for the first time since my diagnosis, totally pain-free. I felt no need to take medication for pain or inflammation. One morning while having breakfast with Jules I turned to him and said, "It's as if the arthritis has vanished." It was a moment I thought would never come.

Feeling so well was the proof I needed that all my research and efforts would work. I had the foundations of a whole-health prescription and a clear path to follow. So far, I knew that entailed keeping my chronic stress in check, continuing to work on balancing my emotions, harnessing the power of my beliefs and expectations, prioritising a whole foods, plant rich, healthy diet, and committing to regular movement. I also knew there would be more insights to come. And I knew there would be tough decisions to make and even tougher circumstantial changes to make, and that there were bound to be set-backs along the way, but I was motivated, determined, and committed.

Knowing there were so many other people with chronic diseases feeling disempowered, hopeless, and helpless, Jules and I, as filmmakers, couldn't help wanting to share this information with the world. After weeks of careful consideration we decided that instead of making a large payment toward the mortgage we had just taken on with the purchase of our new house, we would take the profit from my production company over the course of the next year and use it to make a film. It would be a tough endeavour. I'd have to keep my client production work going at the same time, but it was something we both felt needed to be done. We agreed on one very important condition: making the film would not be done at the cost of my health, nor would it put health pressure on anyone involved in making it. Health was first. Film was second.

With that priority in place, pre-production on *The Connection* began immediately. It was exciting – reaching out to the world's leading experts whose work I'd been closely studying and asking for interviews, and looking for stories of other people who had taken a whole-health approach to the treatment of diseases for which conventional medicine had no answers. There was a sense that fairy dust had been sprinkled around the project as, one by one, the experts started saying yes and the stories began to emerge. Then, surprisingly, and joyfully, I discovered I was pregnant, something Jules and I had not planned on. We had been told that my autoimmune disease might mean difficulty conceiving so this was truly amazing news. The film shoot now had a nine month deadline.

Key Takeaways

1 For whole-health, from top to toe, exercise is a fundamental human need. Regular physical activity is a key to preventing several chronic conditions. The new science of movement also demonstrates that exercise is good for your whole body, including your mind and brain.

2 The latest expert advice is that you need to go beyond just the minimum recommended aerobic exercise throughout the week, and start getting a *variety* of movement types into your week, including cardiorespiratory, resistance, flexibility, and neuromotor exercise. But the important thing is to make sure you move. Remember, doing some exercise is better than doing none.

3 Sitting is the new smoking – the more you sit, the greater your risk of developing chronic illnesses, regardless of whether you're getting the recommended amount of exercise. We need to move more and sit less.

4 While in the past, doctors would have recommended rest and relaxation for those of us coping with chronic illnesses, medical advice is starting to shift and we're now being encouraged to exercise despite the obstacles. Consult your doctor for counsel on what may be suitable for you and remember Theodore Roosevelt's advice to "Do what you can, with what you've got, where you are."

5 The obstacles you face in your everyday life may derail your best intentions to move more and sit less. You'll need to put into place key strategies such as changing your environment, and using planning and motivation techniques to succeed. See the next page for Getting Started tips, and Chapter 10 (Lasting Change) for more information.

Getting Started

THINK of three ways you can move more in your everyday activities. For example:

- *Take the stairs not the elevator.*
- *Take the farthest spot away from your destination in the parking lot.*
- *Walk around while you make phone calls.*
- *Catch up with friends for a walk, not a coffee.*

IF you don't have an important meeting or social event during the day, why not put your exercise gear on first thing in the morning? Wearing the right clothes means one less thing getting in your way later in the day.

IF you're a desk bound worker, consider getting a sit-stand work station. There are a wide variety of options on the market, with new products coming out every day. I wrote this book at a standing work station that I can lower when I get tired and have a variety of chairs (kneeling, saddle and regular) to vary my sitting position, too.

TAKE advantage of the plethora of new smart apps and devices available that will get you moving. I keep a list of recommended apps on my website that I update regularly. I also used a fitness tracking device for a few months to get a feel for how much I was moving throughout my day. It was helpful to set it to vibrate every hour to remind me to get up and move. There are also mobile apps available to help you do this.

Extra Resources

AVAILABLE AT
www.thewholehealthlife.com/resources

LISTEN to extended audio interviews with the experts including:

- *Arthur Kramer (Senior Vice Provost for Research and Graduate Education and a Professor of Psychology & Engineering at Northeastern University. He previously served as the Director of the Beckman Institute for Advanced Science and Technology at the University of Illinois)*
- *Stuart Biddle (Professor of Active Living and Public Health at Victoria University's Institute of Sport, Exercise and Active Living)*
- *Peter Gollwitzer (Professor of Psychology in the Psychology Department at New York University); Gollwitzer's work on closing the intention-behaviour gap is explored in more detail in Chapter 10 (Lasting Change)*

DOWNLOAD my free PDF which outlines a simple technique called "If-Then" planning which helps keep your exercise goals on track. More on this in Chapter 10 (Lasting Change).

MY recommended reading list, which I update regularly, is available on my website. Books relevant to this chapter include:

- *Psychology of physical activity: Determinants, well-being, and interventions (3rd Edition)*, by Stuart Biddle
- *Spark: The Revolutionary New Science of Exercise and The Brain*, by John J. Ratey and Eric Hagerman
- *The First 20 Minutes: The Surprising Science of How We Can Exercise Better, Train Smarter and Live Longer*, by Gretchen Reynolds

Chapter 6

Environment

The Good Life

I was running late for a meeting, stuck on Sydney's notorious Spit Bridge sitting in traffic. It had taken me 20 minutes to travel 100 metres, and I was only half way across. I felt my blood start to boil as I sat completely helpless, unable to move or take action of any kind. It was a classic case of a modern stress response 101. Cortisol, adrenaline, and norepinephrine were all coursing through my body with nowhere to go.

Jules and I had recently moved to a beachside suburb called Freshwater on Sydney's northern beaches. "Freshie" is the birthplace of surfing in Australia, a laid-back place with a friendly village vibe where the ocean sparkles, the people are bronzed, and it feels as if you're on holiday all year round. Our intention was to say farewell to our old inner-city life which had centred on being close to work and nightlife, and instead live closer to our families, enjoy the seaside, and become more like the happy, healthy Freshie locals with sun-bleached hair and healthy glows. We decided to take this significant step so that we could make health more of a priority. But although we'd moved to the beach to live the good life, my office was still located in the inner city. Every day I spent three hours in traffic getting to and from work, and on this particular morning, I was far from living the dream. I'd done an interview from home, so I'd missed the early morning traffic window and was now stuck smack bang in the thick of peak hour.

I was half-way through my pregnancy, and although my arthritic symptoms weren't flaring, my body ached. All the sitting I did during the day aggravated my front-heavy, pregnant body. My hips especially were groaning about the unnatural position I was constantly forcing them into. The move to a new suburb had thrown my usual yoga and meditation routine out of whack, and I was having trouble finding time in my day for all the things I knew I wanted to do – eat well, move more, relax. On top of this, the little house Jules and I bought – our first home – had just flooded after days of heavy rain. It was an absolute mess. We were mortgaged to our limit. What extra money we did have had just been invested in our film *The Connection*. I was about to head overseas to shoot the film, but it was still a long way away from completion.

So there I was, running late, stuck in immovable traffic, body aching, house in ruins, bank balance empty, and soon to have a baby. Worry, powerlessness, and exasperation mixed in a gut-wrenching cocktail and I felt as though I was about to burst. I took in a gulp of air and was about to scream out my frustration when I completely surprised myself by letting out a slow, deep exhale instead. I took in another breath of air, held it for a moment and released it. The traffic wasn't moving, so for another few breaths I closed my eyes and focused. *In. Out. In. Out. In. Out.* Then, like magic, my mood cleared. I became aware of my surroundings: the bright shining day; the school children holding hands on the footpath beside my car; the sailing boats in the water below the bridge.

What on earth had I been thinking? It wasn't so bad. My pregnancy was going great. Despite my aching hips, I had no autoimmune symptoms and the baby was healthy. Jules and I were excited about becoming parents. As for the money worries, well, this is what we knew we were getting into when we decided to buy a house and produce a film. This was always going to be a challenge and it was our job to rise to it.

As I navigated the traffic and made my way to my office, I had a new sense of clarity and had come to an important realisation: I wasn't going to join those healthy, glowing people I saw on Freshwater beach by sitting in traffic for 15 hours every week. I liked my groovy little office in the inner city, but being surrounded by the constant hubbub of people, the thunderous racket of traffic and construction, and tall buildings that blocked sunlight for all but a few brief moments a day wasn't doing me any favours. Taking a whole-health approach to my life meant knowing that everything is connected to everything else, and that included the environment in which I surrounded myself. I knew it was time to close my office and relocate my work life closer to home.

It was a big decision. I'd likely be forgoing job opportunities and production contracts. My best clients would probably change the way they perceived me, thinking I was dropping out of the industry, and good staff would be less likely to want to travel out to the "insular peninsula" on the north side. But I had known for a while that putting my health at the top of my priority list was going to demand some big changes, and this was one of them. Working closer to home would free up time for yoga and meditation, and for planning and preparing good meals. I would have more energy to enjoy my local area and take advantage of living near the beach. The more I thought about it, the easier the decision became. A clean slate became an exciting prospect, and I wanted to make sure that the changes I was making were going to be worth it.

How could I take advantage of the latest science connecting our health to the world around us, and what were the proven things I could do for myself that would make a difference?

Nature Versus Nurture

On February 19, 1979, the Ohio *Lima News* reported the extraordinary story of Jim Lewis and Jim Springer, identical twins who had been separated at birth.[1] Theirs was an astonishing tale that caught the attention of the media around the world. The men were of identical height and weight, as might be expected, but despite having been raised in different families, both men smoked Salem cigarettes, drank Miller Lite beer, hung their keys from their belts, drove the same model and colour Chevrolet, and had the habit of biting their fingernails.

But it wasn't just small habits and brand choices that marked the Jims' similarities. Their lives were full of spooky coincidences. Both had married women named Linda and divorced them. Both were remarried to women named Betty. They had named their first sons James Alan and James Allen, and each had a dog named Toy. They both served as part-time sheriffs and had taken up carpentry as a hobby. They even vacationed at the exact same beachside location in Florida. All this similarity and yet the men had never met.

Their stranger-than-fiction story meant the two Jims were destined for media stardom. More important, their story piqued the interest of University of Minnesota psychologist Thomas Bouchard, who in 1979 launched a major scientific investigation that attempted to untangle the effects of genes versus the effects of environment on a person's development. Because identical twins develop from a single fertilised egg that splits in two, they share the same genetic code. Any differences between these human clones must therefore be due to environmental factors. So the opportunity to study identical twins raised apart presented a unique opportunity for Bouchard and his team of researchers. Over the years, they gathered exhaustive information from more than 80 pairs of separated twins, including the Jims, in order to explore the eternal question of nature versus nurture.

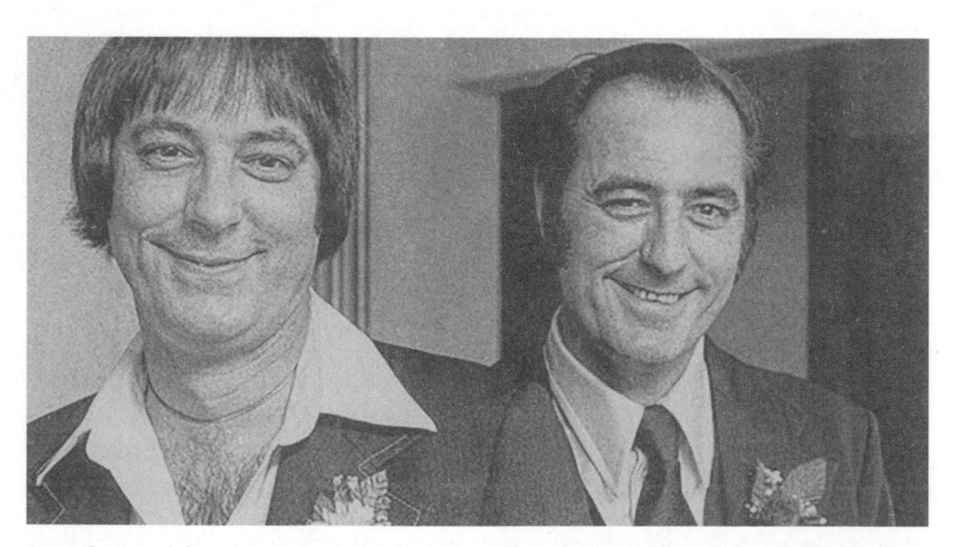

James Springer (left) and James Lewis (right) pose for a photo after being reunited. *Credit: The Lima News*

In 1986, before the first results of the study were published, science journalist Daniel Goleman got the scoop on the research team's conclusions and in a controversial article in the *New York Times* wrote that genetic makeup was more influential on personality than parenting.[2] Goleman revealed what the researchers would soon share with the world: that more than 50 percent of our personality is the result of genetics, and that the overall contribution of a common family-environment component was negligible.[3] Over time the research, which has come to be known as the Minnesota Study of Twins Reared Apart, has been picked apart by the critical eyes of other scientists, and the nature versus nurture question continues to generate heated debate.[4] But when you hear the story of the two Jims, and read the conclusions made by Bouchard and his team, it's easy to be swayed into thinking we are at the mercy of genetic forces with the power to continually shape our daily thoughts, feelings, choices, habits, health, and wellbeing.

Before you give in to this fatalistic viewpoint though, I'd like you to consider another example of identical twins whose story isn't quite so media-friendly, but whose case was reported in a medical journal in 2012. These sisters were raised in the same family and for the first four years of their lives grew and developed normally. But tragedy struck when one twin developed leukaemia. Although there was no cancer on either side of their family going back four generations, cancer of this nature is generally considered genetic. You would expect that because they were genetically-matched, if one twin developed the illness, the other would too. But while one remained healthy, the other continued to deteriorate. By age seven, the sick twin required a bone marrow transplant, made possible because of stem cells donated by her healthy sister, and throughout her life, she continued to suffer ill health. When she was 25 years old, her thyroid was removed after it was discovered to be cancerous. At 29 she developed type 2 diabetes. Because she had spent most of her life on hormonal medication, it's not surprising she grew to be 12 centimetres (almost five inches) shorter than her identical twin sister. Thankfully, the story has a happy ending: by the time she was 33 years old, the sick twin had recovered enough to become a mother and gave birth to a healthy baby girl.[5]

By considering a case study like this, the notion that our genetic destiny is fixed and unchangeable is called into question. We are forced to consider the impact of the other 50 percent of Bouchard's equation – the "nature" part of "nature versus nurture," that is, the subtle and often-unseen forces of the environment around us.

To explore this further, let's look at recent research on identical twins being done by Tim Spector, whom we met in Chapter 4 (Food). You will recall that in addition to being at the forefront of gut bacteria research, Spector is a professor of genetic epidemiology at King's College London and the custodian of the Twins UK Registry. Spector, a rheumatologist, wanted to understand why when one twin developed rheumatoid arthritis, the other rarely did. "When we looked at identical female twins with the disease, 85 percent of the women never developed their sister's disease," Spector told the *Sydney Morning Herald* after the release of his book *Identically Different: Why You Can Change Your Genes.*[6] The Twins UK Registry, which has information collected from 12,000 twins, reports that for most diseases studied, there was rarely more than a 50 percent chance of both identical twins getting the same disease.[7] "The reason for such disparity is the epigenetic differences between them," Spector said.

Epigenetics is a relatively new field of study that looks at how chemical changes to our genes caused by our environment can alter the way our genes are expressed. Genes are stretches of DNA that sit in almost every cell in your body. They contain instructions for producing proteins that control every bodily function. We inherit half of our DNA from each of our parents. And if your parents, grandparents, or other relatives have an inheritable disease or condition, you have a greater risk of getting that disease or condition. But through the study of epigenetics, scientists now know that your genes can be switched on and off. And while for the most part every cell in your body contains exactly the same genes, and that won't change, being exposed to external conditions can flip the gene switch one way or another.

Minute differences while you're developing in your mother's womb, differences in lifestyle, environmental exposures, infections, and other life events can all influence whether or not certain genes are activated.

Just because you have inherited the gene for childhood leukaemia for example, does not mean you will necessarily develop childhood leukaemia. In the case of the identical twin girls whose health histories were so different, researchers looked at their DNA and discovered that although the sisters had the exact same genes, the way in which those genes were *expressed* was very different. In fact, several recent studies have identified the existence of epigenetic differences between identical twins, which helps explain Spector's observations.[8]

By studying epigenetics, scientists are able to explore how factors like the neighbourhoods we live in, the schools we attend, the people around us, the money we earn, the food we eat, and our life circumstances can have a profound influence on our health and wellbeing. Even the father of twin research, Thomas Bouchard, acknowledges the importance of environmental influence. "Identical twins, I often say, can be compared to two renditions of a piano concerto played by musicians with different styles and skill levels. The written piece of music constitutes a set of specific instructions, yet each version, while clearly identifiable, carries the unique stamp of its performer. Similarly, twins, while created from the same genetic instructions, bear the indelible marks of their development under unique circumstances," he wrote in a paper published back in 1997.[9] So rather than it being a case of nature *versus* nurture, the evidence actually shows that it's a matter of nature *and* nurture.

In 2004 when I was first diagnosed with an autoimmune disease, my doctor indicated the illness was caused by bad genetics and that beyond taking immune-suppressing medication, there wasn't much more I could do. I felt disempowered and hopeless. But thanks to this new research on epigenetics, I now know that my story doesn't begin and end with my DNA. When I learned that subtle environmental forces could push and pull me below the surface of my conscious awareness to influence my health and wellbeing, I felt a sense of hope. Although I can't change my DNA, I can, to a large extent, control the environment in which I live.

Mindless Eating

In April 1998, Chicago theatre-goers attending a matinee screening of Mel Gibson's action movie *Pay Back* got a nice surprise. They were offered a free soft drink and a bucket of popcorn. What wasn't so nice was that the popcorn had been cooked five days earlier and was stale. Researchers from the University of Illinois were doing an experiment to see what influence the size of the popcorn bucket would have on the amount people ate. Despite that the popcorn was so stale it squeaked, the show-goers couldn't leave it alone. During the movie, the researchers observed people reaching into their buckets, taking a couple of bites, putting the bucket down, then picking it up again a few minutes later and having a few more bites. As the credits rolled and people left the theatre, each container was weighed to see how much popcorn had been eaten. It turned out that people who had been given large buckets of popcorn ate an average of 53 percent more stale popcorn just because it came in a bigger bucket.[10] Since then, many more popcorn studies have followed, and the results are always the same. It doesn't matter what city they are in or what kind of movie is showing, whether the movie-goers are hungry or full, or whether the popcorn is fresh or 14 days old – people eat more when they are given a bigger container.[11]

Brian Wansink was the man who led that study and many others like it. He is now a professor of marketing and the director of the Food and Brand Lab at Cornell University where he and his team are dedicated to studying why we eat what we eat and how triggers around us, such as people, packages, dinnerware, product names, labels, lights, smells, distractions, and containers, can unconsciously influence what we put into our mouths. I spoke to Wansink while he was travelling across Europe advising on cafeteria and supermarket design that will encourage people to eat less and make healthier choices without realising they are doing so.

Wansink's work explores the principles of *mindless eating*, a term that refers to the fact that we are aware only of about 10 percent of the 200 choices we make about food every day.[12] In other words, we are subtly and unknowingly influenced by our environment when we're determining when to eat and how much to eat. "It's not just, 'Am I going to have cereal A or cereal B for breakfast?' It's how much we're going to have, where do we finish it, how much milk we put on it, or whether we add sugar. The list goes on. The thing is, most of these little decisions we make are so quick and they're so micro that we don't even realise we're making those decisions. And so that's why the environment around us – whether it be the size of our cereal bowl or what the person is doing next to us, or the lighting and sound level in a room – all can bump us to eat too much or to pour or serve much more than we otherwise would," Wansink said.

At this point, you might be thinking you don't fit the profile of being a mindless eater and that you're immune to the effects of your environment because you're more self-aware than the average person. But what is really interesting about Wansink's research is that it demonstrates how we are *all* susceptible to mindless eating. In the popcorn studies, for example, the vast majority of people felt that the size of the container hadn't influenced how much they ate. "When the movie was over and they were leaving, we would ask, 'Hey, you ate about 50 percent more than the person with the smaller bucket. Do you think the size of the bucket had anything to do with it?' They'd say, 'No.' We'd then say, 'Oh, are you really hungry?' They'd say, 'No.' We'd say, 'Was the popcorn really good?' They'd say, 'No, it's terrible.' We'd say, 'Why do you think you ate so much more?' These people were speechless," said Wansink, laughing.

Okay, so now you may well be thinking, this is great, now that you know about the traps of mindless eating, you'll be more careful in the future. But what astonishes me about Wansink's research is the finding that simply being aware of these environmental influences isn't enough to counter their power. In 2005, Wansink spent 90 minutes explaining his research on mindless eating to 65 intelligent, motivated graduate students. During his lecture he told them that if he served them Chex Mix (a party snack mix) in a large serving bowl they would eat more than if he instead presented them with two small bowls. He lectured to them, showed them videos, asked them to go through a demonstration, and separated them into groups to discuss strategies they could use to prevent this from happening. Six weeks after their 90-minute mindless eating coaching session, Wansink invited the same students to a Super Bowl party at a local sports bar, complete with (surprise!) free party snacks. On arriving, half the students were led to one room where they were presented with a large serving bowl of Chex Mix, and the other half were led to a different room where they were presented with two small bowls. Although intelligent and thoroughly educated about the danger of large serving bowls, the students eating from the large bowls served themselves 53 percent more Chex Mix and ate 93 percent of what they were served.[13] At the end of the evening when the students were asked if the size of the serving bowl had influenced how much they took, all but two denied the possibility. "The bigger message that we're trying to get across with a lot of these studies is that, as rational as we are, most of us don't want to think we're fooled by something as simple as the cues around us.... That's why making a change rather than knowing the change is where we see the biggest, greatest results with people," Wansink said. Put simply, it's easier to change our environment than to change our minds.[14]

The research coming out of Wansink's Food and Brand Lab demonstrates that healthy environmental changes don't need to be expensive or complicated to be effective. A 2015 analysis of 112 studies that had collected information about healthy eating behaviours found that most healthy eaters made healthy choices because a restaurant, grocery store, school cafeteria, or spouse made foods like fruits and vegetables visible and easy to reach (convenient), took care that they were enticingly displayed (attractive), and made them seem like obvious choices (normal).[15] Wansink, who calls this the C.A.N (Convenient, Attractive, Normal) approach, says the key is to deliberately engineer our environment so that we mindlessly eat *well*. "What we need to understand is what we can do as individuals, what we can do as parents, what we can do in schools, in restaurants, and grocery stores to nudge ourselves to eat just a little bit healthier and a little bit better without having to keep a checklist of calories, without having to keep a daily food diary, and to do this in a natural way that doesn't interfere with what we really want to do, which is to live life, have fun, and enjoy ourselves."

5 Mindless Eating Tips

(Courtesy of Professor Brian Wansink)

1 Put your fresh fruit bowl visually on display on your kitchen counter or table. Replenish it regularly.

2 At the supermarket, don't walk down the cookie and sweets aisle. If it goes into your shopping cart, sooner or later it will go into your mouth.

3 Clear the junk food out of your pantry and put it in a different place (such as your laundry) for those special occasions. Or better yet, clear it out entirely. If it's not there, it can't be eaten.

4 Pre-cut your fruit and vegetables and put them in attractive containers so they're readily accessible when you're hunting for a snack.

5 Find at least two takeaway restaurants near your home and office where you know you can reliably buy convenient, healthy takeaway for those times when you get caught out and need nourishment in a hurry.

Remember the **C.A.N** approach and make healthy foods:

CONVENIENT: the easy, obvious choice
ATTRACTIVE: displayed in an appealing way
NORMAL: the default, most abundant option

Nature that Nurtures

In early September 2005, a dozen Tokyo businessmen were plucked from their usual jobs in large companies and taken to a cedar forest near Liyama in northwest Japan. For three days and two nights the men immersed themselves in the woody scents of the forest and walked at a leisurely pace among the red-brown bark and evergreen leaves of trees reaching up to 70 metres tall. The men were participating in the practice of *Shinrin-yoku,* a Japanese term coined in 1982 that translates in English to "taking in the forest atmosphere" or "forest bathing." Essentially, forest bathing is where mindfulness meets nature, and in a country that also coined the term *Karoshi* (death by overwork), the practice is becoming increasingly popular. Throughout the Tokyo businessmen's three-day forest bathing trip, scientist Qing Li from Nippon Medical School took blood samples which demonstrated that the experience had a profound effect on their immune systems. The activity of their natural killer (NK) cells, a component of the immune system that fights cancer, increased by about 50 percent.[16] The trip marked the beginning of a series of studies led by Li where men and women went on three-day forest bathing trips around Japan so researchers could investigate the effect of the forest experience on immune function.[17]

We've long known that spending time in nature can help improve mood and relieve anxiety, stress, and depression.[18] There is something magic about being in a leafy forest, and now, thanks to the growing body of work led by both Li and Yoshifumi Miyazaki from the University of Chiba in Japan, scientists are starting to unravel how the enchantment works on a molecular level. They've found that, overall, participants in the forest bathing trips experience a 12.4 percent decrease in levels of the stress hormone cortisol, a 7.0 percent decrease in sympathetic nervous activity, a 1.4 percent decrease in blood pressure, and a 5.8 percent decrease in heart rate compared with people in an urban environment. In addition, the forest bathers also report better moods and lower anxiety, which is reflected by a 55 percent enhancement of parasympathetic nervous system activity, a biological measure of the relaxed state we feel after being in the great outdoors.[19] These health benefits of forest bathing have been shown to last as long as 30 days after the participants returned to their urban lives.

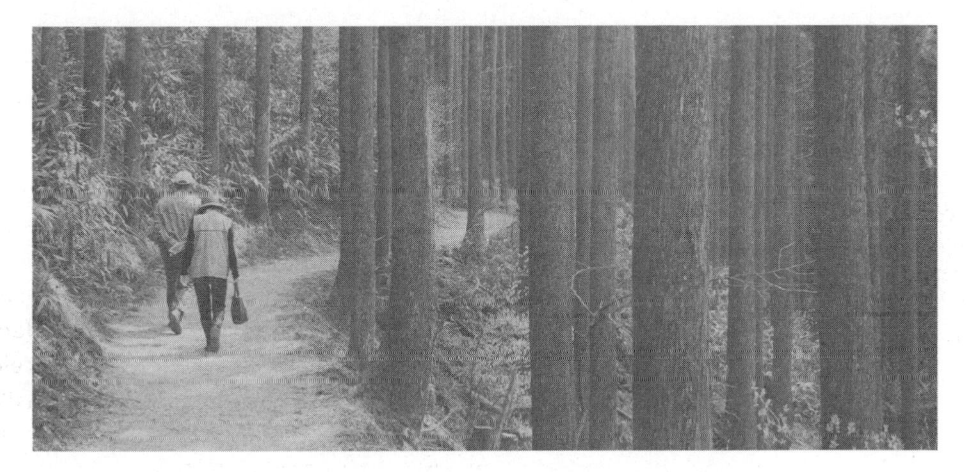

People walking in a forest in Japan. *Credit: elwynn / shutterstock.com*

With compelling evidence like this, it's little wonder that nearly a quarter of the stressed-out Japanese population living in mostly urbanised cities is embracing forest bathing, with between 2.5 million and 5 million visitors walking the country's 48 Forest Therapy trails every year.[20] Miyazaki believes that because humans evolved in nature, it's where we feel most comfortable, even if we don't always know it. "Throughout our evolution, we've spent 99.9 percent of our time in natural environments," he told *Outside* magazine. "Our physiological functions are still adapted to it. During everyday life, a feeling of comfort can be achieved if our rhythms are synchronised with those of the environment."[21]

Never before have humans been so removed from nature. Fifty-four percent of us now live in urban areas, and that number will rise to 66 percent by 2050.[22] With the allure of job opportunities, schools, hospitals, and entertainment, we are drawn ever closer to each other and increasingly live in built-up environments. It is little wonder that spending time in nature is also on the decline. A survey in the UK found that 71 percent of adults played outside every day when they were children, compared to 21 percent of children today.[23] Instead of bathing in the great outdoors, the average person is now bathing nine hours a day in the glow of a blue screen.[24] It seems our own wellbeing has suffered as a consequence[25] because coinciding with this increasing urbanisation is a worldwide increase in the prevalence of mental disorders.[26] In fact, when scientists looked at the brains of people living in cities, they found a distinct neural signature. City dwellers have increased activity in the amygdala, the brain's stress centre.[27]

Fortunately, we may not have to travel to the forests of Japan for the antidote. A research team at Stanford University in the US compared the effects of taking a walk through parkland area near the university with a stroll along a three lane main road in Palo Alto. Brain scans of the walkers showed that those who went on a 90-minute walk through the natural environment reported lower levels of rumination (worrying) and showed reduced neural activity in an area of the brain linked to risk for mental illness, compared with those who walked through an urban environment.[28] In the UK, researchers attached a portable EEG machine, which measures brain activity, to participants taking a 25-minute walk through three different environments. Their walk took them first through a busy shopping zone, then into a green space, and then into a busy commercial zone.[29] Analysis of their brain activity showed evidence of lower frustration and arousal when they moved into the green space zone.

As researchers start to see that nature makes our brain and immune system happy, the medical community is starting to consider how it can put these newest principles of wellness science to good use. One pioneering program in the US is encouraging doctors to "prescribe nature" to patients. Led by Washington-based paediatrician Dr. Robert Zarr, the D.C. Park Prescription program trains physicians to help kids at risk for chronic disease and obesity to connect with nature.[30] Tourism and government bodies are also starting to see the ecotourism opportunities for forest therapy. In the US, the Association of Nature and Forest Therapy Guides & Programs offers guided forest therapy walks, and is working to develop a global network of guides skilled in connecting people with the healing power of forests.[31] South Korea is also embracing the concept of healing forests. Chungbuk University offers a "forest healing" degree. A hundred-million-dollar healing complex is under construction next to Sobaeksan National Park.[32]

The Scent of Influence

You might think the evidence gathered by Qing Li from Nippon Medical School about the effect of wilderness walks on the immune system of stressed-out city dwellers would be enough to convince him of the health benefits of forest bathing. But the Japanese scientist wanted to go even further to isolate exactly what it was about being in the forest that had such a profound effect. Li suspected the trees themselves were important and specifically wondered if it was something about the scent of the forest.

The aromatic substances given off by trees to prevent them from rotting or being eaten by some insects and animals are called phytoncides and during his experiment Li found several different phytoncides in the forests that were absent from the cities.[33] He extracted essential oils from Japanese Hinoki cypress trees and put his theory to the test by having a dozen men stay for three nights in a hotel room where the room was vaporised with the scent. The results showed a 20 percent increase in NK cells during their three-night stay. They also had decreased levels of the stress hormones adrenaline and noradrenaline. Li concluded that the smells of the forest and decreased stress hormone levels at least partially contributed to the immune system boost during forest bathing.[34] He found similar results when he took the experiment into the laboratory and studied the effects of wood oils extracted from cypress and white cedar on NK cells in a petri dish.[35]

Other Japanese researchers have also demonstrated that the aroma inside a room built from Japanese cedar suppressed the activation of sympathetic nervous activity, which may help explain why we might feel relaxed and calm in certain timber rooms.[36] The smell of oil extracted from prickly ash and pine have also shown anti-tumour properties,[37] and oil from mountain pine has shown anti-oxidative properties.[38] "This is a very big effect, bigger than people get with pharmaceuticals," Li said in the *Outside* article. "In fact, I use a humidifier with cypress oil almost every night in the winter."

Although these experiments are very small, I wouldn't be surprised if word of Li's research soon gets out to the entrepreneurs of the world and we start seeing forest-scented essential oils "With phytoncides!" being offered as the next big thing in spa experiences and products. Certainly there is already a lucrative aromatherapy industry that goes back to ancient times, but compelling as the research findings are, it's far too soon to conclude that *all* essential oils have healing properties.[39]

Let There Be Light

There's something fundamentally disheartening about being in a windowless room all day long, and it's not surprising that most people prefer sunny and light environments to overcast and dark environments.[40] In 2014, a research team from the University of Illinois at Urbana-Champaign set out to discover why. They found that compared to workers in offices without windows, those whose workplaces had windows received 173 percent more white light exposure during work hours and slept an average of 46 minutes more per night. Workers whose workspaces did not have windows reported lower scores than their counterparts on quality of life measures and were less inclined to exercise. They also had poorer outcomes in measures of overall sleep quality, sleep efficiency, sleep disturbances, and daytime sleepiness.[41] These are not one-off findings: another recent study found that lack of exposure to natural light in the workplace is associated with poor sleep and depressive symptoms.[42]

Scientists are still trying to untangle the exact biological mechanisms by which light affects our health. So far we know that light is a key influence on our sleep[43] and in the next chapter I'll be looking specifically at how exposure to bright light at the right or wrong time of day can affect our circadian rhythm.

In addition to its ability to affect our sleep, daylight can positively influence our health through at least one other known biological pathway – vitamin D production, which occurs in your body when sunlight touches your skin, and which in turn has been linked to many health outcomes, such as reduced risks of cancer and cardiovascular disease.[44] Vitamin D has also been shown to improve mood via the production of the "happy hormone" serotonin, which explains why it can feel so good to get out in the sunshine.[45]

Of course, current public health warnings focus on the increased risk of skin cancer that comes from getting too much sun. And with good reason – there is vast evidence that too much sun is a risk factor for melanoma.[46] The legacy from the "tanned is beautiful" culture of the first half of the 20th century has been an epidemic of skin cancers.[47] But what is not being effectively communicated in the "beware of the sun" message is that many people are actually suffering from the harmful effects of *not getting enough* sunshine. Fifty-four percent of the world's population is considered at risk of vitamin D deficiency,[48] a situation now recognised as a pandemic.[49] Lack of vitamin D is associated with autoimmune diseases, complications in pregnancy, mental illness, and heart disease.[50] Vitamin D deficiency is also linked to several cancers including colon, breast, and prostate cancer.[51] It's important to remember that in most cases vitamin D deficiency is established as being *linked* to these illnesses and not established as the *cause* of the illness. Researchers are still debating which comes first, the illness or the deficiency.[52] There are some foods that naturally contain vitamin D, including oily fish such as wild-caught salmon, mackerel, and herring,[53] but unfortunately, taking a vitamin D supplement may not be the solution. Evidence for benefits that may be reaped from population-wide vitamin D supplementation is weak,[54] and there is some evidence that *high-dose* supplements may even be harmful.[55] The good news is that in a systematic review of other studies, researchers found that even if you regularly apply sunscreen, it won't entirely block your body's ability to produce vitamin D,[56] so there is still every reason to slip, slop, slap when you head outside to enjoy the great outdoors to boost your natural vitamin D production.

The Rising Din

In the days when pre-historic humans were roaming the African savannah, a loud noise often signalled a potential threat, so it's little wonder that even in our modern times, noise activates our fight or flight stress response.[57] Times have changed since then; our world is now loud. From traffic and aircraft noise to your neighbour's party or the sound track of your favourite action movie, even the constant flow of chimes, buzzes, dings, and dongs from your smart devices can put you on high alert.

This rising din is associated with all manner of health complications, the most obvious being noise-induced hearing loss. In the US for example, it's estimated that nearly one-third of the population is exposed to noise levels deemed harmful to hearing and that 104 million people are at risk of hearing loss because of excessive noise. Tens of millions more may be at risk of heart disease and other noise-related health effects.[58] And the problem is expected to get worse. The World Health Organization recently warned that 1.1 billion teenagers and young adults around the world are at risk of hearing loss from their personal audio devices.[59]

Environmental psychologist Arline Bronzaft is a leading expert on the effect noise has on your health. She's famous for a study she published in 1981 conducted at a public school in Manhattan's Washington Heights neighbourhood in which some of the classrooms faced directly out to an elevated subway track. Every four and a half minutes the students heard a train rattle by, and the teacher had to stop teaching until it passed. Bronzaft compared the performance of the kids in the noisy classroom to their peers on the opposite, quiet side of the building and found that the kids who were constantly interrupted by the noise of the trains were nearly a year behind in their reading skills. After the study was published, the school took steps to dampen the sound, including installing rubber pads on the tracks and noise-absorbing ceilings in the affected classrooms. A year later, reading levels had equalised.[60]

Exposure to excessive noise is also associated with stress, sleep disruption, annoyance, and heart disease. Excessive environmental noise has significant economic ramifications too. One report estimated that in the United States, reducing environmental noise by just five decibels would lower hypertension cases by an estimated 1.2 million and coronary heart disease cases by 279,000, resulting in associated cost savings and productivity gains exceeding $3.9 billion annually.[61]

Coming to Our Senses

If you've ever found yourself in a typical hospital, nursing home, or other healthcare facility either as a patient, visitor, or professional, you'll know the feeling of unease that can overcome you the minute you step foot on a ward. Florescent overhead bulbs create sickly grey tones that bounce light off sterile surfaces. Sealed windows make the air feel stale. The hum of air-conditioning to compensate for the stagnant air is a constant background drone that mingles with the round-the-clock dings and pings of technology. Day and night there is movement and activity, creating a sense of busyness, tension, and urgency. Despite the fact that these are places for rest and recuperation, the ambient noise, light, smells, and general hubbub of activity often leaves anyone who enters feeling drained and tired. I've spent many nights in a hospital bed and never once had a good night of rest, which as you'll read in the next chapter, is the very thing a sick person needs for a speedy recovery.

Often doctors' offices, clinics, and other health departments aren't much better. The babble of daytime television blasts in waiting rooms and instead of art, pharmaceutical posters adorn the walls. The technology used for diagnostic machines like MRIs and CT scanners is imposing and frightening. Harried staff sit behind formidable desks while they "fit you in" for another appointment and hand you a bill.

When you actually stop to think about these environments, you don't need to read an academic research paper to know they're not particularly conducive to recovery, health, and wellbeing. Even so, there is abundant evidence showing this to be exactly the case.

It all started in 1984 with a seminal study performed by Roger Ulrich, Professor of Architecture at Chalmers University of Technology in

Sweden. A suburban hospital in Pennsylvania provided the ideal location for what would become his landmark study investigating the effect of the environment on our health. Ulrich was curious about the restorative effect a window view might have on hospital patients recovering from gallbladder surgery. The hospital's design was ideal for a controlled trial because the windows down one side of the recovery wing looked out on a small stand of leafy green trees and the windows on the other side of the wing looked out on a featureless brown brick wall. When Ulrich painstakingly compared patients' medical records over a number of years, he found clear evidence that the patients with the tree view had shorter postoperative hospital stays, got along better with their nurses, and even took fewer painkillers.[62] At a time when hospital design was focused on keeping surfaces sterile and making space for the latest whizz-bang technology, Ulrich's was a breakthrough study because it was the first to use strict experimental controls and quantified health outcomes to measure the influence of our surroundings on healing. The findings suggest there may be a benefit in considering the emotional needs of patients in the design of the space in which they convalesce.

While the study did raise eyebrows at the time, it eventually inspired an entire movement called "evidence-based design," which takes advantage of this and subsequent research showing that simple things like good air flow and sound, views of nature and daylight, pleasant lighting, improved floor layouts, and single-bed rooms rather than multi-bed rooms, can reduce infections and pain for patients, reduce staff stress, and even improve budget bottom lines.[63] For example, in a coronary ICU at Karolinska Huddinge University Hospital in Sweden, researchers replaced sound-reflecting tiles that caused excess noise with sound-absorbing tiles that created a quieter environment, and found that patients not only slept better, they also had other positive biological markers, less need for beta blocker medication, and were not as likely to be rehospitalised.[64]

When the management at one Florida hospital was having problems with patients cancelling their MRI appointments at the last minute, they decided to get a little creative. They renamed the department Seaside Imaging, and turned the space into a relaxing beach-themed environment.

Three dimensional murals were painted on the walls throughout the waiting and changing rooms, hallways and floors were redesigned to look like beachfront boardwalks, beach cabanas replaced ordinary changing booths, and chairs were replaced with wooden rocking chairs and folding lounge chairs. Patients were given terry robes in place of hospital gowns and even the MRI machine was transformed into a giant sandcastle. The sound of ocean waves and fresh ocean fragrances infused throughout the department completed the makeover. (The video on their website is great fun to watch.[65]) The result of the transformation was a 50 percent reduction in appointment cancellations.[66] A formal analysis hasn't been published in a peer-reviewed journal, but Seaside Imaging's director told *Fast Company* magazine that the number of patients needing sedation dropped from six percent to two percent after the seaside renovation; that's a reduction of two thirds.[67]

Taking all this into consideration, it's little wonder that the concept of healing environments has come to have a significant influence on building and development projects worth billions of dollars.[68]

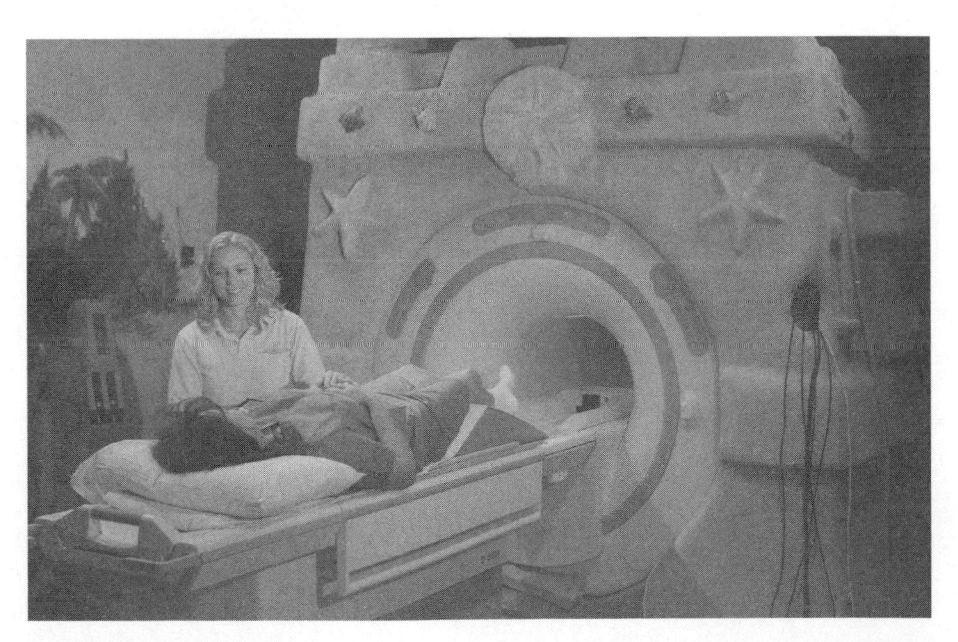

Sandcastle shaped MRI at Seaside Imaging Center. *Credit: Celebration Health*

Mind Your World

In his 1971 book *The Closing Circle*, American biologist Barry Commoner, one of the founders of the modern environmental movement and among the world's best-known ecologists in the 1960s, 70s, and 80s outlined four key laws of ecology, the first of which is that "Everything is connected to everything else."[69] This idea was very much with me as I read through the evidence showing how my surroundings influence me. Whether I was aware of it or not, everything around me, from the sunlight that touched my skin to the aromas in the air I breathed, were all elements woven into a subtle and intricate web of relationships. The more I read, the more I understood that these unseen forces were etching themselves into my very DNA, switching on and off key epigenetic levers that were influencing my health.

At first, when I started taking all this in, I felt vulnerable and exposed. When I had medical appointments I felt powerless over the dreariness of waiting rooms and consultation rooms. In Sydney's bumper-to-bumper traffic, I felt trapped and impotent. Even my local supermarket became a symbol of something that had power over me. Apart from choosing a nice, newly-renovated hospital in which to have our baby in a few months' time, I didn't see that there was much I could do. But my decision to move my office out of the inner city and closer to home marked the beginning of an important shift in my thinking, and over time I started to see there were in fact many things I could do to design the environment around me to help encourage good health.

At home I began to change my food environment so I could nudge myself to eat less and eat better. Small things – like having an out of the way place to store food items containing ingredients of questionable nutritional value, having a fresh fruit bowl prominently on display in my kitchen, and having a fairly steadfast rule never to walk down the candy and cookie aisle at the supermarket – have made a real difference in my eating patterns. We've also made subtle changes to our lighting environment at home which I'll describe in the chapter on sleep.

The changes I made to my office environment have also made an impact. As I mentioned in the last chapter on movement, I now work at a sit-stand desk, a change that has greatly reduced the amount of sitting I do during my day. I also now split my time between a home office, where I've written this book, and an office in the heart of Manly on Sydney's northern beaches. It takes 10 minutes to ride my bike along the Manly beach front from my home to my office, a huge change from the hour and a half I was spending sitting in Sydney's toxic traffic just a few years ago. There's a whole lot less stressing and a whole lot more healthy living that I can fit into my life now that I'm not sitting in traffic for 15 hours a week.

By keeping in mind the principles of evidence-based design – nature, light, sound, air, space, design, and layout – I'm always looking for new ways I can change my environment to improve my health.

Throughout this book I've written a good deal about the power of mindfulness – of non-judgmentally paying attention in the present moment – and this practice has certainly made a difference to my life and my health. But there are times when being in the moment just isn't possible. Life is busy. Things happen. We get caught up. In many ways, this chapter on the environment has actually been all about *mindlessness*, about learning to recognise environmental triggers and protecting ourselves in advance, about pre-committing to healthy choices, and about being proactive in taking advantage of the subtle forces around us so that rather than letting them influence us in negative ways, we can use them as powerful forces for good in our lives and health.

Key Takeaways

1 Your genes continually shape your daily thoughts, feelings, choices, habits, health, and well-being. But through the study of epigenetics, scientists now know that your genes can be switched on and off by external environmental influences.

2 Your everyday choices and behaviours that influence your health such as when to eat and how much to eat, are subtly and unknowingly influenced by your environment. Even being aware of the environmental forces pushing and pulling you one way or another isn't enough to counter their power. You need to change the environment around so you will be automatically nudged in the right direction.

3 At a time when most people live in urban environments, researchers are discovering that spending time in nature is not only healthy for mental wellbeing, but it also makes your brain and immune system happy.

4 Whether you're aware of it or not, everything around you, from the sunlight that touches your skin, to the aromas in the air you breathe, and the noises that flood your ears, is woven into an intricate web of relationships that have the ability to get under your skin to change your physiology and influence your health.

5 Though places such as hospitals and clinics are supposed to be where we go for rest and recuperation, the overwhelming noise, light, smells, and general hubbub of activity often leaves anyone who enters feeling drained and tired. Simple things like good air flow, gentle sounds, views of nature and daylight, pleasant lighting, improved floor layouts, and single-bed rooms rather than multi-bed rooms, can have dramatic beneficial impacts on health outcomes.

Getting Started

TAKE a walk through your home and make a list of the changes you can easily make in order to shift it towards being a more health-giving environment. Inexpensive ideas include putting up a vibrant poster or artwork, buying a soft lamp for a room so you don't have to use a harsh overhead light, shifting furniture around to make it less cluttered, and using an oil burner or aromatic humidifier to produce calming fragrances. Consider elements such as natural and artificial light, smells, air flow, noises and furniture layout.

THINK of three things you can change in your kitchen to nudge yourself to eat better. For instance, you might place a freshly filled fruit bowl on your kitchen counter, clear your pantry of junk foods, or pre-cut your fruit and vegetables to make them easily accessible and convenient for the week ahead.

TAKE a look at your desk at work and consider ways you can make it a more pleasant set-up that can nudge you towards being healthier. Ideas include placing a vibrant plant on your desk, removing any tempting candy jars, moving your desk closer to a window, or getting a sit-stand work station.

SCHEDULE a walk through a green environment this week. It could be in a forest if there's one nearby or just your local park. Pay attention to the sights and smells around you and take note of your mood before and after the experience.

IF you or someone you know is convalescing after an illness, make the environment more therapeutic. For example, you could place a beautiful flower arrangement or an uplifting piece of art or photograph by the bedside. If you can, insist on having a single-bed hospital room with a window view.

CHECK out Professor Brian Wansink's website, *www.slimbydesign.org* which offers a four week course to help you improve your eating environments at home, work, in restaurants, in the grocery store, and at your child's school.

Extra Resources

AVAILABLE AT
www.thewholehealthlife.com/resources

LISTEN to extended audio interviews with the experts including:

- *Brian Wansink (Professor of Marketing and the Director of the Food and Brand Lab at Cornell University)*

MY recommended reading list, which I update regularly, is available on my website. Books relevant to this chapter include:

- *Born Together – Reared Apart, The Landmark Minnesota Twin Study,* by Nancy L. Segal
- *Identically Different: Why You Can Change Your Genes,* by Tim Spector
- *Playing the Genetic Hand Life Dealt You: Epigenetics and How to Keep Ourselves Healthy,* by Craig Hassed
- *Healing Spaces: The Science of Place and Wellbeing,* by Esther Sternberg
- *Mindless Eating: Why We Eat More Than We Think,* by Brian Wansink
- *Slim by Design: Mindless Eating Solutions For Everyday Lives,* by Brian Wansink

Chapter 7

Sleep

Storm

In February 2013, I was driving in a rental car between New York and Boston with my film crew. My dream of making a feature documentary about the latest research in mind-body medicine was becoming reality, and we were on an 11-day whirlwind tour of the US. I was six months pregnant and my aim was to get as much production on *The Connection* done as possible before the new arrival, after which time I strongly suspected the film would take a back seat to other priorities.

My crew and I were looking forward to a much-needed full night of sleep. After the 14-hour flight from Sydney to Los Angeles, we immediately flew into San Francisco, and without any chance to adjust to the time zone difference, launched straight into production and interviewed two experts: Dean Ornish, whose lifestyle programs have been beneficial for people with heart disease and prostate cancer, and David Spiegel, a leading researcher from Stanford who is renowned for his work on the effects of social support on health and the progression of illness, especially cancer. Then we took a seven-hour flight to New York where we interviewed Jon Kabat-Zinn, the expert on mindfulness featured in Chapter 1 (Stress). After traveling and working in three very different time zones in just three days, we were exhausted.

To pull off this ambitious project on my self-funded budget, this time in Boston with my film crew was critical. Over the next few days, we would interview five of the sixteen people that would make up the heart of the film. With so much riding on the Boston leg of the shoot, you can imagine my dismay when I started getting emails and calls from some of the people I'd lined up to interview saying they were cancelling. They apologised but stressed the danger of going outside during a storm. I was dumbstruck. In Australia, a storm generally lasts for half an hour or so, after which there's a bit of cleaning up to be done and some power lines to repair. Why would a storm require people to cancel their interviews?

It turned out that Nemo, the approaching winter storm, would be one of the severest in recorded history, bringing with it hurricane-force winds and nearly 25 inches of snow. The city of Boston was buried. Hundreds of thousands of homes lost power. Airports were shut down and travel bans were enforced. Massachusetts Governor Deval Patrick declared a State of Emergency and issued an executive order prohibiting people from using public roads or risk a penalty of one year in prison. Eighteen people died. It was catastrophic.

We arrived at our hotel room in Boston one day before the storm hit and I soon realised that all my key interview opportunities could very well be lost. I will be forever grateful to Ali Domar, an associate professor at Harvard Medical School and leading expert in the mind-body connection and the treatment of infertility, who braved the storm front to meet me for an interview. If you look at the extended video of my interview with Domar, which is available on my website, you'll notice in the wide shot that she's positioned next to a double bed in my hotel room instead of the Harvard location we'd initially planned. What commitment. What a woman.

As the storm rolled in and the city shut down, I felt immense pressure. I had put all the savings from my production company into the US shoot and I didn't have the money, time, or resources to extend it. I had no wiggle room.

In the not too distant past, this is exactly the kind of situation that would have been disastrous for my health. The old version of me would have been tearing my hair out with worry. I would have been frantically making phone calls long into the night, sending emails, begging the weather gods to change their minds, and turning to caffeine and comfort foods to "get me through it." Instead, I saw that I had an opportunity to put to the test all that I had been learning about minimising chronic stress,

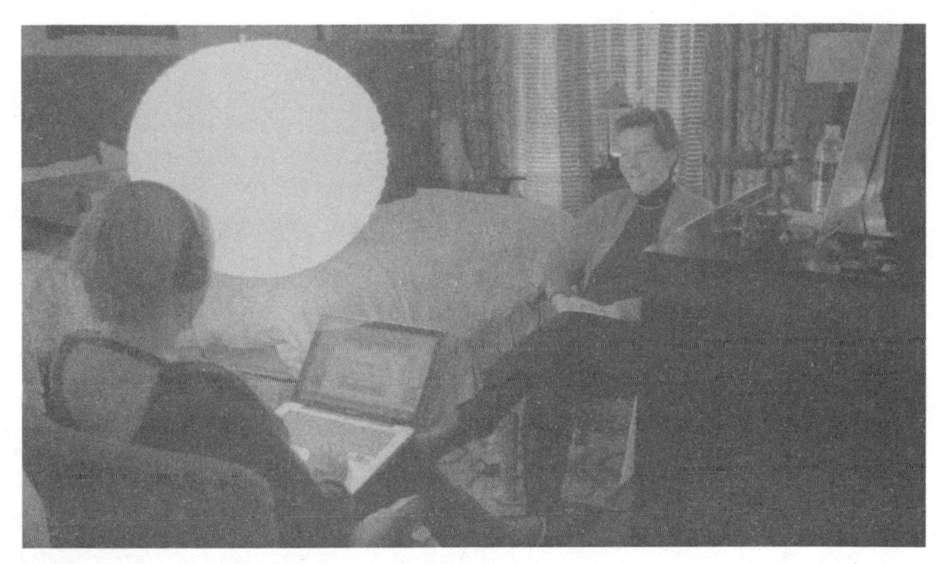

Ali Domar, associate professor at Harvard Medical School during an interview for *The Connection* documentary, 2013.

about being mindful of my intense emotions, about prioritising eating well, and about moving my body even when times got tough. The reality was, there was nothing I could do about the storm, and it was an immense weight off my shoulders to be able to just let it all be. I organised massages for the crew, took the opportunity to meditate and practise yoga, and most important after all the travel we'd been doing, I went to sleep.

The Myth of Productive Wakefulness

By the end of his life, Thomas Edison, a prolific inventor and businessman, held 1,093 US patents for innovations. These included an early version of the microphone, record player, and movie camera. On January 27,1880, Edison was granted US patent 223,898 for "An electric lamp for giving light by incandescence."[1] He had invented the first commercially practical incandescent light bulb. He illuminated the night and the world was forever changed.

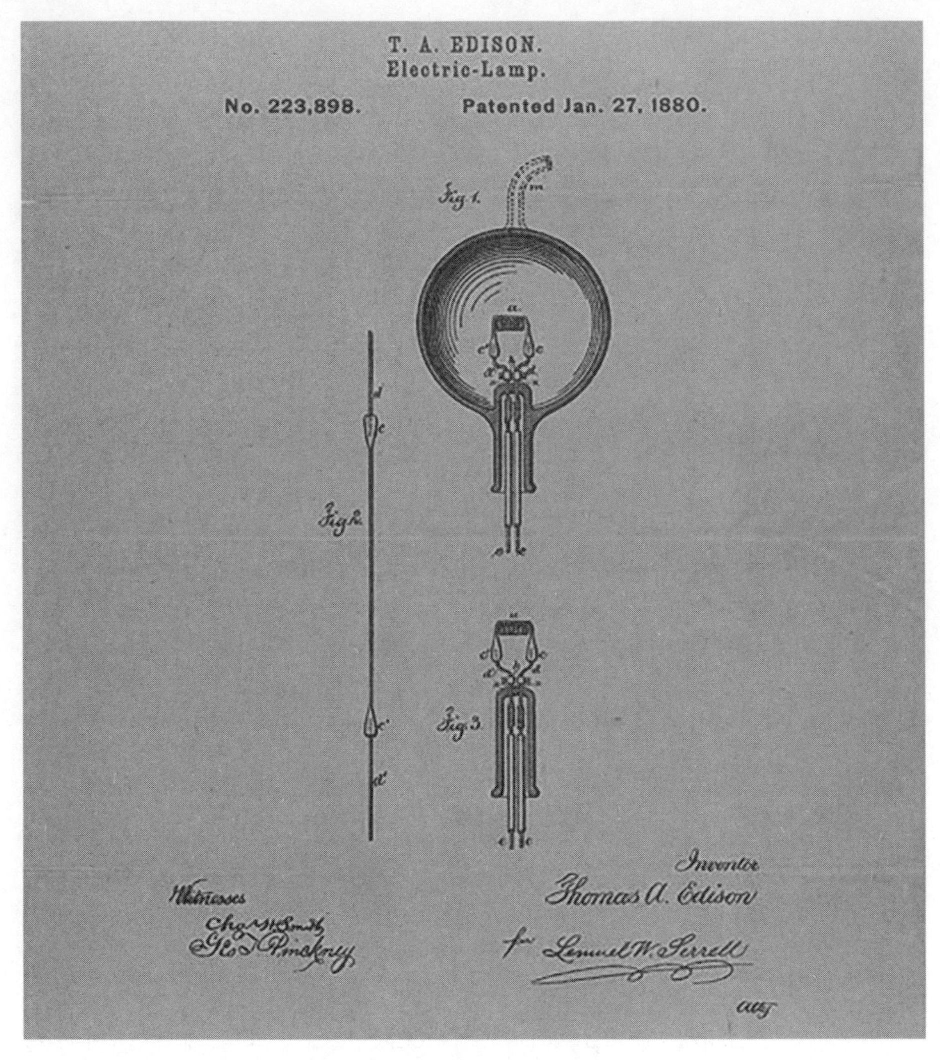

Thomas Edison's Patent Application for an improvement in electric lamps, 1880. *Credit: Records of the Patent and Trademark Office; Record Group 241; National Archives.*

It may not come as a surprise that Edison, the father of artificial light, was also a committed opponent of sleep. The great inventor was a media celebrity and used his platform to enlighten Americans on his approach to self-advancement through ceaseless work and minimal sleep. In a 1908 interview he gave to the *New York Times*, Edison boasted of having not slept more than five hours a night for 40 years, of having trained his wife to do the same, and of having put 100 of the men who worked in his laboratory through a two year test by limiting them to four hours sleep a night. "After all, sleep is only a habit; there is nothing to prove that men really need it," he said.[2] As Alan Derickson writes in his book *Dangerously Sleepy: Overworked Americans and the Cult of Manly Wakefulness,* "Edison spent considerable amounts of his own and his staff's energy in publicizing the idea that success depended in no small part in staying awake to stay ahead of the technological and economic competition." In Edison's way of thinking, sleep was a sign of laziness, and he wore his brand of heroic wakefulness as a badge of honour.[3]

Of course, Edison is not alone in waging a personal war on sleep. Stories in the popular media about the modern day treadmill-pounding, number-crunching, smart phone-wielding titans of the corporate and political world fortify the message that sleep is merely an obstacle to getting more done. US President Barack Obama goes to bed at about 1:00am and is up at 7:00am to hit the gym, but doesn't always get those six hours of sleep.[4] High-profile chief executives such as Marissa Mayer at Yahoo! and Pepsi's Indra Nooyi are said to function on four hours a night.[5] Donald Trump claims to stay a step ahead of his competition by surviving on anywhere between 90 minutes and four hours of sleep each night.[6] "Don't sleep any more than you have to," he wrote in his 2004 book *Trump: Think Like a Billionaire: Everything You Need to Know About Success.* The message we get from some of the world's richest, most powerful and productive people is loud and clear: in the words of Trump, "How can you compete against people like me if I sleep only four hours? It can't be done. No matter how brilliant you are, there's not enough time in the day."[7]

While Edison, Trump and their seemingly indefatigable comrades would have you believe that sleep is wasteful and unproductive, research actually shows that the time you spend sleeping – a time you might think all systems are powered down – is actually when your brain and body go to work to perform some of their most vital functions. As it turns out, the processes that take place while you are asleep are essential for optimum immune function, hormone regulation, healthy metabolism, memory, attention, problem-solving, and emotion regulation.[8] Sleeping for six hours or less each night makes you four times more likely to get a cold than someone who sleeps more than seven hours a night.[9] Sleep deprivation is linked to an increased risk of obesity, diabetes, heart attack, hypertension, stroke,[10] and total mortality risk.[11] Sleep disorders like insomnia, sleep apnea, and Restless Legs Syndrome (RLS) are associated with increased morbidity and mortality.[12] This may be in part because sleep deprivation can hasten the process of cellular ageing.[13]

It's not just your physical health that suffers when you're not sleeping enough. Your mental health is also challenged by lack of sleep, which is linked with mood disorders and anxiety.[14] When researchers experimentally disrupted people's sleep cycles they observed a significant deterioration in mood, which goes toward explaining why a high prevalence of anxiety, depression, and other mood disorders is reported among shift workers whose sleep rhythms are constantly challenged.[15]

Sleep deprivation doesn't just potentially shorten your life by increasing your risk of disease and putting your mental health in jeopardy, it also makes you a danger to yourself and to those around you. In one Harvard study, sleep-deprived medical interns at a US hospital made more than double the number of errors at night, a result that has been replicated multiple times.[16] When you're sleep-deprived you're also far more likely to be involved in a traffic accident.[17] Researchers in Australia and New Zealand found that being sleep-deprived can have some of the same hazardous effects as being drunk.[18] In the study, people who drove after being awake for 17 to 19 hours performed worse on driving tests than those who had a blood alcohol level of .05 percent, which is the legal limit for drunk driving in Australia. It is even more unsettling to learn that some of the worst disasters in our history (including the Chernobyl nuclear power plant explosion and the Exxon Valdez oil spill) may have been prevented if key personnel had simply slept more the night before.[19] With all this in mind, it's little wonder that the US Centers for Disease Control and Prevention considers insufficient sleep a serious public health concern.[20]

Despite what some of the most powerful people in the world would have you believe, foregoing sleep does not make you more productive or successful. You may have heard of the 10,000 hour rule, made famous by author Malcolm Gladwell in his book *Outliers*.[21] The idea is that it takes roughly 10,000 hours of practice to achieve mastery in a field. The concept has its basis in a study conducted in the early 1990s by K. Anders Ericsson, a professor of psychology at Florida State University who looked at the practice habits of violin prodigies and found that by age 20, the most elite performers had averaged more than 10,000 hours of practice, while the less able performers had only clocked 4,000 hours of practice during their lifetimes.[22] This study is often used to make the case for practice over innate talent as the underpinning of greatness. But a key factor in the results of the seminal research is often overlooked. In addition to time spent practicing, Ericsson also found that *sleep* was a major factor in influencing peak performance. The top performers slept on average eight hours and 36 minutes a night, about an hour more than those who didn't quite make it to the top. The virtuosos were also more likely to take a nap during the day, especially before public performances. There's more on the power of napping in the break out box later in this chapter.

Ericsson's research is even more compelling when you consider the results of newer studies conducted at the Stanford Sleep Disorders Clinic and Research Laboratory. In 2004, researchers demonstrated they could improve the brain function of Stanford undergraduate students by getting them to sleep more.[23] In 2011 they followed up by having elite basketball athletes increase their average sleeping time from 6.5 hours to 8.5 hours a night. When they looked at the players' on-court performance measures, the results were staggering. The athletes had improved their free throw shooting by 11.4 percent and their three-point shooting by 13.7 percent. Every player who participated ran more quickly than before the intervention, improving their sprint drills by an average of 0.7 seconds. The players also reported feeling less fatigue, more energy, and improved mood. In just a few months, they had attained the sort of performance boost usually achieved only after years of training or by using performance-enhancing drugs.[24]

Although researchers have established that the average adult needs somewhere between seven and nine hours of sleep a night, many of us aren't getting even close to that much.[25] The US National Health Interview Survey of more than 250,000 people found that almost 30 percent of adults were sleeping less than six hours a night.[26] A global survey of 35,327 people found that one in four people say they don't sleep well, and more than one in ten people reported feeling "very sleepy" or "dangerously sleepy" during the day.[27] Another study found that kids around the world are being affected too, and are losing on average 37 minutes of recommended sleep every night.[28]

It's time we challenge the adage "if you snooze, you lose." I confess I used to be like my ambitious friends and family members who sacrifice sleep in hopes of getting ahead in the world. I thought I would be a cut above the rest for pulling all-nighters in pursuit of accomplishment. I wore the number of days I worked straight without time off as a badge of honour, using my lack of sleep as a way of telling the world that I was going somewhere and making something of my life. But after falling ill, and the more I learned about the latest science that links our mind, body, and health, the more I realised the folly of this approach. It's not just about achieving good personal health. It's also about performing at my best and sleep is now up there among my top priorities.

How Much Sleep Do You Need?

In 2009 a rare genetic mutation was discovered that allows some individuals to sleep less than 6.25 hours a night with no negative effect.[29] Unfortunately, it's thought that this super power is limited to less than one percent of the population.[30] For the rest of us, sleep researchers don't seem to agree on exactly how much we should sleep.[31] From time to time news stories carry headlines like "Why Seven Hours of Sleep Might be Better than Eight,"[32] but these findings don't necessarily translate for every person. Simply put, some people need more or less sleep than others. Depending on our age and gender, most of us need somewhere between seven to nine hours of sleep every night. Toddlers need around thirteen hours, including a daytime nap. Teenagers need around nine and a half hours, and women tend to need more sleep than men.[33] But keep in mind that the amount of sleep you need from day to day will also vary. Studying for exams, preparing for a major presentation at work, training for a marathon – these kinds of activities all demand more from you, and as a result, you'll need more sleep.[34] See the "Getting Started" section at the end of this chapter for a simple way to work out how much sleep you need.

The Benefits of Napping

Though the prodigious Thomas Edison would have been loath to admit it, he likely got far more sleep than he claimed. Edison was, in fact, a notorious cat napper, with nap cots in his lab and library, and this may have been one of the secrets to his productivity and success.

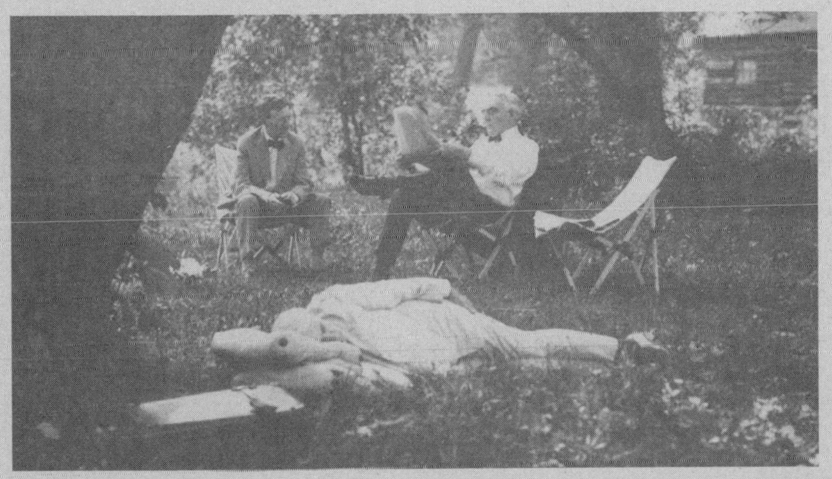

Thomas Edison napping under a tree. United States President Warren G. Harding is reading the newspaper, with Harvey Firestone seated, 1921. *Credit: The Henry Ford*

We now have substantial evidence that documents the invigorating effects of short naps, especially for people who are having trouble getting enough sleep at night such as teenagers, shift workers, and people with sleeping disorders.[35] Even if you've had enough sleep during the previous night, studies show that a short nap can also improve your mood, alertness, and performance.[36]

Generally, it's thought that mid-afternoon is the ideal time to nap because it coincides with the average person's peak daytime sleepiness.[37]

To avoid feeling groggy after waking from your nap, experts recommend keeping your nap to just 20 - 30 minutes, which prevents you from going into deep sleep.[38]

Why Do We Sleep?

When you think about it, sleep doesn't really make sense from an evolutionary-survival-of-the-fittest standpoint. After all, during sleep we're unconscious, at times partially paralysed, and hardly on red alert for any wild animals looking to make us their next meal. And yet we humans spend about a third of our lives asleep, which means that if you live to 90, you'll have slept for a total of 30 years during your lifetime.[39] Although biologists have scoured the earth, to date they have found no clear evidence of any animal species that does not need some form of sleep, so we can conclude that sleep must serve some kind of vital need.[40] But why, when it's so risky, do we spend such a significant part of our lives lying semi-dormant, with our eyes closed, oblivious to the world around us?

It was sleep research pioneer Nathaniel Kleitman, a professor of physiology at the University of Chicago, who made the first tentative steps toward answering this question. Before the 1930s, the scientific community wasn't much interested in sleep and its potential to affect our lives and health. But in 1938, Kleitman and his research assistant, Bruce Richardson, descended into Mammoth Cave in Kentucky for an experiment that grabbed the interest of the media and captured the imagination of the American public.[41] For 32 days, they lived in the cave, 140 feet below ground, without the influence of noise or sunlight to disturb them.

At that time, it was commonly understood that most people sleep and wake on a 24-hour cycle, spending about eight hours each day in the Land of Nod, and the other 16 hours a day at work or play. Kleitman and Richardson wanted to know whether this 24-hour sleep-wake rhythm was a fixed and unchangeable internal body clock or if by depriving themselves of environmental cues they could switch to a 28-hour sleep cycle.

Delightful black-and-white newsreel footage from the time shows the earnest young scientists sleeping on specially-fashioned beds designed to keep the rats at bay. With orchestral music of the period playing dramatically underneath the narration, the newsreel shows the welcoming party entering the cave to greet the men at the conclusion of the experiment, crossing a subterranean river, and working its way through "jungles of stalactites and stalagmites." Lit by the ghostly flicker of an oil lantern and dressed in layers of clothing to ward against the cold, a very serious Kleitman tells the camera, "This is in no way a stunt, or an act of endurance or perseverance, but a bonafide scientific experiment. We hope the results of which we have obtained will be of benefit to science."[42]

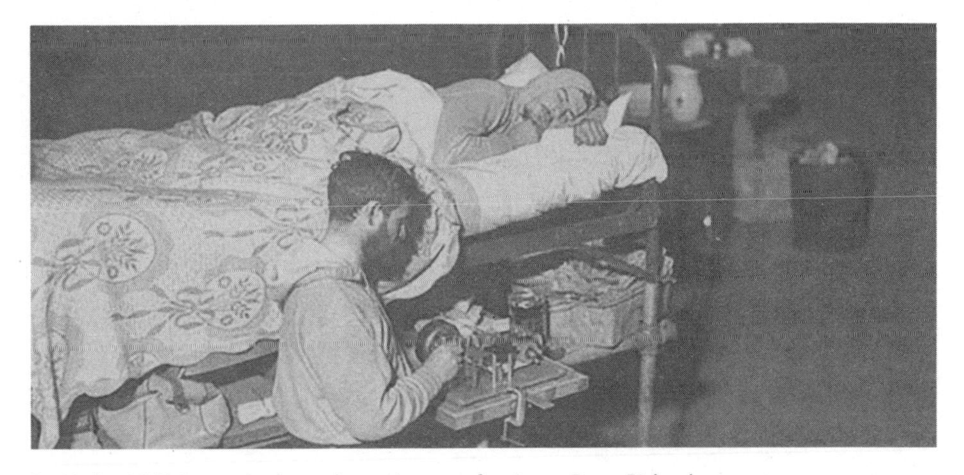

Dr. Nathaniel Kleitman checks on the restiveness of assistant Bruce Richardson during the 1938 sleep experiment in Mammoth Cave. *Credit: The University of Chicago Medicine*

Despite the media attention, and although their beards were impressive, their scientific results were inconclusive. Richardson adapted to the new cycle in just a week but Kleitman, who was 20 years older, did not. Nevertheless, the Russian-born Kleitman went on to blaze the trail for modern sleep research by subjecting himself to further weird and wonderful experiments, including keeping himself awake for 180 consecutive hours to study the effects of sleep deprivation, spending two weeks in a submarine, and living north of the Arctic Circle.[43]

Despite his efforts to legitimise sleep science through these adventurous experiments, it wasn't until 1953, when he and one of his students, Eugene Aserinsky, reported the discovery of rapid eye movements during sleep that Kleitman was finally taken seriously by his fellow scientists. By attaching electrodes to Aserinsky's eight-year-old son while he slept, they found that sleep was not a totally passive state during which the brain was switched off like a lamp; rather, the brain remains actively involved with various processes.[44] The finding, which was as significant as the discovery of a new continent in the brain, opened previously unexplored territory to scientific investigation. Kleitman's work inspired a new generation of researchers, and over the last 60 years the mysteries of sleep's purpose have begun to reveal themselves.

We now know, for example, that the brain controls two distinct types of sleep: Slow-wave sleep (SWS), known as deep sleep, and Rapid Eye Movement sleep (REM), also called dreaming sleep. Most of the sleeping we do is of the slow-wave variety and it is characterised by large, slow brain waves, relaxed muscles, and slow, deep breathing. Slow-wave sleep is considered restorative because it helps your mind and body recuperate after a long day.[45] Rapid Eye Movement sleep is not well-understood, but is considered so important that some researchers describe it as a third state of consciousness.[46] To an observer, REM is utterly bizarre. A dreamer's brain becomes highly active while at the same time the muscles are partially paralysed; breathing and heart rate can become erratic. In a typical night, a person will alternate between REM and SWS four to six times, with each cycle lasting 90 to 110 minutes.[47]

Mental Spring Cleaning

Although there is a growing understanding of the biochemistry and the neurobiology of sleep, its exact function and purpose remains a mystery.

One breakthrough study was led by neuroscientist Maiken Nedergaard at the University of Rochester in 2013.[48] By studying the waking and sleeping brains of mice, she discovered that during sleep the brain activates what might be thought of as a waste disposal system, clearing out harmful proteins that build up between brain cells. "You can think of it like having a house party. You can either entertain the guests or clean up the house, but you can't really do both at the same time," Nedergaard told BBC News when her research was first published.[49]

Like the lymphatic system, which clears waste from our bodies, the brain's glymphatic system clears waste such as beta-amyloid (a protein associated with Alzheimer's disease) from our brains.[50] When our brains don't have enough time to rest properly, toxins build up, increasing the risk of neurodegenerative disease. Given that sleep disruption has been closely associated with diseases like Alzheimer's disease and dementia,[51] it may well be that too many of us have been doing too much entertaining and not enough cleaning up afterwards.

Sleep Interrupted

Of course, *knowing* that we should be getting more sleep, and actually *getting* more sleep, are two completely different things. There are many reasons you might not be sleeping enough. It might be that you're too hot or too cold, or that you have an uncomfortable bed. It might be that you're sleeping next to a partner who snores or fidgets and keeps you awake. Maybe it's your noisy neighbours or your young kids who need you during the night or wake you early in the morning. Maybe you're over-stimulated after watching a TV show or playing computer games, or perhaps you're being affected by eating too much or too late, or drinking caffeine or alcohol. Maybe it's worry about work, family, or money. Or it might be that you're suffering from chronic pain, or a sleep disorder such as sleep apnea or Restless Legs Syndrome. It may be any combination of things.

Estimates are that about one third of us will suffer from sleeplessness at some point in our lives.[52] In fact, insomnia is not only the most prevalent sleep disorder, it is also the second-most prevalent mental disorder after anxiety and ahead of depression.[53] And increasingly, insomnia is becoming paired with other chronic conditions such as anxiety, depression, fibromyalgia, diabetes, epilepsy, and Parkinson's disease.[54]

When you have difficulties falling asleep or maintaining sleep, or if you wake up too early for at least a month, your insomnia is considered chronic. If you're like up to one in five people around the world who suffer from this horrendous sleep disorder,[55] you'll know that this also comes with daytime consequences such as fatigue, attention deficits, and mood instability.[56]

I used to be one of them. I would lie in bed awake worrying over things that had happened in my past or might happen in the future. I'd stress about my To Do list and fret about deadlines. I'd worry about other people's problems and the problems of the world in general. My overactive mind and heightened emotions would cause all these worries to circle around in my head until I could not rest. The more I told myself I should be sleeping, the harder it became to actually sleep. Sometimes I found myself lying in bed listening to the morning chorus of birds, having not slept a wink all night. The effects of my sleeplessness on my mood and productivity the next day were shattering. I had trouble concentrating. I was super sensitive, stressed, and generally ineffective. I had no doubt that my sleeplessness also contributed to my poor health, and I knew that to overcome my sleep problems, I needed to know where I was going wrong.

We know that sleep is governed by two internal body systems processes – homeostatic sleep drive and the circadian biological clock.[57] Your sleep drive is essentially your need to sleep. Provided you're well-rested, when you wake up in the morning, your sleep drive will be low. But as a consequence of the accumulation during the day of a neurotransmitter in your brain called adenosine, your need to sleep will steadily increase. This chemical is not produced while you're asleep, so the longer you sleep the lower your levels of adenosine and the more refreshed you feel in the morning.[58] Interestingly, caffeine can fool your brain into thinking there are low levels of adenosine, which is why it can help pick you up after a rough night.[59]

The second governor of sleep is your internal circadian biological clock which, aside from regulating functions such as hunger, hormone production, and body temperature, is also critical in sleep. Most central to sleep is your 24-hour cycle of alertness. Throughout the 24-hour day, your body goes through an alternating cycle of sleepy and alert periods. That familiar 3pm slump is actually part of this natural cycle.

Your body's production of the hormone melatonin, the master of your biological clock, is critical to your ability to sleep. Melatonin is sometimes called the "vampire hormone" because it sleeps during the day and rises at night. About an hour after melatonin levels start to rise, your alertness will start to decline and you will begin to feel sleepy.[60] Artificial blue light – such as the light emitted by our computers and mobile devices – is a major disruption of melatonin production. There's more information on this later in this chapter.

If you are like most average, healthy, well-slept adults, these two biological sleep rhythms – your sleep drive and the 24 hour cycle of alertness – will work in harmony to allow you to fall asleep at a regular time, to sustain a solid period of quality sleep, and to feel rested and alert when you wake. Unfortunately, in the modern world that never sleeps, we've abandoned 200,000 years of evolution. Thanks to long work hours, commuting, shift work, artificial light, artificial stimulants, television, and smart devices, our natural sleep rhythms have been thrown into confusion.

5 Common Sleep Disruptors

CAFFEINE

A 2016 review found that overall caffeine typically prolongs sleep latency (the time it takes to fall asleep), reduces total sleep time and sleep efficiency, and worsens perceived sleep quality.[61] The stimulant effects of caffeine work by blocking an important sleep chemical called adenosine, which builds up in our body all day long.[62] From the moment we wake up, the adenosine levels in our brains accumulate until we eventually succumb to sleep. This chemical is not produced while we are asleep, so the longer we sleep, the lower the levels of adenosine and the more refreshed we feel in the morning. Caffeine fools the brain into thinking there are low levels of this sleep chemical. But if we're still under the influence of caffeine when we go to bed, we may have trouble initiating sleep. Over time we can build up a caffeine tolerance[63] and although we all metabolize caffeine differently,[64] this changes as we age.[65] One study showed that caffeine consumed even six hours before bedtime could significantly disrupt sleep[66] and another study showed that the equivalent of two cups of coffee at 7:10am in the morning could disrupt sleep efficiency and duration at night.[67]

LIGHT

The light around you influences hormone secretion, heart rate, alertness, sleep propensity, body temperature, and gene expression.[68] It's particularly interesting that the production of the sleep hormone melatonin is highly sensitive to light.[69] Melatonin production is inhibited as soon as your eyes detect light, making you feel more alert and awake. When you turn out the lights, the subsequent release of melatonin makes you feel drowsy. Research shows that artificial blue light can mimic the effects of the natural blue light of daytime and can thus suppress the production of melatonin. Researchers also found that practising meditation produces high levels of melatonin, which may be why meditation is helpful for people with insomnia.[70]

ALCOHOL

Alcohol is used by more than 1 in 10 people to self-medicate sleep problems.[71] While having a drink or two can have an initial sedative effect, there is a catch – when you fall asleep after consuming alcohol, what follows is a period of fragmented and disturbed sleep, as well as early morning awakenings.[72] Researchers call this the "rebound effect."[73] Often the headache and dry mouth associated with excessive drinking is enough to deter people from overdoing it, but a small 2010 study found that even having just one glass of wine each night could disrupt participants' sleep cycles.[74]

ANXIETY

Nearly 50 percent of people who struggle to have a good night's sleep also have anxiety.[75] When you're stressed and anxious, you produce hormones like cortisol, adrenaline, and noradrenaline that tell your body to prepare to fight or flee. As we learned in Chapter 1 (Stress), it makes no difference if our worries are real or imagined; any kind of worry can trigger this response. Unfortunately these stress hormones are designed to put us on high alert, so they also interfere with your melatonin production and mess up your circadian rhythm.[76] After all, if your life is on the line, the last thing you should be doing is sleeping. If you suspect that anxiety is keeping you awake at night, please see a professional as soon as possible.

NICOTINE

If you're a smoker, nicotine probably makes you feel good. You may even have a "calming" cigarette before bed because it makes you relaxed and happy. Unfortunately for you, cigarette smoking has been widely recognised as a behaviour that interferes with sleep[77] and the more you smoke, the more it affects your sleep. If you're a smoker, you're more likely to have difficulty falling asleep; and when you do sleep, your sleep is more likely to be fragmented and of poorer quality.[78] Because you haven't slept well, you're also more likely to be sleepy the following day.[79] This is because nicotine is a stimulant that causes an increase in adrenaline and boosts your heart rate, blood pressure, and breathing rate.[80] Nicotine also stimulates your brain by causing it to produce a chemical called acetylcholine.[81] Smokers frequently report having trouble getting to sleep and staying asleep, as well as feeling sleepy during the day.[82] While quitting smoking will come with a period of withdrawal, during which you might have even more trouble sleeping, these effects will eventually pass.[83]

Social Jet Lag

In 2006, an international collaboration of people formed a new society that called for "an uprising against the tyranny of early rising."[84] The B-Society, as they called themselves, represents the interests of the "B people," or late risers, who perform at their best later in the day and prefer to go to bed later at night. The organisation, which now has more than 10,000 members from 50 different countries, advocates "making a flexible society, which can accommodate different types of families, ways of working, and circadian rhythms."[85]

In a lengthy e-mail exchange, B-Society's founder Camilla Kring wrote from her home city of Copenhagen and explained that the organisation's advocacy efforts are to represent those who are burdened with the disadvantage of living in a time zone not their own. "We need to break free from an eight-to-five society and its lack of respect for B-people's circadian rhythms. Quality of life, health, infrastructure, and productivity would all improve if we offered people work hours matching their circadian rhythms. In a knowledge-based society, getting up early in the morning is no longer what is important. Instead it is about working when you are most productive," she wrote.

Radical as this may seem, Kring's arguments are based on the latest sleep science, particularly research conducted by German scientist Till Roenneberg at Ludwig-Maximilian University in Munich, a leader in the field of chronobiology (the study of our biological rhythms). Roenneberg's research, which draws on data collected from more than 55,000 people, demonstrates that even though we all sleep and wake according to a cycle of roughly 24 hours, each of us has a different *chronotype*, or timing of our biological clock. You may be a "lark" who likes to go to bed early and get up early, you may be an "owl" who struggles to get out of bed in the morning, or you may be like the majority of people and perch somewhere in the middle.[86]

Where you sit on the lark-to-owl scale depends on a number of things, including when the sun rises and sets in your day, your age, gender, and your genetics.[87] It's estimated that about 50 percent of your natural sleep preferences are determined by genetics, which is why whole families can tend toward one preferred sleep pattern or another. But this internal clock is not fixed throughout your lifespan.[88] For example, as you age, the tendency to prefer waking earlier increases, which is why older people tend to go to bed earlier and wake earlier.[89] On the other hand, teenagers tend to be night owls whose ideal circadian rhythm has them going to bed in the wee hours and waking up late in the morning.

With a growing body of research illuminating the link between poor sleep and poor health, researchers like Roenneberg are starting to investigate the importance of understanding a person's chronotype and identifying the times of day during which they function best. It's been found, for example, that many teenagers are forced to operate on a social clock that is counterproductive to their natural rhythms, and are suffering severe negative health effects as a consequence.[90] Night owls are more prone to depression[91] and more inclined toward substance abuse,[92] possibly because they rely on uppers and downers (such as caffeine and alcohol) to help them cope with a biological clock that is out of synch with society's clock. When researchers scanned the brains of night owls in 2013, they found they had diminished white matter, a type of tissue that facilitates communication among nerve cells.[93] Being a night owl is also linked to an increased risk of developing type 2 diabetes.[94] Roenneberg also demonstrated that "living against the clock" may be a contributing factor to the growing epidemic of obesity.[95]

Given that only an estimated 10 percent of the global population are morning larks, and roughly 20 percent are night owls, Roenneberg believes that many of us are suffering from the effects of accumulated sleep debt resulting from chronic sleep deprivation or a kind of "social jet lag."[96] I was delighted when, despite that he was taking some well-earned time off on his farm just outside of Munich, Roennenberg agreed to have a chat with me over Skype. "Let's use an example. We all know that if we work in a factory and the owner of the factory provides us all with just one shoe size, most people would be rather unhappy. They would either have too much room in the shoe or get blisters because the shoe is too small. That is what's happening today – people ask us to come to work at a certain time because they don't recognise there are individual differences in shoe size. It's as simple as that. If we can make society understand the importance of sleeping the right amount at the right time for each individual, then nobody would have to wear too small a shoe and we would do much better."

The message about the importance of paying attention to our natural sleep rhythm is starting to get through to some movers and shakers who are taking on board the research findings. By 2014, approximately 1,000 schools in the US had successfully implemented a delay in start times, and that list has grown steadily longer; the result has been wide ranging physical and mental health benefits, as well as improvements in academic achievement.[97]

Despite these tentative steps toward changing social structures, the research on chronotype is still very new and it's not likely we'll see sweeping society-wide changes anytime soon. Kring from the B-Society wrote passionately to me about the challenges her organisation faces in changing the system. I could imagine the twinkle in her eye when she wrote, "I know it will be a long journey. Maybe it will B a fight for a lifetime."

What I take away from this is that it is up to me to manage my social and biological clock. I've determined that I'm an owlish person. In an ideal world, I'd hit the hay at about midnight and rise at 8:00am or 9:00am. I find my stride in the late afternoon and early evening, which is when I'm at peak creativity, productivity, and alertness. Unfortunately, with the demands of my home life and work schedule, this is not a practical schedule to keep. The result is that I'm often challenged to get enough sleep. But there is good news if you're like me and don't have the luxury of manipulating the world to suit your chronotype. Roenneberg explained there are certain things you can do to adjust your schedule and at least make it a bit easier to, for example, get up earlier or stay up later. While your internal clock does play a major role in determining your sleep time preferences, so too does the amount of light you're exposed to during the day.[98] By being more strategic about light exposure, you can tweak your internal clock. "I'm very lucky to have good sleep," he said. "I also try to be on my farm as much as possible, which lets me be outside during the day. I can tell you whenever I'm here, I fall asleep very early and I wake up by myself very early, so it's quite remarkable how this easy change of light exposure will change our sleep habits."

I've implemented a number of strategies. Most important, we have almost no blue light in our house after sundown. The bulbs in our lamps at home have an orange filter. (This is explained further in the Digital Detox section below.) On the occasions when I watch television, I aim to switch it off an hour before I intend to sleep, but generally I use my evening hours to practice some yoga, do my household chores while I listen to an audio book, read, or take a long bath. If I'm working on my computer in the evening, I wear rather daggy-looking orange tinted glasses that filter out blue light. The results of these changes have been dramatic. I usually feel sleepy much earlier than I used to and fall asleep much more quickly. I'm in bed by 10pm at the latest most nights, with lights out at around 10:30pm. I find it remarkable that these simple steps can make such a big difference.

A Nightly Digital Detox

We live in a world that never sleeps. Smart phones. Smart tablets. Smart televisions. An Internet that operates 24 hours a day. With the push of a button, at any time, we are instantly in contact with friends, family, and total strangers all over the world, or fully immersed in the latest updates from the office. When everything and everyone is always switched on, it can be hard to switch off.

But it's not just the hyper connection of modern living that we need to be mindful of. Researchers are increasingly concerned about the effect that artificial blue light at night has on sleep.[99] Photoreceptors in your eyes connect directly to the areas of your brain that regulate the production of melatonin, the sleep hormone. In 2001, it was discovered that exposing the eyes to light in the blue end of the visible spectrum suppresses the production of melatonin.[100] Essentially, when you use a device that emits blue light (computers, televisions, phones, tablets etc.) during the evening or night, your brain thinks it is daytime, and your natural rhythm, which evolved over thousands of years, is thrown off course.[101]

One study led by Charles Czeisler, a professor of sleep medicine at Harvard Medical School, found that people who read electronic books before they went to bed took longer to get to sleep, had reduced levels of melatonin, and were less alert in the morning.[102] Another study from researchers in Berlin showed that exposing healthy subjects to 30 minutes of blue light an hour before bedtime delayed the onset of REM sleep by 30 minutes.[103]

There are some fairly simple strategies you can use to reduce your exposure to blue light before bed. The most obvious is to avoid using devices that emit blue light, starting after sundown. But there's another solution that may not require you to forego all your modern evening entertainment luxuries. A number of recent small studies tested whether giving people orange-tinted glasses, which block blue light, helped their sleeping difficulties. The results are promising; significant improvement was observed in both sleep quality and mood.[104] Participants weren't too put out by having to wear their orange glasses around the house, either.

Based on this encouraging research, one of the solutions to our chronic sleep difficulties may well be simple and cost-effective. The orange glasses I bought on eBay cost about US$3.00. I wear them at night if I'm working on my computer or tablet. We've also replaced the bulbs in our lamps at home with orange or red ones from our local hardware store.

Some researchers are calling for mandatory filters to be standard on devices that emit blue light.[105] But in the meantime, the tech world is also starting to catch on. Software such as F.lux adjusts a computer display's colour according to its location and time of day. Newer devices often have a setting that allows you to adjust the colour of the screen. There are also a host of smart lamps coming onto the market, so it won't be long before you'll be able to customise your home to suit your natural biological rhythm.

For Vanity's Sake

It turned out that the enforced two-day break during the Boston snowstorm gave my film crew and me the opportunity to fill our empty tanks and restore the stamina we needed for rest of the US shoot. In the end I was able to reschedule all but one of the interviews I'd lined up, and even then, I discovered there was another researcher I could interview on the same topic back home in Sydney. As the storm cleared, the city of Boston and its surrounds was blanketed in a picturesque layer of fluffy white snow. In fact, I could not have designed a more charming back drop to depict the story of Ann Salerno, a leading children's kidney doctor who used a mind-body approach to overcome her infertility. The images we shot with her and her young family playing in the snow were some of the best in the film.

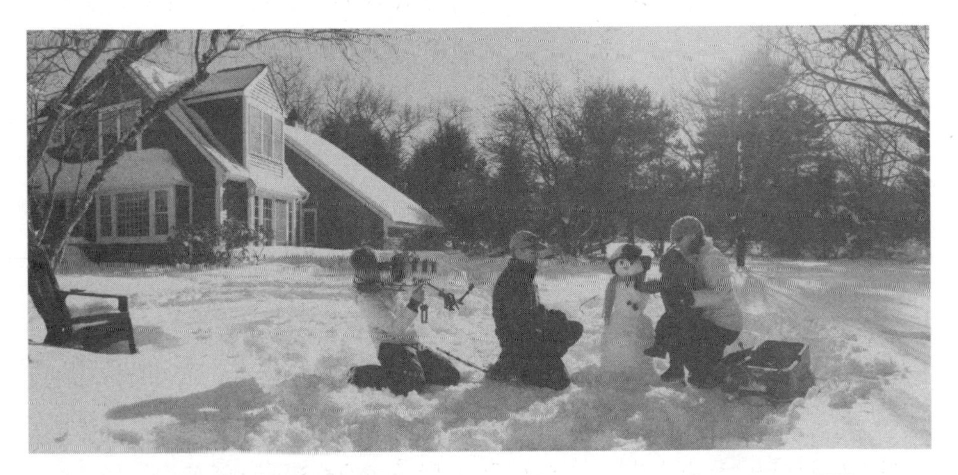

Filming in the snow with Ann Salerno during production of *The Connection* documentary, 2013.

These days, I'm happy to report that the changes I've made in my life in order to get more sleep have made a world of difference. My chronic insomnia is a thing of the past. The mindfulness and meditation I practice have had a particular effect in this area. If I meditate before bed, I fall asleep straight away. It's interesting that preliminary research suggests that Jon

Kabat-Zinn's Mindfulness-Based Stress Reduction may be as effective as pharmacological drugs in helping people recover from insomnia.[106]

Don't get me wrong. I'm far from perfect, there are plenty of nights when I either don't get enough sleep because of circumstances beyond my control, or I choose to stay up late because the benefits are worth the consequences the following day, but these instances are the exception and not the rule. Overall, I rate my sleep as excellent, and I'm sure this has been a major contributing factor in my good health.

These days when I chat with friends, colleagues, and family members, I am continually struck by how many of them seem totally exhausted. Whether it's because they are the parents of young kids, have been partying too much, are hard at work climbing the career ladder, or have just taken on too much, there is a pervasive sense of heaviness and fatigue among them. It's as if there is a society-wide agreement that the first thing we should sacrifice in an effort to keep up with the pace of modern life is our sleep.

When I look at the swollen and red eyes, dark shadows, and pale skin of the chronically sleep-deprived people in my life, I often wonder what it would take to convince them of the importance of sleep. For that reason, I end this chapter on this final note: if not for your metabolism, if not for your brain health, if not for your mental and physical health, and if not to increase your effectiveness and productivity, then I urge you to get more sleep simply for the sake of your vanity.

In 2015, a group of 30 British women agreed to be photographed and to have their skin examined, first after having had a night of eight hours of sleep, and then after having had only six hours of sleep for the next five nights. English fashion model Jodie Kidd was among them. Researchers counted the number of wrinkles, enlarged pores, brown spots, and red areas, and found that the women who had less sleep had up to double the number of fine lines and wrinkles and up to three-quarters more brown spots in the form of dark circles under their eyes.[107] While the experiment was not published in a peer-reviewed academic journal and was done to promote a bed manufacturer, Swedish research has also demonstrated that chronic sleep deprivation makes you appear less attractive because of drooping eyelids, reddened and swollen eyes, darker circles under the eyes, paler skin, more wrinkles and fine lines, and droopier corners of the mouth.[108] Considering that the Jodie Kidd study documented the appearance changes after just five nights of poor sleep, imagine the effects of sleep deprivation over a lifetime. Research like this certainly provides a new take on the idea of "beauty sleep."

Key Takeaways

1 Despite what some of the world's most influential people would have you believe, getting enough sleep is a vital human need. Sleep deprivation doesn't just potentially shorten your life by increasing your risk of disease and putting your mental health in jeopardy, it also makes you a danger to yourself and to those around you. And it's not just about good health, it's also about performing and looking your best.

2 Depending on your age and gender, most adults need somewhere between seven to nine hours of sleep every night. You'll require more than usual if you need to catch up on lost sleep or are going through a physically or mentally demanding time. See the following Getting Started section for a simple way to work out how much sleep you need.

3 Some of the known disruptors of sleep include caffeine, not enough light exposure during the daytime, too much blue light after sundown, anxiety, alcohol and nicotine.

4 You may be suffering from "social jet lag" if you are forced to operate on a social clock that is counterproductive to your natural rhythms. Once you know where you perch on the owl-lark scale you can manage your social and biological clock. See the following Getting Started section for the link to a questionnaire that can help you determine whether you're an owl, a lark, or somewhere in between.

Getting Started

TRACK your sleep by keeping a diary for a week and take note of when you go to bed, how soon you fall asleep, how many hours you sleep, and anything that may be disturbing your sleep. A template to get you started is available for download from my website. See the following Extra Resources page for details.

WORK out how much sleep you need. This month, schedule a week that you can dedicate to sleeping. Go to sleep when you're tired and get up in the morning when you feel refreshed, without an alarm. Limit your caffeine and alcohol consumption as well as your exposure to blue light after sunset. During the day, get out into the sunlight and exercise. After a week or so you should have paid off any accumulated sleep debt and you'll start finding your natural rhythm. Please note that if you do all this and you're still experiencing trouble sleeping, it might be time to talk to a doctor or experts at a sleep clinic.

WORK out if you're a night owl or morning lark. Sleep researcher Till Ronneberg has made the questionnaire that he uses in his studies available for the public online. Search for the Chronotype Study from the Worldwide Experimental Platform - www.thewep.org./chronotype-study

SET the screen on your blue-light emitting electronic devices to turn orange after sunset. Newer devices have this in the settings or you can download software such as F.lux.

PLACE lamps around your home with orange or red globes that you can use after sundown instead of blue-light emitting lights.

My Favourite Sleep Tips

HAVE a comfortable mattress, bed linen, pillow, and payjamas.

MAKE your bedroom completely dark, with as little artificial light as possible (think block-out blinds and no glowing light from electronics).

PRACTICE deep breathing or meditation before bed.

IF you're feeling anxious, write your worries down, and at the end of your writing session note three things you can do about those worries to stop them from going around and around in your head. Don't be afraid to seek professional help if your anxiety is causing chronic insomnia.

TAKE a warm bath before bed (this helps with temperature regulation).

SPRINKLE some lavender on your pillow; its scent has been shown to help with insomnia.[109]

GET as much natural daylight as you can during the day.

REDUCE your exposure to blue light from screens and overhead lights after sundown.

EXERCISE every day, ideally outside.

Extra Resources

AVAILABLE AT
www.thewholehealthlife.com/resources

LISTEN to extended audio interviews with the experts including:

- *Till Roenneberg (Professor of Chronobiology at the Institute of Medical Psychology at Ludwig-Maximilian University in Munich)*

DOWNLOAD the sleep diary template if you'd like to keep track of your sleep for a week.

MY recommended reading list, which I update regularly, is available on my website. Books relevant to this chapter include:

- *Internal Time: Chronotypes, Social Jet Lag, and Why You're So Tired,* by Till Roenneberg
- *The Complete Guide to a Good Night's Sleep,* by Carmel Harrington
- *Night School: The Life-Changing Science of Sleep,* by Richard Wiseman

Chapter 8

Healthcare

A Baby is Born

It was nine at night and I was getting ready to turn in after painting walls all day. Jules and I were trying to finish the shoestring budget renovations we'd been forced into after our house flooded, but my soon-to-be-born baby had other plans. My waters broke. As the labour sensations came on, I focused on my breath, counting beats and relaxing my mind and body. *In – two, three, four, five. Out – two, three, four, five.*

We made our way to the hospital and a dull ache in my lower back began growing stronger. A midwife explained that my baby's spine was pushing against mine in what is called a "posterior position." I tried yoga poses and hot baths, and Jules helped me to keep focusing on breathing. *In – two, three, four, five. Out – two, three, four, five.*

Night fell away, the sun came up, and fatigue set in. I had been awake for 27 hours and could no longer focus on my breath. The baby had not turned and the pain in my back broke through. It was like someone was stabbing me in my spine for 90 second intervals every few minutes. Consuming. Excruciating. Brutal.

A new midwife came in after a change of shift and examined me. The next thing she said was terrifying. "This could take another *six* hours." In that moment a switch flipped. Every part of my mind and body screamed. *Make it stop. Make it stop. Please, make it stop.* I asked for an epidural, a procedure that would block the pain signals being sent to my brain.

The 10-minute wait for the anaesthetist to arrive was torture, but once the epidural began to take effect, I nearly decided to name my unborn child after him. *The wonder of modern medicine.*

The day turned to afternoon; 32 hours had passed since my last restful sleep. But things had to keep moving. It was time to push. After 45 minutes there was no progress and a sense of uncertainty lingered in the room. My doctor, who had been monitoring my pregnancy closely, arrived and took control. He had delivered more than 5,000 babies and his confidence and positivity gave me renewed resolve. He timed his words of encouragement with the waves of contractions, willing me to push the baby out. Jules held my hand. But after another 45 minutes, the uncertainty returned. My body was worn out. My doctor, who knew I was hoping to avoid a cesarean section, took my hand and looked directly at me, focusing my attention on no one but him. "Shannon, you are strong. You are going to have a baby today." I believed him. I summoned the last of my energy and at 4:58 pm, my son was born; an amazing little alien with huge ocean blue eyes and a bewildered expression. He was placed on my chest for our first embrace. I had a vague sense that my entire life would never be the same again. I also intuitively felt that the experience wasn't over and soon discovered why.

At first there was a trickle of blood, then a gush. I was haemorrhaging. Jules took our son, and suddenly three other people were in the room working to stop the bleeding. I was jabbed with a needle and started throwing up convulsively. An oxygen mask was put over my face. An intravenous line was put in my arm. Someone started vigorously massaging my womb, trying to stimulate it to contract and stop the flow of blood. I felt dizzy and out of my body. There was nothing I could do. Then, as though an autopilot had taken over, I defaulted to my training and started counting with my breath. *In – two, three, four, five. Out – two, three, four, five.* Around me, the experts were rapidly responding to my doctor's instructions. I knew they would get things under control. I zeroed my attention in on my new family, a spotlight on them in the corner of the room. There was my baby. There was my husband. Everything would be fine.

It is a testament to the skills of the medical professionals who treated me during my postpartum haemorrhage that I am still around.

In another era, a trauma like mine might have meant I didn't get to see my son, whom we named Theodore, grow from being a little alien into the bouncing beautiful toddler he is today. When I think back to my experience in childbirth and the other experiences I've had in the medical system before and since, I can't help reflecting on the interactions I've had with these experts, how they've made me feel. Whether it was my obstetrician's rallying encouragement, "Shannon, you are strong. You are going to have a baby today," or the midwife's pessimistic prediction, "This could take another six hours," the words they spoke had a profound impact on me.

The importance of these relationships with our healthcare providers cannot be overstated. The patient-provider relationship depends on trust. As patients, we put our health in the hands of these experts, and the experts, in turn, are tasked with making momentous and potentially life-changing recommendations.

In 2013, Dignity Health, one of the five largest health systems in the US conducted a nation-wide survey on the power of human kindness in healthcare. They found that 87 percent of Americans feel that kind treatment by a physician is *more important* than other key considerations in choosing a health care provider, including average wait time before appointments, distance from home, and the cost of care. In fact, 72 percent of Americans would be willing to pay *more* for a physician who emphasised kindness when treating patients.[1] In our efforts to be well, clearly many of us feel getting the care we need is about more than simply seeking expertise and technical competence from our healthcare providers. So, what is it that makes a doctor or other healthcare professional *good*? And how do we go about finding the right people to help us with our health?

The System

In the files of hospitals, clinics, and doctors' offices all around Australia, there are hundreds of forms that have my name and date of birth at the top. If you were to compile all that data with their check boxes and symptom lists, the unfortunate story of a young woman diagnosed with various autoimmune diseases over a number of years would begin to unfold. The plot would involve endless blood tests, urine tests, scans, and examinations. There would be prescriptions for medications, referrals for more tests, second opinions, and endless appointments.

What this information wouldn't reveal is the emotional story of my experience in the healthcare system. It wouldn't reflect my frustration with sitting in waiting rooms for hours on end when doctors ran late. It wouldn't document the indignity of sitting on an examination table in a flimsy gown with an open back. It wouldn't capture the tears that welled in my eyes countless times after an exchange with a doctor who saw me as little more than a set of test results with which to match the appropriate diagnosis and prescription for medication.

Because of the way our healthcare systems are structured, the quality of the patient experience rarely enters the minds of key influencers, planners, and managers. Patients are often treated as parts on an assembly line that need to be kept moving in order to meet bottom lines, time windows, and "key performance indicators." As one cardiologist wrote in the journal *Global Advances in Health and Medicine,* "There is no incentive today for physicians to sit with patients and listen to their stories. Instead, physicians do procedures and prescribe treatments – as quickly as possible to maximise reimbursement. Diagnoses and procedures, not outcomes, drive reimbursement. The payment for inserting a pacemaker or performing an angiogram is much higher than the payment for a preventive cardiology office visit."[2]

A New Way

While I was in the US filming the interviews for *The Connection,* I made a special trip to Arizona to meet Andrew Weil, a professor of medicine and public health from the University of Arizona. As my film crew and I made our way to Weil's home in the stunning burnt-orange desert just outside Tucson, I confess to feeling a tad nervous. This was a man who had twice been on the cover of *TIME* magazine;[3] a publication that in 1997 named him one of the 25 most influential Americans and in 2005 one of the 100 most influential people in the world.[4] His 11 books have sold more than 10 million copies worldwide.[5] Unlike all the other experts I'd spoken to, it wasn't that Weil was a researcher on the cutting edge of health science that drew me to the desert, it was that Weil was leading a new movement of healthcare professionals who want to find a better way of doing things.

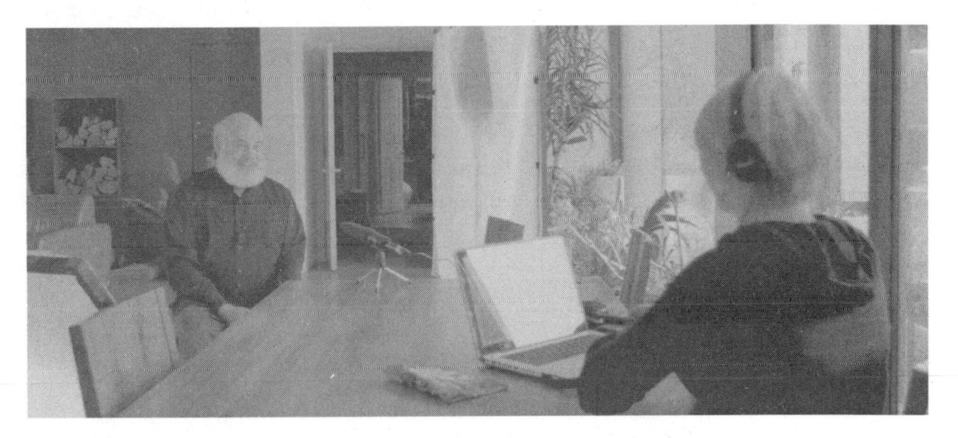

Dr. Andrew Weil being interviewed by Shannon Harvey during the production of *The Connection* documentary, 2013.

Weil, who is considered a pioneer of "integrative medicine," founded the Arizona Center for Integrative Medicine at the University of Arizona, which aims to transform healthcare "by training a new generation of health professionals and by empowering individuals and communities to optimise health and wellbeing through evidence-based, sustainable, integrative approaches."[6] The Center has now graduated more than 1500 fellows from 15 different countries. "One day we'll be able to drop the word *integrative*, this will just be good medicine," he told me, explaining that the central premise he's trying to get medical professionals to understand is that we need to take a whole-person approach to healthcare. "That means that you have to look at patients as not just physical bodies. They're also mental, emotional beings, spiritual entities, community members; and those other dimensions of human life are highly relevant to understanding health and illness. And you ignore them at your peril, as both a practitioner and a patient," he said.

With his robust publishing empire, commercial line of vitamins, minerals, and supplement formulas, as well as a chain of restaurants, Weil has his critics. Indeed, when I got home and went to my local department store I found Weil's face staring at me from the label of a line of cosmetics that promised: "Whether you need to sleep well, reduce your skin's stress or boost your natural defenses against the changes of time, Dr. Andrew Weil for Origins™ will help improve your body, mind and spirit."[7] He's also been subject to criticism for promoting yet-to-be-proven regimens over evidence-based medical practices.

That said, we are living in the age of illness, and the system is broken. Something has to change, and the validity of Weil's key message cannot be dismissed. "Integrative medicine is a system that focuses on the innate healing potential of the human organism and regards patients as whole persons, not just physical bodies; that emphasises the patient-practitioner relationship as central to the healing process, pays attention to all aspects of lifestyle, and is willing to use all available therapies as long as they show reasonable evidence for efficacy and aren't going to cause harm," he said.

The second part of Weil's argument - that good medicine should focus on all aspects of lifestyle - was one I felt I had already started to grasp in my own recovery journey. I was convinced of the importance of stress reduction, emotional balance, a healthy diet, regular exercise, better sleep, and changing the environment around me so that it was optimised for healthy living. These were all things I could be doing for myself in order to take charge of my chronic illness.

But what of his first and final points, that the patient-practitioner relationship is central to the healing process? And that *all* available therapies can be considered as long as they cause no harm? I knew that many of the interactions I'd had at clinics, doctors' offices, and hospitals hadn't been particularly uplifting. Were the frustrations I'd experienced as a patient in the medical system affecting the outcome of my treatments? I'd also had such mixed experiences with alternative and complementary therapies that I was left feeling unsure about whom to trust and where to turn.

The Doctor is the Medicine

Ted Kaptchuk's background is not typical of someone who holds the title of Professor of Medicine and Professor of Global Health and Social Medicine at Harvard Medical School. While many of his colleagues were peering through microscopes in windowless laboratories before achieving prestige at the esteemed university, Kaptchuk was a few miles down the road operating an acupuncture clinic alongside fellow "healers" on a street commonly referred to as Quack Row.[0] He'd opened the clinic in 1976 after studying Traditional Chinese Medicine (TCM) in Asia for four years. For decades, Kaptchuk saw patients who turned to him to treat everything from bronchitis to arthritis. In that time he witnessed the dramatic positive effects of his treatments. In 1994, Kaptchuk wrote a seminal textbook about TCM called *The Web That Has No Weaver: Understanding Chinese Medicine* which today still sits on the book shelves of acupuncture practitioners and TCM students around the world.[9]

Despite his fame among complementary therapy enthusiasts, there was something bothering Kaptchuk about his work. He told *Harvard Magazine* that patients who came to him got better, but sometimes their relief began even before he'd started the acupuncture treatments. He didn't doubt the value of the therapy, but he suspected there was something else about the care he gave his patients that helped encourage their health improvements.[10] Kaptchuk eventually went to Harvard wanting to solve that mystery, and became one of the most prolific placebo researchers in the world. In 2011, Beth Israel Deaconess Medical Center invited him to create the Harvard-wide program called Placebo Studies and the Therapeutic Encounter.[11]

One of Kaptchuk's breakthrough studies was published in 2008, when he demonstrated that the care and concern shown for patients during treatment can have a significant impact on their recovery. The study recruited 262 people suffering from irritable bowel syndrome, a chronic, gastrointestinal disorder that causes frequent abdominal pain and diarrhoea or constipation. He divided the volunteers into three groups, the first receiving no treatment and the second two groups each receiving fake acupuncture involving the use of trick needles. People in one of the sham acupuncture groups were treated by practitioners who purposely adopted a warm, friendly manner and expressed empathy by saying things like, "I can understand how difficult IBS must be for you." They communicated an air of confidence and positive expectation and at times spent 20 seconds in thoughtful silence while feeling their patient's pulse or pondering the treatment plan. The other fake acupuncture group received little attention from their therapists, who merely introduced themselves and stated they had reviewed the patient's questionnaire and knew what to do. After six weeks, the patients in the group who received the most personal care were the ones who reported experiencing the greatest symptom relief as well as the greatest improvements in disease severity and quality of life.[12]

The study was a step toward explaining in Western scientific terms one of the reasons so many people report feeling better after having acupuncture. It hinted that something about the connection between a suffering patient who expresses discomfort and an empathetic health expert may in and of itself trigger a therapeutic response, independent of the actual treatment being administered. In other words, the doctor can be the medicine.

When a patient sees their doctor, nurse, or other health professional, a special and unique interaction takes place. This connection is at the very heart of the latest research on the doctor-patient relationship.[13] Through their words, attitudes, and behaviours, healthcare providers can communicate critical information that can have a profound impact on their patient's health – for better or for worse.[14] For example, one study of patients with hypertension found a correlation between empathetic nurses and improved symptoms and quality of life.[15] Another study demonstrated that doctors are far more effective at treating various symptoms such as cough, sore throat, tiredness, abdominal pain, and muscular pain if consultations are conducted in a positive rather than a negative manner.[16] In fact, a review of research studies about the effectiveness of empathy in general medical practice found it is of "unquestionable importance."[17]

This research was taken to another level in 2010 when Kaptchuk demonstrated that the patient-provider interaction could be effective even when the patient *knew* the treatment was fake. Patients with irritable bowel syndrome reported their symptoms improved after a caring and considerate doctor or nurse explained that placebos could be effective and powerful, then instructed them to take pills from a bottle clearly labeled "Placebo. Take 2 pills twice daily."[18]

The "Knowing Effect"

The power of patient-provider interactions becomes even more important when we consider research demonstrating that the effects of a variety of real treatments are significantly reduced and sometimes eliminated completely if patients don't know they are receiving them. Fabrizio Benedetti, the neuroscientist we met in Chapter 3 (Belief), studied this "knowing effect" extensively. In one experiment he studied 42 patients who had undergone thoracic surgery. This is one of the most difficult surgical procedures to handle because it is extremely painful for the patient post-operatively. Their chests are cut open so the surgeon can gain access to their heart, lungs, or throat, and when their anaesthesia wears off, the simple act of breathing can be extremely painful. In Benedetti's study, 21 patients were given morphine by a doctor who explained their pain would subside within a few minutes. The remaining 21 patients received morphine secretly via a pre-programmed machine, without a doctor or nurse in the room. Both groups were given the same amount of the powerful opiate, but those who knew they had received it reported significantly less pain than those who didn't know.[19]

These are not one-off findings either. One study demonstrated that the effects of drugs that cause the airways of asthmatics to either widen or contract were enhanced when patients were told they'd received the drug.[20] Benedetti also showed that when patients with high anxiety levels were *not* told they had been given the tranquillising drug diazepam, the drug was totally ineffective.[21] "We studied morphine, we studied buprenorphine, we studied tramadol, we studied metamizole. All these painkillers were less effective if they were given with a hidden injection," the Italian scientist told me during our chat over Skype.

Incredibly, studies show that even dental surgery patients who were injected with a saline solution, but told they were being given pain medication, received the same pain relief as patients who were secretly injected with six to eight milligrams of morphine. Only when the hidden morphine dose was increased to 12 milligrams was the pain-relieving effect stronger than with the placebo.[22] "This is quite interesting because it shows that treatments have two components – pharmacological components and psychological components. If you eliminate the psychological components, you can bet that the total effect of the treatment would be much smaller," Benedetti said.

This research highlights that being fully informed and understanding what treatments we receive and why we receive them is a critical component in any therapy. How we respond is dependent not only on the actual treatment, but also the responses triggered in us by the interactions we have with our providers. This understanding gives strength to Andrew Weil's argument that the patient-practitioner relationship is central to good medicine. "Whenever you give a treatment and there is a positive response, it's impossible to know how much of that response is due to the direct effect of the treatment and how much is an indirect effect that's mediated by the mind," Weil said. "There's no way you can ever draw a line and say 'On this side are the intrinsic effects of treatment, and on this side are the mind-mediated effects.'" Weil believes that it's not only impossible to separate these effects, but foolish to do so because the central tenet of good medicine is to trigger the body's own healing mechanisms. "To me, the placebo response is the meat of medicine, that's what you're trying to make happen," he said.

When Words Hurt

In 1934, Walter Cannon, the famous Harvard physiologist who first identified the fight or flight response, received an intriguing letter from Australian pathologist John Cleland who had a keen interest in the diseases of indigenous Australians. Cleland described his experience with a tribesman in central Australia who had been injured in the fleshy part of his thigh by a spear he believed was enchanted. The fine and robust man slowly pined away and died, though the wound had not caused any complication that Cleland could detect.[23] Cleland sent this story in response to Cannon's request to physicians and anthropologists around the world for authentic accounts just like the one Cleland had witnessed. Cannon hoped to use the anecdotes to formulate a theory about the physiological explanation for sudden, unexplained death resulting from a voodoo curse. His paper on the subject, published in 1942,[24] was the foundation for many subsequent studies as scientists grappled to understand what is now called the "nocebo effect."[25] You will recall from Chapter 3 (Belief), that the nocebo effect is when you have a negative response to a harmless substance you believe is harmful, as happened to the young man who collapsed after "overdosing" on sugar pills.

Through the work of Dimos Mitsikostas, the head of the neurology department at Athens Naval Hospital in Greece, we start to see that Walter Cannon may have been onto something when he hypothesised that the fear of death could trigger a physiological response that could go as far as precipitating death itself.[26] Mitsikostas, who has extensively reviewed decades of nocebo research, concluded that negative suggestion causes people to experience negative symptoms in treatments for everything from headache, to multiple sclerosis, fibromyalgia, Parkinson's disease and depression.[27] In trials for Parkinson's disease, as many as 65 percent of people given a placebo report negative side effects as a result of their treatment.[28] Mitsikostas's reviews have estimated that anywhere from 4 percent to 26 percent of patients who receive placebos in trials discontinue their use because they *think* they are experiencing adverse effects.[29]

When I think back to the interactions I had 11 years ago with the specialist doctor who first told me he suspected I had lupus, I distinctly remember his prognosis. He explained I had a very serious condition, and if the disease progressed my immune system might start attacking my organs or I could end up in a wheelchair. Given that much of the nocebo research has only taken place in the last few years, it's unlikely the specialist realised the potential negative impact of his words and the downward spiral they would trigger.

When I mentioned my experience to Weil, he said I was not alone in being what he called "medically hexed." "Many patients have been told by doctors in one way or another that they're not going to get better," he said. "Often doctors haven't meant to do that, and may even be unconscious of what they've said, but I think this is an area that needs correction, that doctors need to be aware of how powerful their words are and to use them to promote healing rather than hinder it."

There is now clear evidence that the words and actions of our healthcare providers can be deeply powerful. While I'm not for one moment suggesting that we should not be well-informed about our medical conditions and the potential side effects of treatments, as a journalist I know all too well that information can easily be spun one way or another depending on how it is presented. I wonder what path I might have taken had my doctor explained that having an autoimmune disease is by no means a terrible diagnosis, and that many people with these sorts of diseases continue to live healthy and fulfilled lives? I wonder how things would have turned out if instead of giving me a prescription for drugs that "may or may not work," he had handed me information on safe and comprehensive lifestyle changes I could do for myself and that have been shown to make a difference for people with lupus?[30] How would I have felt about my diagnosis and my prognosis? Would it still have been a 10-year journey toward recovery?

I don't want this to come across as a wholesale criticism of doctors, nurses, and other healthcare providers because there are some worthy and meaningful efforts to incorporate this new evidence into clinical practice. For example, beginning in 2015, when aspiring doctors in the US take the Medical College Admission Test, they need to prove not only their knowledge of science, but also demonstrate an understanding of the human and social components of health. "Being a good doctor is about more than scientific knowledge. It also requires an understanding of people,"[31] president and CEO of the Association of American Medical Colleges Darrel Kirch said when the new requirement was announced.

There are also a growing number of programs available to help encourage kinder, gentler, more empathetic doctors. A series of online courses for physicians called "Empathetics" has been developed and, so far, rolled out to 2,000 residents (doctors in training) at Massachusetts General Hospital and other Harvard teaching hospitals.[32] The program draws on the emotions research done by Paul Ekman that we explored in Chapter 2 (Emotions), and teaches doctors "how to show up, not what to say," according to Helen Riess, the program's chief scientist and chairman.[33] Evidence suggests the program is working. A 2012 study of medical residents found that those who had taken the empathy course were judged by patients as significantly better at understanding their concerns and making them feel at ease than were the doctors who had not done the training.[34] With further evidence showing that over 80 percent of malpractice claims are correlated to low physician empathy,[35] that patients who experience empathetic care have better medical outcomes[36] and are more likely to follow their doctor's recommendations,[37] and that communicating empathetically increases clinician job satisfaction and reduces burnout,[38] putting the "care" back into "healthcare" makes sense on all sides.

Sense and Sensitivity

In 2013, Daniel Jacobs raised $50,000 on the fundraising website Indiegogo for his app called *Placebo Effect,* which is "designed to help people harness the power of placebos in their own lives by delivering you a virtual placebo."[39] Despite the scepticism of researchers at the forefront of placebo breakthroughs, Jacobs is just one of a growing legion of online entrepreneurs trying to find ways to monetise the new evidence. What I find even more interesting is that these online entrepreneurs are not alone in taking advantage of the power of the patient-provider placebo effect. In fact, it's common practice for doctors to knowingly prescribe medicines they know are not effective in order to meet their patient's expectations of being given a treatment. A UK survey of primary care practitioners found that three out of four doctors use placebos at least once a week.[40] A systematic review of 22 studies from 22 countries found that between 41 percent and 99 percent of physicians and nurses had used placebos.[41] The most frequently prescribed placebos are antibiotics, sedatives, painkillers, and vitamins.[42] Our healthcare providers prescribe them not because they think the treatment itself will have an active effect, but because they want to meet their patients' expectations for an effective treatment.

I have no issue with anyone – be they a doctor, nurse, massage therapist, acupuncturist, or my own mother – who shows compassion, kindness, care, attention, and empathy when I'm feeling sick. At the end of the day, when I consider all that I've experienced in my journey through the medical and alternative health systems, all I'm really after is to be cared for by someone who understands that a conversation is as important as a prescription, that I am more than the sum of my test results, and that my own body's innate healing mechanisms are as important as state-of-the-art procedures. But, as with so much of what you've read in this book, my words come with a caveat. When you read about the body of evidence being accumulated, it's easy to get excited about the potential promise of the patient-provider placebo effect. You might start thinking that if compassionate doctors using saline injections, and caring experimental scientists using fake acupuncture needles can trigger a physiological response, then the same biological mechanisms can be triggered by *any* practitioner of conventional, complementary, or alternative medicine, and therefore, that they can all be considered positive for your health.

I have two major concerns with this line of thinking. First, it assumes that these sometimes-untested treatments will not have any harmful effects. With disturbing regularity herbal products with exotic sounding names have been shown to be contaminated with drugs, toxins, or heavy metals, or have been revealed to lack the listed ingredients.[43] These treatments can interact with prescribed drugs, cause serious side effects, or be unsafe for people with certain medical conditions. It's important to know that in most countries complementary therapies and products (including everything from over-the-counter vitamins, herbs, and oils, to treatments involving energetic healing, reflexology, or kinesiology) are not regulated in the same way that the conventional medical and pharmaceutical industry is.

The global wellness industry is a US$3.4 trillion market, or 3.4 times larger than the worldwide pharmaceutical industry. The market for complementary and alternative medicines is valued at US$187 billion a year.[44] Some of this is generated by huge multinational, multibillion dollar businesses. Some is generated by well-meaning practitioners operating over a local fish and chip shop who are genuinely making a difference in people's lives. When they express empathy, devote their time to us, and encourage us to find meaning in our pain, more often than not, they make us feel better, the importance of which cannot be overstated.

But this leads me to my second concern about exaggerating the potential of the new science of the patient-provider interaction. Researchers note that empathetic care is effective in addressing people's *subjective* feelings or *perceptions* of their illness such as reducing their pain, anxiety, nausea, dizziness, or fatigue. Kaptchuk himself takes great care to draw attention to this in a 2015 piece he wrote for the *New England Journal of Medicine* where he highlighted one of his own studies that found that while placebos can dramatically relieve asthma symptoms, they are no match for real drugs when it comes to objective measurements such as lung function.[45] "Placebos may provide relief, but they rarely cure," he wrote.[46]

These days, when I'm considering *any* treatment, it takes a lot to win my trust. I never make health decisions based on brief news reports where the story has been condensed. I'm wary of generalisations that don't come with references or qualification. I rarely trust second-hand interpretations of research findings unless they are offered by a highly credible expert who has weighed up all the available information. Now when I go to an appointment with a new doctor, physiotherapist, masseuse, or any person who will be treating me and giving me health advice, I ask myself: beyond giving me the best possible diagnosis and treatment, how will this person help trigger my body's natural healing response?

Key Takeaways

1 When it comes to optimal healthcare, people need to be seen as more than just physical bodies, the sum of their test results, or items on a spreadsheet. Good medicine should focus on all aspects of lifestyle as well as the patient-provider relationship, and should integrate with other treatment options that sit outside the conventional system – provided they are safe.

2 How you respond to a treatment is dependent not only on the treatment itself, but also on the responses triggered by the interactions you have with your healthcare providers. Through their words, attitudes, and behaviours, healthcare providers can communicate critical information that can have a profound impact on your health – for better or for worse.

3 Being fully informed and understanding what treatments you are given and why you're given them is a critical component in any therapy.

4 While it's tempting to get excited by the new research on the power of the patient-provider placebo response, it's important to remember that the findings do not mean that any interaction with any healthcare provider can trigger a biological healing response. It is mostly effective in addressing subjective feelings or perceptions of illness such reducing pain, anxiety, nausea, dizziness or fatigue.

Getting Started

When you consider that your health is on the line, the patient-provider relationship is one of the most intimate and important relationships you may ever have. Establishing a trusted relationship and finding the right healthcare team should be a priority.

Here are five steps to consider when you're looking for a new care provider:

TAKE some time to evaluate and write down what your needs are and what you expect from a provider. What blend of experience and personality traits are important to you? I look for four Cs – Credentials and competence, plus communication and compassion.

DO your research. I use a combination of taking recommendations from other providers I respect, word of mouth from friends and family I trust, and of course, Internet research, including reading the practitioner's own website and other people's comments and reviews.

THINK of your first meeting like an interview. Is there mutual respect and understanding? Will the provider treat your care plan as a partnership and include you in the decision making-making process? Are you more than test results on a screen? Will you feel comfortable being open and vulnerable with this person?

REMEMBER that it's a two-way relationship. Think of your provider as being more like a coach, rather than a friend. Ask yourself, are you going to be like an elite athlete and listen to, respect, and comply with your coach in order to get the best performance?

IS this expert available to you? The person you prefer may be the best practitioner in the world, but if he or she can't see you for a month, or can't return calls when you're in the midst of a medication reaction or a flare-up, they're not going to be much help to you. Do they have competent staff who can follow-up for you or send you lost prescriptions, without your having to chase them down? Do they have a waiting room full of other patients and do they run perpetually late? And if they do, is this a problem for you?

Extra Resources

AVAILABLE AT

www.thewholehealthlife.com/resources

ACCESS extended audio and video interviews with the experts including:

- *Andrew Weil (Founder and Director Arizona Center for Integrative Medicine, Professor of Medicine and Public Health, Jones-Lovell Endowed Chair in Integrative Rheumatology, University of Arizona)*
- *Fabrizio Benedetti (Professor of Physiology and Neuroscience at the University of Turin Medical School and at the National Institute of Neuroscience, Turin, Italy)*
- *Damien Finnis (Associate Professor at the University of Sydney Pain Management Research Institute, Royal North Shore Hospital and the School of Rehabilitation Sciences, Griffith University)*

MY recommended reading list, which I update regularly, is available on my website. Books relevant to this chapter include:

- *Placebo Effects: Understanding the mechanisms in health and disease*, by Fabrizio Benedetti
- *Meaning, Medicine and the 'Placebo Effect,'* by Daniel E Moerman
- *Health and Healing*, by Andrew Weil
- *The Patient Will See You Now: The Future of Medicine is in Your Hands*, by Eric Topol

Chapter 9

Relationships

A Little Help from my Friends

Theodore's early arrival caught us off guard. While I convalesced in hospital, Jules enlisted a small troop of friends and family who rallied together to finish off the house repairs. When we came through the front doors for the first time with our newborn, the house had metamorphosed from the sawdust ridden-mess it had been just a few days before. Gone were the work tools and paint buckets, and in their place were bouquets of flowers and handwritten cards from well-wishing friends offering pearls of wisdom for this new phase of our lives.

Being the thorough journalist that I am, I was naturally inclined to read several books written by experts before I became a parent, but a head full of the latest scientifically-validated advice did little to prepare me for the reality of motherhood. Still recovering from the postpartum blood loss, and suffering from the chronic sleep deprivation that comes with caring for a newborn, I needed all the help I could get. When I was in the thick of this hazy chaos, I read an article featuring one of Australia's greatest athletes, Cathy Freeman, who described the first 20 months of motherhood as being harder than winning gold at the Sydney 2000 Olympics.[1] I knew exactly what she meant.

We were only five weeks into our new lives before Jules and I faced our first major work-life balance challenge. A video shoot my company had been commissioned to do had to go ahead on the same day a feature documentary Jules had directed was to premiere at the Sydney Film Festival. The premiere was a major career achievement for Jules, and of course we needed to be there. The video shoot would provide income necessary to pay our bills and keep *The Connection* film in production. There was no choice - we had to do both.

It was going to be a long day. Production would start at 6am and finish at 6pm, with Jules and me directing simultaneous crews and conducting back-to-back interviews throughout the day. By 7pm we'd have to be red carpet ready and at the cinema. All this with a baby who did not yet understand the difference between night and day, and who needed to be breast-fed every few hours. Given what we'd been learning about health and balance, the situation was less than ideal, but it was also unavoidable. There was only one thing we could do to get through it: we called in our support crew.

At 4.30am on the morning of the shoot, Jules's mum, Alice, arrived to be with our peacefully-sleeping newborn. She would bring him to me later in the day when he needed to be fed. Our production crew included some of our closest friends, many of them parents, who knew what we were up against. They handled the location scouting, prop gathering, and gear wrangling in the lead-up to the shoot and didn't blink an eye when I had them clear the room between interviews so I could express breast milk. The shoot took place in a two-bedroom apartment we'd rented that was one block away from the cinema. When the shoot was over, we cleared everyone out and the apartment became home base for our family for the night. We arrived at the cinema with just moments to spare and found the audience brimming with family members and friends who had come to support Jules on his big night. It was an extraordinary day and an even more extraordinary night, made possible only because of the extraordinary people in our lives.

The Loneliness Epidemic

On February 13th 1972, the French scientist Michel Siffre descended into Midnight Cave near Del Rio, Texas for a six-month, NASA-sponsored experiment. Siffre had dedicated his career to studying how the natural rhythms of human life are affected by living "beyond time."[2] With electrodes attached to his head to monitor his brain activity, Siffre isolated himself from natural sunlight and human interaction for 205 days. I came across Siffe's work when I was looking at the research on circadian rhythms for the sleep chapter in this book. Although the experiment did give NASA insights into the challenges that would be faced by long range space travellers, the results of this particular cave experiment actually revealed something far more significant about our need for human connection.

In the harrowing account of his experience he wrote a few years later for *National Geographic Magazine*, Siffre described how on day 77 his memory started to fail and he could not recall anything that occurred the previous day, or even the events of the morning. Just two days later, his sanity started to crack and he reported being "overcome with despair with feelings of overwhelming self-pity." By day 86, he was suicidal and the "long loneliness" was "beyond all bearing." For a while, Siffre found companionship in a mouse he called Mus that occasionally rummaged through his supplies. On day 170, he attempted to use a casserole dish to trap Mus in order to make a pet of him, but accidentally killed him. He wrote, "I stare at him with swelling grief. The whispers die away. He is still. Desolation overwhelms me."[3] Although the old film footage of Siffre emerging from the cave shows a smiling man greeting the awaiting media with no apparent ill effect,[4] Siffre would later report that long after his stay in Midnight Cave he suffered "psychological wounds I do not understand."

Since Siffre's 1972 experiment, scientists have continued to study the effects of isolation on people, and a physiological explanation that can help explain what happened to Siffre during and after his ordeal is starting to emerge.

After just a few days, extreme isolation disrupts sleep cycles, induces anxiety and hallucinations, and causes a rapid decline in mental performance.[5] People who are socially isolated show elevated blood pressure, more inflammation, and higher levels of the stress hormone cortisol.[6] Having fewer interactions with family and friends is correlated with an increased likelihood of catching the common cold, more rapid cognitive deterioration, and a greater risk of developing hypertension, heart disease, cancer, liver disease, diabetes, and emphysema.[7]

In one large study of 2,835 women with breast cancer, those women with the fewest social connections before their breast cancer diagnosis were twice as likely to die of their cancer as were the women who started off with strong social connections. The women in this study who continued to go through the cancer journey alone were four times more likely to die of breast cancer than those women who gained the support of 10 or more friends during their treatment.[8] Repeatedly, studies indicate that social seclusion leads to an earlier death.[9] In fact, in a 2015 comprehensive review of the data on isolation and loneliness, researchers analysing the results of 70 independent studies concluded that loneliness is on par with other major risk factors like lack of exercise, obesity, addiction, and mental illness that routinely make the list of public health concerns.[10]

Although these studies and statistics highlight an important factor that cannot be ignored as we try to understand the underlying causes of the chronic illness epidemic, they don't actually tell the full story. Facts and figures just cannot convey the feeling of loneliness and what that feeling does to the mind and body.

In 2004, when I first began to experience the symptoms of my autoimmune disease, I was just starting out in journalism. At that time, there was an unwritten law for people trying to get their foot in the door - *You have to do your time.* If you wanted to make it in the industry, you had to cut your teeth by reporting from a regional office, outside of the main hubs. My first break meant that I was based in a town called Burnie in North West Tasmania. Although it is a stunning part of the world with a wild coast line, some of the freshest air on earth, and on the whole a polite and friendly community, it is also a very isolated place where outsiders will always remain outsiders. One woman I met had lived there for 30 years, raised her four grown children there, and was still treated like a visitor.

Fortunately, at first I lived with a group of other young people who had moved there for job opportunities, and we had a blast making our own fun together. But they soon found new jobs and moved away and I found myself living in a studio apartment by myself. What followed was loneliness. Deep, pervasive, omnipresent loneliness. Sure, I spoke with colleagues every day and had amiable conversations with people, but being physically present in the company of others is not the same as being emotionally connected.

I was surrounded by people, but deeply alone. It was as though I was on the edge of a great uncrossable chasm looking across to where other people were talking to each other, laughing, and having a good time. I have no doubt that these feelings of isolation and loneliness were a significant contributing factor to my illness.

The irony of all this is that I was far from alone in feeling alone. Despite the rise of communications technology, and the rapid globalisation that was expected to foster social connections, people are becoming increasingly more socially isolated. The quantity and quality of our relationships are deteriorating, with trends toward reduced intergenerational living and an increased number of single person households.[11] In fact, we live in an era where affluent nations have the highest rates of individuals living alone since census data collection began, and those rates are projected to increase.[12] Over the last two decades in the US, there has been a three-fold increase in the number of Americans who report having no person in whom they can confide.[13] For 15-30 percent of the population, loneliness is a chronic state.[14] To put this into context, if you were reading this on a crowded bus carrying 50 people, chances are that as many as 15 of your fellow passengers would be feeling lonely. Especially among the elderly, loneliness is predicted to reach epidemic proportions by 2030.[15]

All You Need is Love

Imagine if as a college student in 1939 you had agreed to be part of a study dedicated to unlocking the secrets of a life well-lived. Imagine if from that moment on, every two years or so for as long as you lived you were poked and prodded with virtually every medical test and psychological tool at the researchers' disposal. Imagine if 267 of your classmates agreed to do the same thing. Then imagine, over the course of seven decades, as your whole group was studied throughout college, World War II, careers, marriages and divorces, through parenthood and grandparenthood and into old age, what kind of data would be gathered, and what sorts of insights all that information would give us about the keys to a happy, healthy, and meaningful life. This is exactly what the men of the Harvard Grant Study agreed to do. Now in their 90s, they can see the results of their generosity, patience, and candour in one of the longest and most comprehensive studies of human development ever undertaken.

Before I tell you what the study found, I want to highlight that the study did have some shortcomings. For a start, all of the subjects were white, privileged men who were students at what was then called Harvard College. Although their identities have been suppressed, we do know that by the time they were middle-aged, four of the men had run for the US Senate, one had served in a presidential cabinet, and one was elected governor. And it was revealed that President John F. Kennedy was a Grant Study participant.[16] There was also a best-selling novelist and a Fortune 500 CEO among them. At age 45, the average income of the men was the equivalent of US$180,000 by today's standards. All this accomplishment from a group of just 268 men is a distinct sign of their privileged position in life. But although the Grant Study scrutinises a very particular subset of the US population, it nevertheless paints a detailed, flesh-and-blood portrait of our journey through life and how the things that happen to us, the way we respond to them, and the choices we make, influence our health and happiness from college to old age.

In 2012, George Vaillant, the Study's director for 40 years, wrote *Triumphs of Experience,* a book that summarised the result of more than seven decades of material and the work of the 95 different researchers who, at a cost of US20 million dollars, harvested the data for scientific publication. His conclusions? Any which way Vaillant measured prosperity in life, the answer came down to one thing: love. "In short, it was the capacity for intimate relationships that predicted flourishing in all aspects of these men's lives," he writes.[17]

For example, by the end of World War II some of the Grant Study men who were in the armed services had been promoted to major, while others had remained at the rank of private. To their surprise, the researchers found that physique, social class, and even intelligence did not predict these men's position in the military; rather, the predictor was having enjoyed a warm childhood. Men suitable for advancement in the military, it turned out, were raised in loving homes. Another example is that the men who had good relationships with their siblings when they were young earned an average of $51,000 more per year than the men who didn't get on with their siblings. Having a stable childhood home predicted an average of $66,000 more income each year, and having a warm mother in particular was correlated with a salary boost of $87,000. The 58 men in the study who were identified as having had the best relationships were more likely to appear in *Who's Who*, a US publication of prominent people. When it came to conclusions about marriage, loving people for a long time was a good thing, but divorce wasn't necessarily a problem. It turned out that it was a man's ability to cherish his parents, siblings, children, friends, and at least one partner that proved a far better predictor of his mental health than did a poor early choice in his search for love.

Overall, Vaillant surmised that by far the most important influence on a flourishing life is love. His straightforward five-word conclusion? "Happiness is love. Full stop."[18]

What is Love?

The query "What is love?" consistently ranks among the most-frequently searched items on Google.[19] Unfortunately, love is more easily experienced than defined, especially if you're a scientist and you want to work out why this elusive feeling is so beneficial to our health and wellbeing. There are, of course, many kinds of love. The love a mother has for her child is very different from the love she has for her husband. The special kind of non-sexual intimacy that forms between friends who share deep connections is very different from the lustful, temporary, passionate kind of love that drives sexual desire. There is a mature, comfortable love that develops over time between a couple, a general love of life and for humanity, not to forget the self-love we must have to inspire healthy decisions. The various loves we feel for ourselves, parents, partners, children, friends, relatives, neighbours, country, God, and so on all have different qualities. Love can be blind, misguided, passionate, unreciprocated, secure, painful, and unconditional, but when all is said and done, scientists will tell you that love is basically just chemistry.

At every stage of the human experience of love, your brain and body are flooded with a range of different hormones that influence your behaviour, mood and, as scientists are now beginning to understand, your health. These hormones include dopamine (associated with pleasure and reward), serotonin (the "feel good" hormone), oestrogen (the primary female sex hormone), testosterone (the male sex hormone), and a host of others. But when it comes to the health benefits of love, one particular hormone that circulates throughout your brain is worth singling out: oxytocin.

Oxytocin has many colloquial names including "the cuddle hormone" and even "the great facilitator of life."[20] Essentially, it takes centre stage when it comes to social bonding and attachment, encouraging our relationships throughout life from the moment we bond with our parents to the forming of romantic relationships as adults.[21] It shows up during life's pivotal moments, surging during sexual intercourse, childbirth, and breastfeeding, but it's also around during everyday moments like when you play with your kids.[22] When they sprayed synthetic oxytocin into men's noses, researchers found that the men became more trusting,[23] empathetic,[24] and felt more secure.[25] Other studies show that fathers become more responsive, patient, and interactive with their babies and toddlers after they are given an oxytocin squirt,[26] which is an intriguing prospect for mothers who want to encourage their partners' enthusiasm to entertain the kids for a while.

There are easy, natural ways to get an oxytocin boost. In a study of 55 mums and dads who were observed while playing with their four-to-six month old babies for 15 minutes, researchers detected higher levels of oxytocin in both the parents and the babies.[27] Researchers also found that hugging can naturally increase your oxytocin.[28] Even interacting with your pets can give you a boost. For example, frequent interaction between dog-owners and their dogs is associated with higher oxytocin levels in both species.[29]

As researchers delve ever deeper into the function and purpose of this ubiquitous love hormone, they're also discovering that its role and function goes way beyond petting, cooing, gooing, and cuddles. It turns out that oxytocin also has a significant role as a powerful immune regulator. Oxytocin tunes down the stress response, thus helping buffer its negative effects.[30] It does this in part by suppressing the stress hormone cortisol.[31] It also modulates activity in the amygdala, your brain's stress centre. Under the influence of oxytocin, the parts of your amygdala that tune into threats are muted.[32] This is not to say that oxytocin somehow dulls your senses. It actually heightens your attunement to social cues. You become more attentive to people's eyes[33] and subtle facial expressions.[34] One of my favourite titles for a study I read while looking into all this was called "Oxytocin improves mind-reading in humans," though the researchers were referring to their discovery that oxytocin improves our ability to read and understand the mental state of others rather than uncovering a new sense.[35]

The Elixir of Health

In the 1960s, the town of Roseto, Pennsylvania was an anomaly in the US. At a time when heart disease was on the rise in the rest of the country, no one in the town under the age of 55 had died of a heart attack or showed signs of heart disease. In fact, the local death rate for men over 65 was half the national average. A team of researchers led by Stewart Wolf considered whether this longevity was because of diet, location, family history, or exercise habits. On the surface, nothing appeared radically different from the rest of America. In fact, the town was home to a population of Italian immigrants who worked in quarries and factories, smoked unfiltered cigars, and whose dinner tables were laden with rich Italian food. How then could the researchers explain the good health of the townsfolk?

When they looked beyond these physical factors, researchers found that the Rosetans of the 1960s still held onto their Old World ways. It was typical, for example, to find three generations living under the same roof. And outside the home, community relationships were important; 80 percent of men in the town were members of at least one community group. They would gather in each other's kitchens, play cards, and simply talk.

Wolf's conclusion was that the people of Roseto were nourished by each other. It was their strong family ties and close friendships that accounted for their good health. Over the next decade, the multigenerational homes broke up and the community relationships eroded. By 1971, when opulent houses, expensive cars, and swimming pools appeared, the first Roseto resident under the age of 55 died of a heart attack. By the 1980s, the rate of fatal heart attacks in Roseto was the same as in the rest of the country.[36]

Since Wolf's breakthrough research, the link between social closeness and good health has become well-established. In the same way that social isolation is linked to poor health and an increased chance of death from all causes, studies continue to demonstrate that people who are more socially connected are healthier and live longer.[37]

One of the experts I interviewed for *The Connection* was David Spiegel, a professor of psychiatry and the Director of the Center on Stress and Health at Stanford. He is renowned for his work on the effects of social support on health and the progression of illness, especially cancer. His early work stirred up a storm in the late 1980s because it demonstrated that women receiving treatment for advanced breast cancer who participated in support groups lived longer than women who were not members of support groups. The study, which was published in one of the world's most highly-regarded medical journals, *The Lancet*, was groundbreaking at the time because it was one of the first to demonstrate a clear mind-body-health connection.

In the *Lancet* article, Spiegel reported that the women who were randomly assigned to attend support groups for one year experienced less depression and pain, and lived 18 months longer than those who were not.[38] During our interview he told me of the experience of one woman who said, "Being in this group is like standing at the top of the Grand Canyon when you're afraid of heights; you know it would be a disaster if you fell but you feel better about yourself because you can look." Spiegel explained that the group support helped the women face their illness by improving their relationships with their families, reordering their priorities in life, and communicating better with their doctors who had also taught them self-hypnosis to control pain. "At the end of the first couple of years of the study, we were able to show that we reduced their anxiety and depression and we reduced their pain by 50 percent, so we were feeling pretty good about that," he said.

A major review published by *PLOS Medicine* in 2010 that analysed 148 studies with more than 308,000 participants found that people with strong social relationships had a 50 percent increased likelihood of surviving disease compared to those with weaker relationships.[39] The authors who undertook the review felt that even this estimate of the power of social support was conservative. The editorial accompanying the study declared that the influence of social relationships on the risk of death is comparable with the influence of well-established risk factors for mortality such as smoking and alcohol consumption, and exceeded the influence of other major risk factors such as physical inactivity and obesity.[40]

As they have done with the relationship between social isolation and poor health, scientists are now also starting to unlock some of the biological mechanisms that explain why good relationships are linked to good health. Through brain scans, blood tests, and saliva analysis, researchers have observed greater abundance of powerful "good" hormones such as dopamine, serotonin, endorphins and, of course, our friend oxytocin in people who have strong relationships. These hormones, in turn, boost the immune system, sending signals to decrease inflammation and increase blood circulation and oxygen levels.[41]

A 2014 study regenerated the buzz about the power of social support for women with breast cancer when researchers from the University of Calgary's Department of Oncology demonstrated that being involved in a support group has a positive impact at the cellular level. The researchers were interested in a possible connection between social support and changes in telomeres, which are little cap-like structures at the ends of our chromosomes (like the caps at the ends of your shoelaces) that shorten as we age. They found that the telomeres of breast cancer survivors who practiced meditation or were involved in support groups maintained their normal length, while the telomeres of a comparison group without any intervention became shorter. This information is made even more compelling with the knowledge that shortened telomeres are linked to higher chances of getting cancer and higher mortality for those who do get cancer.[42]

We've known for a while that meditation can affect telomere length,[43] but this study demonstrated that social support can have a similar effect. "We are not just splendid individuals," Spiegel told me. "We define ourselves in part by the people around us, and how they interact with us. It is very different to worry about dying at three in the morning by yourself than it is to talk about it at three in the afternoon with nine other women who have the same problem you do. It makes the stress different. And so I have no doubt at all that it helps people live better, and I think the evidence is accumulating that it helps them live longer as well."

Survival of the Kindest

When you think about it from an evolutionary perspective, the health benefits of being connected to others make a lot of sense. In comparison to other animals, early humans didn't have a lot going for them. In wild Paleolithic days, men and women weren't particularly fast or strong, so individuals needed all the support they could get just to stay alive. Living in social groups meant there were more people to help with the hunting and food gathering, bringing up the kids, and fending off attackers.[44] If you wanted to live long enough to pass on your DNA to the next generation, getting along with others was essential to your survival. This means that in the same way we have basic needs for food, water, and shelter, we also have a basic need for connectedness.

As David Spiegel explains, "The power of group support makes tremendous sense to me. We're social creatures. If you think about it physically, we're pretty pathetic. We're not that big, we're not that strong, we're not that fast. Animals can smell better than we can, see better than we can, and hear better than we can. What have we got? We've got an opposing thumb; that's a good thing, and we've got a big brain. And the brain enables us to form connections with others and build networks of support that help us stay alive, that help us deal with threats, that help us nurture our young, and create stable and relatively safe cultures." In fact, anthropologists have determined that the strongest predictor of a species' brain size (specifically, the size of its neocortex, the outermost layer) is the size of its social group.[45] In other words, we have big brains in order to socialise.

The great evolutionary thinker Charles Darwin, noted for his theories about the survival of the fittest, actually also wrote about the survival of the kindest. "Those communities, which included the greatest number of the most sympathetic members, would flourish best, and rear the greatest number of offspring," he wrote in 1871.[46] Indeed, anthropologists have found clear evidence of humankind's early sense of compassion. For example, a 60,000-year-old cave man, affectionately called Nandy by his excavators at Shanidar in Iraq, is believed to have suffered a violent blow to the left side of his face at some point in his life, one that would have left him partially or totally blind in one eye. The physical evidence also suggested that Nandy couldn't use his lower right arm because it had been fractured in several places and had withered, either from a childhood disease or an amputation later in his life.[47] The experts who analysed Nandy's fossilised remains determined that he lived to be at least 40 years old, which was considerably old for a Neanderthal. His longevity suggests he may have been supported and cared for.[48]

Although modern life is very different from the prehistoric landscape of our early ancestors, and though we're more likely to face the wrath of an angry boss than a hungry cave bear, our desire to be in a loving relationship, to fit in at school or work, to avoid rejection and loss, to share life's ups and downs, to barrack for a sports team, and to gather friends on Facebook is nevertheless hardwired into our genetic programming.

Viewed from an evolutionary perspective, it's really no surprise that investing in social relationships is essential to health and wellbeing. "It is social connection that has enabled us to survive in this world and take over from every other creature. It makes perfect sense to me that social connection can help us manage our emotions, draw support rather than lose it, cope with life-threatening situations, and get assistance when we need it. Social connection, especially in the face of illness, is a very powerful ally," Spiegel explained.

Hands-on Health

On the morning I began my research on the connection between human contact and health, I found myself weeping in front of my computer screen. I had just watched a news story originally broadcast in 1990 by the US ABC program *20/20*.[49] The exposé revealed a modern-day tragedy on a scale difficult to take in. In the 1960s, the communist dictator of Romania, Nicolae Ceaușescu, was on a mission to boost his country's industrial output. He thought the best way to do that was to increase the population so he enacted a decree that restricted contraceptives, banned abortions for women who hadn't had at least four children, and instituted a 30 percent income tax on childless men and women over the age of 25. Within 12 months the number of babies in the country doubled. The Romanian people faced decades of food scarcity, energy shortages, and rampant national poverty so 170,000 children wound up neglected in 700 understaffed institutions.[50]

In the wake of Ceaușescu's 1989 overthrow and execution, the *20/20* television program broadcast a two part series titled *Shame of a Nation* that revealed the magnitude of the children's suffering. The images of babies tied to steel cribs, rhythmically rocking or banging their heads against walls, locked in dimly lit rooms, lying in their own excrement and supervised by staff with little time to hold or comfort them were beyond heartbreaking.[51] Because meal times could be accomplished more quickly with gruel rather than solid food, some were fed watery formulas and were never taught how to feed themselves with utensils. Malnourished and starved of love or stimulation, it is little wonder that Romania's institutionalised children developed profound mental and physical abnormalities. Many of those who survived are the same age as I am. This was not a remote historical event. This happened in my lifetime, and the tragedy hit me like a ton of bricks.

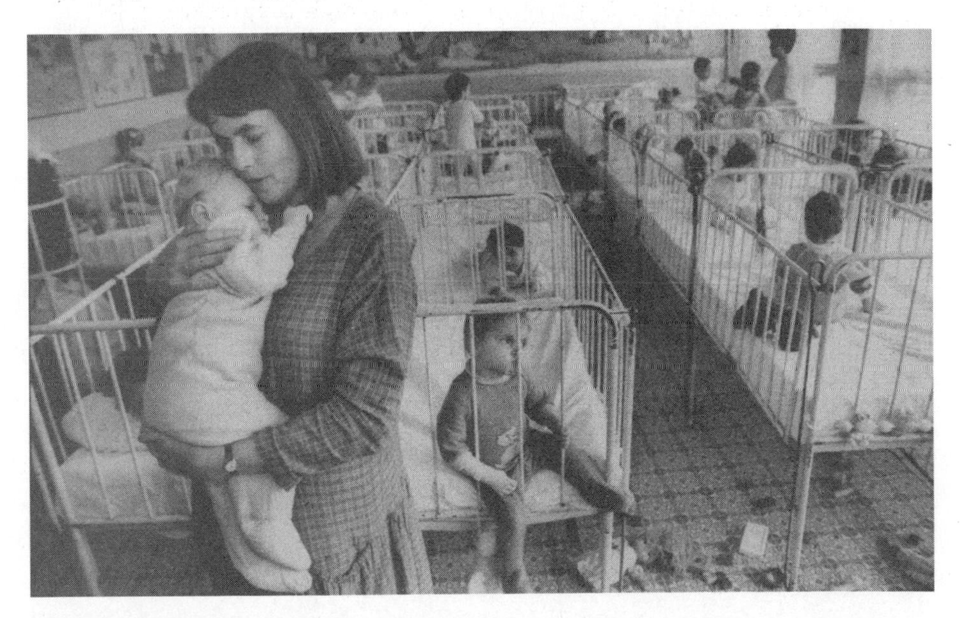

American pediatrician Dr. Barbara Bascom comforts a baby in a Romanian orphanage. *Credit: Taro Yamasaki/The LIFE Images Collection/Getty Images*

Neurologist Mary Carlson and her psychologist husband Felton Earls from Harvard were also moved by the children's suffering revealed in the *20/20* exposé, and they were two of the many foreigners who travelled to Romania to try to help.[52] Carlton had studied under the psychologist Harry Harlow, who first demonstrated the importance of caregiving, companionship, and comfort through a series of controversial experiments with monkeys. Harlow raised monkeys in isolation chambers he called "pits of despair," and recorded developmental abnormalities such as blank staring, repetitive circling in their cages, self-mutilation, and autistic self-clutching and rocking.[53] The published descriptions of monkeys attempting to adjust to these conditions is gut-wrenching, and it's little wonder that Harlow's methods, which remain controversial, are credited with inspiring the animal liberation movement.[54]

When Carlton arrived in Romania, she soon realised she'd stumbled on the human equivalent of Harlow's experiments. "The muteness, blank expressions, social withdrawal, and bizarre stereotypic movements of these infants bore a strong resemblance to the behaviour of socially deprived macaques monkeys and chimpanzees," she wrote in her 1997 paper, which documented the abnormal stress response she had observed in the children.[55]

Researchers are continuing to study the full repercussions of what was, in effect, an unintended social experiment in which an entire generation of children spent their formative years without care, adult social interaction, stimulation, or emotional comfort. A 2015 paper concluded that the Romanian youngsters were not only psychologically traumatised by their ordeal but that their brains did not develop normally. The researchers found reductions in the integrity of white matter in their brains, which helps neurons communicate. These abnormalities are associated with poor language skills and decreased mental ability. But there was some good news in the paper: early intervention, where the kids were looked after by foster parents who were encouraged to develop responsive, committed relationships with them, promoted more normal development of white matter among previously-neglected children, suggesting that a high-quality family environment can put brain development back on track.[56]

Out of all this darkness comes some light as researchers look for clues within the body as to why and how social neglect and isolation can cause such profound emotional and physical problems. It turns out that interpersonal touch, especially the cuddling we receive as infants, is fundamental to human communication, bonding, and health.[57]

Researchers have documented the positive physiological and biochemical effects of touch, including decreases in blood pressure and heart rate, decreases in the stress hormone cortisol, increases in the love hormone oxytocin, stimulation of reward regions in the brain, and reduced activation in stress-related regions.[58] One study of rabbits that were fed high cholesterol diets found that if they were petted, held, talked to, and played with on a regular basis, they had 60 percent less blockage in their arteries than the rabbits that were left in isolation. In other words, positive physical contact was correlated with the animals being better able to eliminate excess cholesterol.[59] In human studies, researchers found that a 30-second hug along with 10 minutes of hand holding reduced the harmful physical effects of stress, including its effect on blood pressure and heart rate.[60] Another recent study found that hugging can reduce our susceptibility to catching a cold during times of stress.[61]

This research is also having an impact outside the lab and in the real world. For example, when babies are born prematurely, they must often be kept in an incubator, which isolates them from human touch, so scientists have been researching "kangaroo care" for premature babies, where skin to skin contact is encouraged between parents and babies. In an analysis of 124 studies, kangaroo care was associated with a 36 percent lower death rate among low birth weight newborns, compared to conventional care.[62] These benefits were still measurable 10 years after the babies were born.[63] Another study gave elderly people the opportunity to massage infants. The volunteers' stress hormones decreased and after a month they needed fewer doctors' appointments, highlighting the benefits for both the giver and the receiver of touch.[64]

Medium-pressure massage is one of the most effective forms of touch. It has been used primarily to treat pain, although it is increasingly used for other problems including job stress, depression, autoimmune conditions like asthma, dermatitis, and rheumatoid arthritis, as well as fibromyalgia, diabetes, and cancer.[65]

Much of this research confirms what many of us already know to be true without the need for scientific verification. Whether it's an enthusiastic handshake, an encouraging pat on the back, a welcoming embrace, a sensual caress, a nudge for attention, or a tender kiss, physical contact can at times convey meaning more powerfully than language.[66] Even the briefest of touches from another person can elicit a strong emotional response. There is nothing like the comforting experience of being touched by our loved ones.

Yet despite its importance for communication, health, and relationships, human touch is becoming increasingly taboo in many cultures. We're actively encouraged to keep our hands to ourselves in fear of being accused of invading personal space, of being misinterpreted, of being sued, or of being accused of child abuse.

When I consider all this research on the power of touch, I can't help thinking back to my lonely time in North West Tasmania, where I felt isolated despite being surrounded by people. I went weeks on end without being touched. If only I had known then that something as simple as human contact could have made a difference - not only to how I was feeling mentally, but also potentially to my physical health.

The Power of Forgiveness

The ancient concept of forgiveness transcends time and culture. It is enshrined in all the great religions as a gesture of supreme value and is the centre of some of the most captivating stories of our time, serving as a core theme in everything from *The Bible* to *King Lear* to *My Name is Earl*. This is because one of the most difficult things to do when we feel wronged is to forgive the person who harmed us. Unfortunately, holding a grudge doesn't affect the perpetrator, it just impairs us from moving on.[67]

In recent years, the concept of forgiveness has moved out of the realm of spiritualism and television plot lines and into the laboratory. We now know that ruminating over hurtful memories and nursing grudges has the potential to harm our health by raising stress hormones and elevating blood pressure.[68] On the flip side, there is an established link between forgiveness and psychological, emotional, and physical wellbeing.[69]

Forgiveness can lower your blood pressure,[70] reduce chronic physical pain,[71] make you less likely to fall off the wagon if you're in rehab,[72] reduce feelings of stress,[73] as well as improve your mood[74] by reducing resentment and vindictive feelings toward someone who has done wrong by you.[75] Practising forgiveness can literally relieve the burden we carry on our shoulders; people can physically jump higher after having forgiven someone.[76]

Think about it this way. Each time you reflect on a time when you've been wronged, your brain will react. If you have a chronic grudge, you could think about it 20 times a day or more and your brain and body will respond by releasing cortisol, adrenaline, and all the stress hormones and physiological responses we discovered in Chapter 1 (Stress). You'll be stuck in a form of fight or flight mode and you won't be thinking clearly. When you forgive, you stop that reaction.[77]

This is not to say that forgiveness is easy. It often takes time, and in many cases is an ongoing process.[78] Nor is forgiveness a panacea to all trauma-induced harm. Forgiveness is not about excusing, exonerating, justifying, condoning, pardoning, or reconciling.[79] It is not about forgetting, but rather about moving on and it requires overcoming resentment, withholding retaliation, and responding to your offender with benevolence.[80]

Viral Friendships

In 2014, Facebook faced a storm of protest when it revealed it had conducted a secret experiment in which it manipulated information posted on 689,003 users' home pages. The social media giant found it could make people feel more positive or negative through a process called "emotional contagion." Researchers from Cornell University filtered the news feeds of users (that is, the flow of comments, videos, pictures, and web links posted by other people in their social network) and discovered that the emotions expressed by our friends via social networks can influence our own moods.[81]

The public reaction from lawyers and politicians was outrage.[82] One UK politician, Jim Sheridan, even called for a parliamentary investigation into how Facebook and other social networks manipulate our emotional and psychological responses. What Sheridan didn't realise is that emotional contagion goes way beyond social media, and that research also shows that anyone has the ability to change public mood. In fact, we can "catch" emotions expressed by our leaders, spouses, parents, siblings, colleagues, friends, and neighbours.[83]

Researchers found that conflict can be contagious too, and can spread from a dispute between two people and rapidly become a swarming mob of unrest.[84] Suicidal thoughts can also be contagious, causing suicide clusters in communities.[85] In one utterly bizarre case study of what researchers call "mass hysteria," a "laughter epidemic" broke out in 1962 in what is now Tanzania, Africa. The laughter began in a mission-run boarding school for girls in the village of Kashasha and quickly spread to other villages. A thousand people were affected and 14 schools were shut down. While this all sounds like a barrel of laughs, the researcher who studied the phenomenon believes it was extensive stress, not bliss, that affected the victims.[86]

It's not just emotions that may be contagious. Two of the leading researchers in this field are Nicholas Christakis from Yale University and James Fowler from the University of California, San Diego. They came up with a way to draw on records from the famous Framingham Heart Study, a three-decade-long analysis of medical records from a community in Massachusetts, and found that we are highly influenced by the people around us in many different aspects of our lives. In one study, they found that friends, and friends of friends, had similar levels of obesity. That is to say, if you have a friend who is obese, the chance that you are also obese increases by 45 percent. If a friend of a friend (two degrees of separation) is obese, your added risk of becoming obese is about 20 percent; and if a friend of a friend of a friend (three degrees) is obese, your risk is about 10 percent. They've found similar results for smoking,[87] depression,[88] happiness,[89] and cooperative behaviour.[90]

While the Fowler and Christakis social contagion studies were huge hits in the media (inspiring a popular book, talks, and TV appearances), mathematical experts questioned the statistical methodology on which they based their conclusions. Critics believe the evidence is weaker than what may have at first appeared, so it may be a bit of a stretch to say that you started putting on weight solely because your daughter's best friend's mother did.[91]

I'd like to highlight that this debate is not around whether or not peer influence exists or even whether it may be more important than we previously realised, but rather around how powerful its effects are. And while we still don't fully understand exactly when, where, how, and why some things seem to catch on, a variety of experiments offer clues. For example, we tend to unconsciously mimic the facial expressions, voices, movements, and behaviours of people around us.[92] Contagious behaviours, such as yawning, laughing, or crying, can be triggered by seeing, hearing, or even thinking of another person's behaviour.[93] We also have an innate human ability to empathise with others. For example, by imagining ourselves in the position of someone who is experiencing depression we might take on some of those stressful and negative emotions as if they were our own. Being around someone who is in a dark mood might easily affect our own mood. We also tend to gravitate toward people with whom we share things in common. For example, our friendships may be based on a mutual love of gourmet food, or taking time out to go for a cigarette break. Birds of a feather do indeed flock together.[94]

Our cues of what is socially acceptable are also taken from the people around us. For example, our idea of an acceptable weight or an acceptable portion size might change when we compare our waistline to the waistlines of our friends or notice how much they eat. As we discovered in Chapter 6 (Environment) when we looked at Brian Wansink's research on mindless eating, these subtle influences can push and pull us subconsciously in ways that influence our health and wellbeing.

While all this brings a whole new level of meaning to the expression "You make me sick," as Christakis and Fowler point out in their book, *Connected: The Amazing Power of Social Networks and How They Shape Our Lives,* "Our health depends on more than our own biology or even our own choices and actions. Our health also depends quite literally on the biology, choices, and actions of those around us."[95]

The good news is that there is no reason the "social contagion" phenomenon can't be harnessed for positive health outcomes. For example, a study of people who wanted to lose weight showed that if they enrolled in a weight-loss program with friends, they were more likely to complete the program, lose weight, and have kept the weight off 10 months later.[96] Another study showed that the spouses of people enrolled in a weight-loss program were also more likely to lose weight, even though they weren't officially participating in the program.[97]

One group of researchers used this information in a truly remarkable way to persuade more people to eat more fruit and vegetables. They identified friendship groups in work places, then singled out the social leader within each group as a "peer educator" who was trained and paid $1800 to spend two hours per week telling their friends in the group about the health benefits of eating fresh produce.[98] Considering that parents' food choices strongly influence the food choices of children and adolescents, programs like this have exciting ripple effect potential.[99]

Crossing the Chasm

There's a scene in my film *The Connection* depicting a group of women playing with their babies in a park on a warm summer's day. As dappled light shines through flickering leaves, soft shadows dance on their smiling faces. It's a picturesque, heartwarming scene, and one of my favourite sequences I've ever directed. Although Shing Fung Cheung, my Director of Photography, created some pretty images that day, it's not the actual pictures themselves that make this scene special. It's what this moment represents in my own health journey. We shot that part of the film about eight months after Theodore was born. We filmed in my local park and, gorgeous as they are, the mums and their bubs are not a group of hired actors; they are my own mother's group.

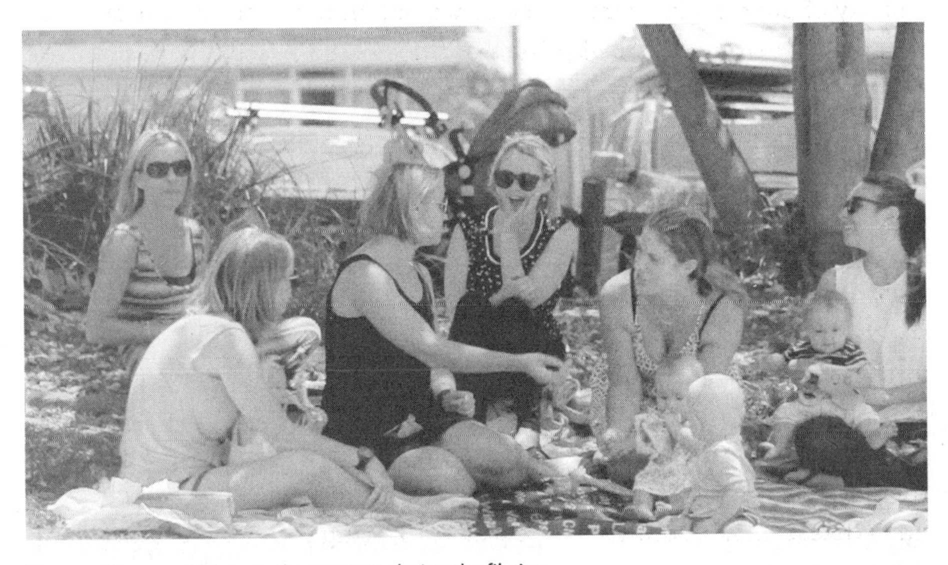

Shannon Harvey with her mother's group during the filming of *The Connection* documentary, 2014. *Credit: Shing Fung Cheung*

By this point in my health journey, my life was unrecognisable from what it had been when I first fell ill. By making relationships in my life a priority above and beyond my work, I found a way to cross the chasm of loneliness I felt when I lived in Tasmania. Now, I was living in a part of Sydney where family and friends were minutes instead of an airplane trip away. Jules and I worked hard on our relationship and spent hours each week talking with each other openly and with open minds. I was making an effort to see my friends regularly and scheduling catch-ups so they would happen automatically. Every interaction began and ended with a warm embrace.

These days, I get my daily dose of oxytocin from the frequent cuddles that come with having a thoughtful and empathetic three-year-old toddler in my house. I also look outside my home for opportunities to connect with others. Rather than looking at my phone when I'm at the grocery store check out, I often ask the cashier how she or he is doing. A recent experience with a nurse I hadn't met before who was doing a blood test for me resulted in a beautiful exchange of personal life experiences and both of us ending up in the tears of human connection.

When I spoke to a midwife recently about some of the experiences that came with the birth of Theodore – traumatic labor, difficulty breast feeding, long-term sleep deprivation – as well as my family history of mental illness, she responded by saying that I was a classic candidate to develop postnatal depression. But I didn't come close to feeling depressed. It's particularly noteworthy that throughout those first few months of becoming a parent and trying to get a handle on the whole work-life-parent thing, my autoimmune disease *didn't* flare. I have absolutely no doubt that the love and support from family and friends I had during that time, and continue to have, is the single most important reason for my speedy recovery from the labour and a key factor in the good mental and physical health I enjoy today.

Key Takeaways

1 At a time when loneliness has been found to be on par with other major risk factors that routinely make the list of public health concerns such as lack of exercise, obesity, addiction, and mental illness, we're living in a world where we're becoming increasingly more socially isolated.

2 Intimate relationships are a key in predicting a flourishing life. In the words of the Grant Study researcher George Vaillant "Happiness is love. Full stop." The link between social closeness and good health is also now well-established. People who are more socially connected are healthier and live longer.

3 Whether it's through massage, hugging, holding hands, an encouraging pat on the back, a welcoming embrace, a sensual caress, or a tender kiss, interpersonal touch is fundamental to human communication, bonding, and health.

4 Ruminating over hurtful memories and nursing grudges have the potential to harm your health. On the flip side, there is an established link between forgiveness and psychological, emotional, and physical wellbeing. Forgiveness is not about forgetting, but rather about moving on.

5 The extent to which "social contagion" can influence your health and wellbeing is starting to be better understood. From our daily mood to our waistline, the subtle and not so subtle influence of those around you can push and pull you in one way or another without you even realising it.

Getting Started

SCHEDULE time to nurture your relationships. I suggest having at least two regular catch-ups with a friend or relative that happen automatically at a reoccurring, unchanging time. For example, I meet my best friend for lunch once a month and my mother's group for drinks on the second Thursday of every month.

CONNECT with a group. Think of one thing you love doing and find others who regularly meet to enjoy it too. It could be anything from joining a book club or a singing group, to playing a weekly game of cards or a sport.

MAKE a list of safe and appropriate ways to boost your physical contact with others. You might hold hands with your loved ones while you're walking, or give your family members a hug when you see them off for the day. At work, you can high-five your colleagues when something good happens. In fact, handshakes and fist-bumps can all be part of a healthy workplace. You can also book yourself in for a massage with a registered therapist.

TAKE the questionnaire available for download from my website to measure your level of social support.

TRY Loving Kindness Meditation (LKM). This is a technique used to increase feelings of warmth and caring for yourself and others. It boosts positivity and life satisfaction and reduces symptoms of depression and illness.[100] You can download instructions from my website. See the following Extra Resources section for details.

IF you're feeling lonely, isolated or depressed, I urge you to get some help so you can learn to reconnect with others. It's interesting that a review of interventions to reduce loneliness showed that changing harmful thinking patterns was the most effective way to reduce loneliness.[101] You might like to check out the organisation Beyond Blue if you don't know where to start. www.beyondblue.org.au

LEARN to forgive. Through the Stanford Forgiveness Project you can learn how to release unwanted hurts and grudges. http://learningtoforgive.com

Extra Resources

AVAILABLE AT
www.thewholehealthlife.com/resources

WATCH extended video interviews with the experts including:

- *David Spiegel, Professor of Psychiatry and the Director of the Center on Stress and Health at Stanford University*

DOWNLOAD the social support questionnaire.

DOWNLOAD instructions and a guided audio recording for practising Loving Kindness Meditation (LKM).

CHECK OUT my recommended reading list. Books relevant to this chapter include:

- *Triumphs of Experience: The Men of the Harvard Grant Study,* by George Vaillant
- *Living Beyond Limits: New Hope and Help for Facing Life-threatening Illness,* by David Spiegel
- *Connected: The Amazing Power of Social Networks and How They Shape Our Lives,* by Nicholas Christakis and James Fowler
- *Love 2.0: How Our Supreme Emotion Affects Everything We Feel, Think, Do and Become,* by Barbara L. Fredrickson
- *Love and Survival: 8 Pathways to Intimacy and Health,* by Dean Ornish
- *The Roseto Story: An Anatomy of Health,* by John G Bruhn and Stewart Wolf

Chapter 10

Lasting Change

A Film Release

It was four o'clock in the afternoon on the 11th of October 2014. I was standing in front of a brightly lit electronic information board at London's Heathrow airport. Like more than 73 million other people who pass through the busiest transport hub in Europe every year, I had navigated the array of security cues, the tedium of passport control, and steered through the chaotic terminal where the rich perfumes of duty-free stores mingled with the scents of fast food and Asian takeaway. I blocked out the mechanical loudspeaker voice calling out the imminent departures, the cries of an overtired toddler, and the tittering of overexcited teenagers, and scanned the constantly-updating information board broadcasting the details of countless flights heading in different directions all over the world. At last I found what I needed. Flight CX11 to Hong Kong. The first stage of my 15-hour journey home to Sydney.

I had been away from Jules and Theodore for a month, travelling from Sydney to Melbourne, Boston, San Francisco, Los Angeles, Tucson, New York, and London on a film screening tour to promote *The Connection*. In the past three years, there had been countless long days and nights of research, pre-production, production, post-production, pick-up shoots, and more post-production. When Theodore was a newborn, I used the hours he slept to research and write. As he got older, my mother-in-law, Alice, helped care for him while I worked with my editor to get the film out of the edit suite and into the world so people could see it. My mother, sister, and best friend made me endless cups of tea and offered words of encouragement and constant kindness. I had asked huge favours of colleagues who had worked on the film in good faith and with enormous generosity.

Jules and I chose not to use a traditional distributor for the film. We'd worked on several other projects that had gone down the conventional release model but had been pulled from cinemas after just one week, or had vanished from stores after a month, never to be seen again. We felt the information in *The Connection* was too important to sit in a warehouse gathering dust, and we wanted to be free to work with community groups and healthcare professionals, and to reach as many people as possible. This meant that all the money I'd made from my small production company over the last few years had been spent on the film, and as we got close to the end of post-production, I'd had to borrow more money to finish it. Jules had provided the sole income for our little family while I worked full time, for no salary. And now, three years of financial, personal, and professional struggle were reaching their culmination. In four days, *The Connection* would officially be released into the world.

This was by far the most ambitious and important thing I'd done so far in my career. It was a busy, challenging, scary time and with so much at stake, along with the added new pressure of being a parent, you might think this would have been the perfect opportunity for my autoimmune disease to rear its ugly head. But I had never been healthier.

As I made my way to the departure gate at Heathrow, I felt rested and calm, balanced, strong, and well. I looked around at my fellow passengers and noticed how stressed-out some of them seemed. Their grey, tired, and harried faces were so familiar to me. I'm sure I had carried the same tense expression on my own face just a few years ago when I was making my way back from Samoa after covering the tsunami – a story that never made it to air. That, too, had been a big deal in my career. But it had left me in agony and bedridden with an arthritic flare-up all through my body. So what had changed between then and now? How had I managed to stay healthy? How had I somehow kicked my lifetime habit of allowing other priorities to dominate my healthy behaviour goals?

Every Day Counts

At the University of California, Riverside a sign on a laboratory door reads "The Termanator Lab." Although the lab is just 85 kilometres (50 miles) east of Hollywood, those working inside are not making a blockbuster movie. The scientists within are working on one of the most extensive studies of longevity ever conducted. In 1921, Stanford University psychologist Lewis Terman enlisted a group of 1,528 bright boys and girls who would be studied for the next 80 years. Howard Friedman, a professor of psychology at the University of California, Riverside, has been the custodian of the Terman data for more than two decades, enlisting the help of other researchers and graduate students to help process and analyse the vast amount of material collected to see who lived long, who died young, why some were healthy, and why others became ill. Rather than describing themselves simply as involved in "Dr. Friedman's longevity project developing the Terman data," his colleagues declared themselves to be *The Termanators*. Like Arnold Schwarzenegger's character in the famous *Terminator* franchise (at least in some of the movies), they're also on a mission to save human lives – by unlocking the secrets of a healthy, long life.[1]

Like the Harvard graduates in the long-running Grant study (which you'll recall from the previous chapter on relationships), The Termanators are studying the lives of people who were white, bright, and educated and who lived through the Depression, war, and times of prosperity. In the early 1990s, when Friedman and his then-graduate student, Leslie Martin, were interested in finding out why some people seemed more prone to disease, or died sooner than others, they had a rich trove of information to study. They launched The Longevity Project and pored through Terman's records, hunting down death certificates and asking follow-up questions of participants who were still alive. They have now published their findings in over 150 influential and often-cited scientific articles and chapters in leading books and scientific journals.[2]

Some of their results were remarkably similar to those of the Grant study, affirming, for example, that good relationships and social support are fundamentally linked to longevity.[3] But Friedman and Martin also wanted to know what kinds of personalities were linked to good health and a long life, and they were surprised by what they found. It wasn't the cheerful people who liked to tell jokes or laugh a lot who lived long, hearty lives. Nor was it those who devoted themselves to running marathons, or always eating organic broccoli. The healthiest individuals in The Longevity Project were united by a very distinct personality pattern. They were diligent, thorough, hardworking, reliable, responsible, committed, and persevering. In a word, they were *conscientious.*[4]

There's nothing sexy or exciting about conscientiousness being the key to good health and a long life. "Conscientiousness is the Secret" is hardly "click bait" nor does it exactly make for a catchy headline. Telling your friends that your new health mantra is "commitment and consistency" is not going to make them think you've uncovered a profound path to radiant health and enlightenment. But the scientific evidence to support this approach is stunningly robust.[5] Conscientious people engage in a variety of important healthier behaviours. They smoke less, eat healthier foods, and are less likely to abuse drugs and alcohol or drive without a seatbelt.[6] Conscientious people also choose healthier environments, create or evoke healthier situations, and select and maintain healthier friendships and more stable marriages.[7] Conscientious people are also more likely to have more successful, meaningful careers, better educations, and higher incomes, all of which are known to be relevant to health, wellbeing, and a longer life.[8] All in all, people who are conscientious stay healthier, thrive, and live longer.[9]

To look at this from another angle, let's say that one of the healthy things you'd like to do after reading this book is lose some weight. And let's say you're considering going on a diet. If you've taken in the key message from Chapter 4 (Food), you're probably convinced that a healthy diet involves cutting out junk and eating a wide variety of fresh fruit and vegetables, whole grains, legumes, nuts, and seeds. But you might be thinking you still need a little more guidance than that, and you might walk into your local book store for some help. If you do this, you'll be faced with an overwhelming choice of diet advice books. Paleo or sugar-free? High-fat low-carb or low-fat high-carb? In 2014, Canadian scientists performed a meta-analysis (a study of studies) to figure out which diet works best for weight loss. They looked at 48 randomised control trials that included data from a total of 7,286 people who had tried various big brand diets: Atkins, South Beach, Zone, Biggest Loser, Jenny Craig, Weight Watchers, Nutrisystem, Volumetrics, Ornish, and Rosemary Conley. Their conclusion? "The weight loss differences between individual named diets were small with likely little importance to those seeking weight loss."[10] Ultimately, what mattered for weight loss wasn't which diet people went on, only whether they *adhered* to it for the whole study period.[11] So which is the best diet for weight loss? The one you'll stick to.

Will taking a conscientious approach to your health make you boring and stale? According to Friedman and Martin, there's no evidence to support this stereotype. Think about it this way: Jules is an adventurer and enjoys the challenge of high-altitude mountain climbing. A few years ago when he was planning an ascent of Mount Vinson (the highest mountain in Antarctica, and the most remote place on the planet) I was able to quell my worries and concerns not only because I know how careful Jules is and how well he plans, but because his friend, Duncan Chessell, who was leading the expedition is one of the most responsible, thorough, and cautious people I've ever met. He's also completely crazy. He doesn't just go to the summit of a mountain. He goes from the sea to the summit of a mountain, making a six-week sled journey before he even straps on a climbing harness. DC has been to the top of Mount Everest *three times*. He thrives on adventure, discovery, and doing things people say can't be done "just because." There is not a dull bone in DC's body. He is hardly routine or run-of-the-mill, but I trust him with my husband's life. My point here is that it's possible to be conscientious *and* live an exciting life.

It is this approach that got me through the high-stakes release of *The Connection* in such good health. By then I'd learned a great deal about what it took to keep my autoimmune disease in check. I was meditating regularly, which was helping me manage my stress levels. I was using mindfulness to help me see small stressors for what they were and keep them in perspective. And although the people in my life who were the source of my emotional triggers were still very much present, I was using journal-writing techniques to balance my emotions and resolve issues that threatened to be a source of rumination and distress. I was prioritising sleep, healthy eating, movement, and getting outside to enjoy the world around me over and above hitting deadlines. In other words, I was being committed and consistent in my health actions rather than taking the "just get through and recover later" approach I had used in the past.

In our busy modern lives we're all constrained by a finite reservoir of resources such as time, energy, willpower, and money. Unless we live in a magical house that contains a gym, a meditation room, a farmer's market, and a personal staff of nutritionists, trainers, and motivational coaches, *and* all we ever have to do all day long is focus on our health, then there's absolutely no way we can possibly meet all the recommendations made by all the experts I've featured in this book, all of the time. But what we learn from the long-lived men and women in the The Longevity Project is that we can shape our *overall, fundamental patterns of living* to lead a long, healthy life.

If, as a result of reading this book, you're going to make changes in your life, make them sustainable. Think of it as running a marathon, not a sprint. You want to go the distance. If you don't like getting up at 6am to go for a run, don't. You won't stick to it. Instead, go for a regular walk at lunchtime with a friend, or plough a patch of dirt for a home vegetable garden that you'll cultivate over time. If you can't abide positive psychology gratitude exercises, boost your mood every day by taking time out to savour the great outdoors. If you've got chronic gut problems but you've had nothing but bad experiences with medical doctors, keep searching until you get the care you need. When it comes to your health, be discerning, be dedicated, be diligent, be committed, be consistent. Be *conscientious*.

Mind the Gap

By now, I hope you're starting to understand that although there's a lot of science to take in, the actual steps to put this information into action are relatively simple and straightforward. You may be picturing your fridge bursting with fresh fruit and veggies and your pantry resplendent with whole grains, nuts, and seeds. You may be planning to get orange-tinted bulbs for your lamps at home so you can harvest the health benefits of getting more and better sleep. Perhaps you've already looked up local gyms in your area, or started exploring sit-stand desk options. You may even be thinking about starting a meditation practice, or you have purchased a lovely new journal to begin getting in touch with your emotions. You may have every intention in the world of getting started right away on your whole-health life and be looking forward to becoming a whole new you. If so, then great! You are the reason I wrote this book.

Having said that, while it would be marvellous to tell you that all it takes to get healthy or to stay healthy in the modern world is to read a well-informed book, merely having good information won't be enough to keep you on track.[12] The truth is, although the practical takeaways I've outlined are completely within your reach, they're actually much easier said (or in your case, read) than done. Having knowledge and putting it into practice are two entirely different things. From my own trials and tribulations, I'm well aware that *wanting* to be healthy is very different from actually *being* healthy and I know I'm not alone in my struggle.

Every year, between 40 and 50 percent of us will take the New Year New Me pledge.[13] As we count down to midnight on the 31st of December, we'll unite in our aspirations to lose weight, eat better, exercise more, save money, stop smoking, or some other noble step we think will lead to self-improvement.[14] Unfortunately, depending on what it is we've pledged to do, studies show that somewhere between 35 and 89 percent of us will fail, often within the first week.[15] While we truly mean it when we make promises of self-betterment, our good intentions aren't often transformed into action. This is because having an *intention* to change our behaviour is not enough to actually *lead* to behaviour change. Social scientists call this phenomenon the intention-behaviour gap[16] and it's been observed in various domains including in our intentions to exercise more,[17] eat more healthily,[18] be more careful with the disclosure of personal information,[19] and even in our intentions to make ethical purchases.[20] Even if you really *really* want to change your actions it doesn't mean you'll succeed.[21] In fact, meta-analyses show that even a medium-to-large change in intention leads only to a small-to-medium change in behaviour.[22] In other words, when it comes to making healthy changes, really *wanting* to do something does not guarantee success.

So why is there a gap? And can we build a bridge to close it? I spoke with one of the world's leading experts on behaviour change, Peter Gollwitzer, a professor of psychology at New York University who has spent decades studying this very question. He's found that in many cases, people fail to get started with their goal in the first place – an intention is forgotten, confusion about how to act engenders paralysis, or the opportunity to take action passes.[23] As Gollwitzer explained, "When a great opportunity for exercising arises, for instance, on Saturday morning, there's also the shopping you have to do. You promised your children you'd play soccer with them. You promised your wife you'd go for breakfast and so forth and so forth. You are busy. Because you are busy, you overlook the good opportunity to get started on your intention."

In addition, our initial efforts can easily be derailed – we fall prey to temptations, distractions, low willpower, or fatigue.[24] "Let's say you put on your running shoes and you are on your way out to run, there might be a disruption. For instance, an e-mail might come in saying, 'Remember that there is a deadline today for submitting your proposal to so-and-so conference. Let's send it out before noon.' Now, you have your running shoes on, what do you do? You sit down at your computer and write the abstract and send it out. You are disrupted. You're not acting on your intention again," Gollwitzer said.

This second problem, where our efforts get derailed, is one I've faced with regularity. At different times since my arthritic symptoms first developed I found myself bursting with motivation and determination to turn my health around. I'd buy a new gadget (or two), go on a diet, sign up for a 40-day challenge, or whatever the thing of the moment was that promised to shake things up for me and get my health back on track. Often these initiatives would work and I'd feel great, reaping the short-term physical and mental health benefits of my efforts. And of course I fully intended to keep doing whatever it was I was doing. I wanted to get well and stay well. But as time passed, my old habits and behaviour patterns would slowly, subtly, mutinously creep back into my life. Without my even realising it, I'd end up right back where I started.

Battle of the Will

When you step out of the lab and into the real world, you only need to briefly think about what you're up against to see why it can be so hard to make lasting healthy changes in your life – brightly packaged treats calling to you off the supermarket shelves, the constant race against time forcing you to make choices based on speed and ease rather than long term gain, a To Do list as long as your arm on which "move more" comes after more pressing priorities, expertly designed labels with pictures of flawless celebrities that imply radiant health while disguising hidden nasties, the behaviours of people around you that blur the line between what is healthy and what is unhealthy. In this crazy, busy, time poor, distracted world, we inevitably slip up, and when we do, we think of ourselves as flawed and weak-willed. At this point we either deride ourselves into trying harder, or we give up.

Relying on willpower and self-control as a central strategy in getting healthy is not entirely without reason.[25] Having good self-control can influence your success in life as well as your health and wellbeing.[26] But the evidence also shows that self-control alone isn't the key.[27] In fact, some researchers found that self-control only has a small impact in determining your success.[28]

Imagine there's a box of chocolates sitting on your desk. Each time you look up from your computer, you see the chocolates. They call to you. They entice you. They beg you to open them. Let's say that in the course of your day you have looked at the chocolate box 99 times and 99 times you resisted them. But then, at 3pm when you're feeling a tad tired and your boss has just given you another impossible deadline, on the 100th time you look at the chocolates you give in. You immediately feel pleasure. The chocolate is delicious, so you have another. What the hell, they're open now, maybe just one more. This doesn't mean you have no willpower. You had willpower *99 times out of 100*. In fact, I would say you have super powers. The problem isn't that you lack willpower or self-control. The problem is that chocolates were sitting on your desk when you were feeling tired and run down.[29]

There is vast evidence demonstrating that our willpower is like a muscle that can get fatigued. This understanding comes from research done by Roy Baumeister from Case Western Reserve University. He devised a foundational experiment on self-control that showed that if people were made to sit in a room in front of freshly baked chocolate chip cookies they were not allowed to eat, they had less self-control in a subsequent problem-solving task.[30] Baumeister called this effect "ego depletion" and believes it reveals a fundamental fact about the human mind – that we have a limited supply of willpower, and that this supply decreases with overuse. The paper has been cited thousands of times and inspired hundreds of follow up studies. For example, dieters who were asked to suppress their emotions during a sad movie ate more ice cream afterward than dieters who were encouraged to let their feelings flow naturally.[31] Social drinkers are more likely to consume more alcohol than they intend to and drink to excess on days they've experienced more self-control demands.[32] Smokers who were deprived of a cigarette for 18 hours, and were also food deprived, were more likely to give in and smoke a cigarette, even though they'd been offered a financial reward if they were able to resist.[33] It's as if you only have a certain amount of willpower, and once it's been tuckered out, you're left vulnerable to temptation.

In 2010, a team of researchers conducted a meta-analysis that seemed to confirm that ego depletion is a real and reliable phenomenon[34] but the strength and significance of this paper has been debated.[35] Scientists are still trying to work out when, where, why, and how we exhaust our willpower. But while they're still figuring things out, there is nevertheless a clear message in all of this for us: we cannot rely on our willpower alone if we want the healthy changes we make in our lives to last.

This was one of the main flaws in my own wellness endeavours. I thought if I could just stay focused enough, if I could *will* myself to eat better, exercise more and stress less, then I'd get healthier. But time and time again with the first headache, the first deadline, the first emotional argument, this strategy failed. So if the key to healthy behaviour change is not just about boosting willpower and getting more self-control, what is it? What other proven techniques might be helpful as we try to keep our health goals on track?

The "How" of Health

In his book, *The Happiness Hypothesis: Finding Modern Truth in Ancient Wisdom*, social psychologist Jonathan Haidt from New York University uses a compelling metaphor to describe how our mind is divided into parts that sometimes conflict. "I'm a rider on the back of an elephant. I'm holding the reins in my hands, and by pulling one way or the other I can tell the elephant to turn, to stop, or to go. I can direct things, but only when the elephant doesn't have desires of his own. When the elephant really wants to do something, I'm no match for him,"[36] he writes. Haidt's premise is that like a rider on the back of an elephant, the conscious, controlled, reasoning part of our mind has only limited power over what our subconscious, automatic "elephant" mind does.[37]

Much of what we do every day is not actually driven by our conscious thought, but rather by our unconscious instincts, patterns, and behaviours.[38] In 2002, researchers found that people performed almost 50 percent of their behaviours without thinking about them.[39] From self-help gurus to the ancient religions, received wisdom exhorts us to be mindful, deliberative, and conscious in all that we do. But contemporary research in psychology shows that we can also use our unthinking routines to form a foundation for what we do in everyday life.[40]

A habit can develop when a situational cue triggers us to do something automatically.[41] The more we repeat the behaviour, the more automatic the behaviour becomes.[42] For example, you might have a habit of routinely washing your hands after using the toilet, putting on your seatbelt when you get into a car, or snacking on crackers when you're sitting in front of the TV. When you find yourself *doing* before *thinking*, that's the hallmark of a habit.

The cues that trigger a habit can be so powerful that your habits may actually override your intention.[43] Remember the free popcorn eaters from Brian Wansink's research in Chapter 6 (Environment)? In their case, the situational cue of being at the movies was enough to prompt them to eat popcorn even though it was squeaky stale.[44] So how can we break the trance? Given that habits are so inextricably tied to environmental cues, the most obvious habit-breaking solution is to remove the cues that trigger the behaviours. In 2011, researchers reported that by either having people eat stale popcorn in a conference room instead of a cinema, or getting them to eat with their non-dominant hand, they were able to break the habit of automatically eating popcorn regardless of their degree of hunger or the quality of the popcorn. Dropping the cue meant dropping the bad habit.[45] But beware, the same researchers also showed that this can also work in reverse. If you move to a new house for example, you might lose cues that trigger some of your healthy habits.[46]

Understanding habit science is useful not only for breaking unwanted automatic behaviour, it is also helpful in creating healthy routines and behaviours that we don't have to think about. You'll recall that the more we repeat the behaviour with the environmental cue, the more automatic the behaviour becomes.[47] With repetition, the mental effort to initiate a new habit gets easier, and over time the action becomes second nature.[48]

In 2010, the first real-world experiment outside a lab put this principle to the test. Researchers from University College, London asked each of 96 volunteers to choose a healthy eating, drinking, or exercise behaviour they wanted to adopt as a habit. Examples of the behaviours that some participants chose included eating a piece of fruit with lunch, drinking a bottle of water with lunch, and running for 15 minutes before dinner. The results showed that repeating a behaviour in the presence of consistent cues helped their behaviour become more automatic.[49] What is interesting about the study's results, though, is that "missing one opportunity does not preclude habit formation, but missing a week's worth of opportunities reduces the likelihood of future performance and hinders habit acquisition." In other words, it doesn't matter if you mess up every now and then, but you should aim to stick to it in the long run. There's that old conscientiousness chestnut again. But the main takeaway from this real-world habit study was that it well and truly busted the decades-old myth that it takes 21 days to form a habit.[50] It showed that the average time it takes to form a habit is more like 66 days, and varies anywhere from 18 to 254 days. It turns out that forming new habits is also dependent on the individual person and the degree of difficulty of the habit. For example, it's much easier to train yourself to drink a glass of water after breakfast than to go for a daily run. Some healthy behaviours are just tougher to make automatic than others.

So what about those more difficult behaviours that you want to make easy and automatic? What more can you do to boost your chances of making healthy behaviour stick?

Back in 1997, when Peter Gollwitzer was just getting started on some of his pioneering behaviour-change strategies, he recruited 111 university students in Munich for an experiment to see what effect using a simple planning strategy would have with helping people follow through with their intended behaviours. Just prior to their Christmas break he asked the students to name two projects they intended to carry out during the upcoming vacation. He instructed that one task should be difficult to implement and the other easy to implement. For their easy goals, the students chose activities such as finishing reading a novel or buying a textbook. For the difficult tasks, they chose goals like writing a term paper or resolving a conflict with a boyfriend. Gollwitzer also assessed whether they had formed "implementation intentions," that is, whether they had made plans for *when* and *where* they would start working toward their intended goals. When he surveyed them after the break, he found that for the projects that were easy to implement, completion rate was very high (80 percent) regardless of whether the students had formed implementation intentions. What was interesting, though, was that if the students had not planned when and where they would complete the difficult projects, they almost all failed to complete them. On the other hand, two thirds of the participants who formed implementation intentions for their difficult tasks followed through.[51]

Since that first study, Gollwitzer has continued to research the effectiveness of his strategy, finding it to be effective in a number of areas,[52] including helping people stay on the wagon after drug and alcohol detox,[53] develop good sleeping habits,[54] regularly take vitamins,[55] exercise more,[56] attend cervical cancer screenings,[57] get flu shots,[58] and eat more healthfully.[59] Specifically, when it comes to healthy eating, the results from 12 out of 15 studies provided considerable support for using implementation intentions to increase fruit and vegetable consumption[60] which, you'll remember from Chapter 4 (Food), is the main aim of the game.

Unlike a simple intention that merely states a goal like "I want to exercise more," implementation intentions specify the where, when, and how of goal-oriented action. The technique relies on an "if-then" principle.[61]

Here's an example of how Gollwitzer's strategy works:

"If it's 3pm on a Saturday,
then I'll go out for a 30 minute run to the park and back."

The strategy also helps you plan for curve balls
that might derail your efforts:

"If it's raining,
then I will wear my waterproof jacket."

The idea behind this kind of planning is that it helps eliminate the choices you have to make, encourages you stop and think about the obstacles you'll face in reaching your goal, and makes your behaviour automatic. "The nice thing about if-then planning is that it more or less automates your behaviour so you do it even if the individual steps of doing it get more complicated," said Gollwitzer during our interview over Skype. "You just do it automatically. You don't think and say, 'Oh, it's raining today. I don't want to run.' If it's 3pm on a Saturday afternoon, you go for a run no matter what."

There's little doubt that Gollwitzer's planning strategy is effective, but the concept does come with a caveat. When he reviewed 94 studies looking at the effectiveness of implementation intentions across a wide range of behaviours, Gollwitzer found they had a "medium to large" effect in helping people achieve their goals.[62] It's good – really good – but not bulletproof, and while planning in this way is effective in getting us to eat more fruit and vegetables, so far the evidence indicates that the technique has only a small effect in helping us *avoid* unhealthy eating behaviours like eating junk food and snacking.[63] Unfortunately, it turns out that breaking existing unhealthy behaviours is more difficult than initiating new healthy behaviours.[64]

All this speaks to the complexity of behaviour change and why research findings are often a little blurry. Unfortunately it is way too simplistic to conclude that good planning is all we need to guarantee that our health metamorphosis will last. The science of behaviour change is much more complicated than that, despite what some of the latest self-help books would have you believe. Many of the studies demonstrating the effectiveness of Gollwitzer's action planning technique also incorporated other motivational strategies, including positive experiences and boosting self-belief.[65]

In two particularly interesting studies that looked at reducing snacking behaviour in women, Gollwitzer worked with his psychology colleague at New York University, Professor Gabrielle Oettingen, to combine his if-then planning technique with another simple exercise called "mental contrasting," which encourages us to focus on visualising our goals as well as visualising the obstacles that stand in our way. They found that women who visualised the positive reasons for reducing their snacking as well as the challenges they would face in doing so, and who then formed an if-then plan, consumed significantly fewer calories from unhealthy snacks than participants in the control condition who were instructed to simply think about and list healthy options for snacks.[66]

According to Gollwitzer, if we want to give ourselves the best chance of success in breaking our bad habits and making healthy behaviour change stick, we not only have to plan, but we also must have knowledge, intention, and considerable self-regulation, as well as motivational and volitional strategies.[67] In other words, we have to know *what* we want to do, *how* we are going to do it, and as important, we need to also know why we are doing it.

The "Why" of Health

In 1945, Viktor Frankl emerged into the world after spending three years as a prisoner in Nazi concentration camps. In four different camps, including Auschwitz and Dachau, he endured extreme hunger, bitter cold, and savage brutality under the constant threat of being sent to the gas ovens. The once-distinguished Austrian psychiatrist had lost every physical belonging he'd ever owned and been forced to surrender a medical manuscript he considered his life's work. On top of everything, he had to come to grips with the knowledge that his wife, father, mother, and brother had all perished. If ever there was a person who had reason to believe his life was meaningless it was Frankl.

But rather than giving in to emptiness and desolation, Frankl penned his seminal book *Man's Search for Meaning,* which had at its core the premise that even in the most terrible situations a person still has the freedom to choose how they see their circumstances and thus create meaning out of them. "Woe to him who saw no sense in his life, no aim, no purpose, and therefore, no point in carrying on. He was soon lost," he wrote.[68] Frankl believed that the way a prisoner viewed the meaning in their life affected their mental state and therefore their longevity. And despite his own suffering, he dedicated himself to lifting the spirits of his fellow prisoners.

More than a half century after it was first published and at the time of his death in 1992, Frankl's book had been reprinted 73 times and translated into 24 languages, had sold more than 10 million copies and was still being used as a text in high schools and universities.[69] In a 1991 survey for the Library of Congress, readers were asked to name a book that made a difference in their lives and *Man's Search for Meaning* was among the top ten, keeping company with the Bible.[70] The book, and Frankl's theories about logotherapy (his belief that striving to find meaning in our life is our primary, most powerful motivating and driving force), have also inspired hundreds of studies into how and why having meaning and purpose can influence our health and wellbeing.

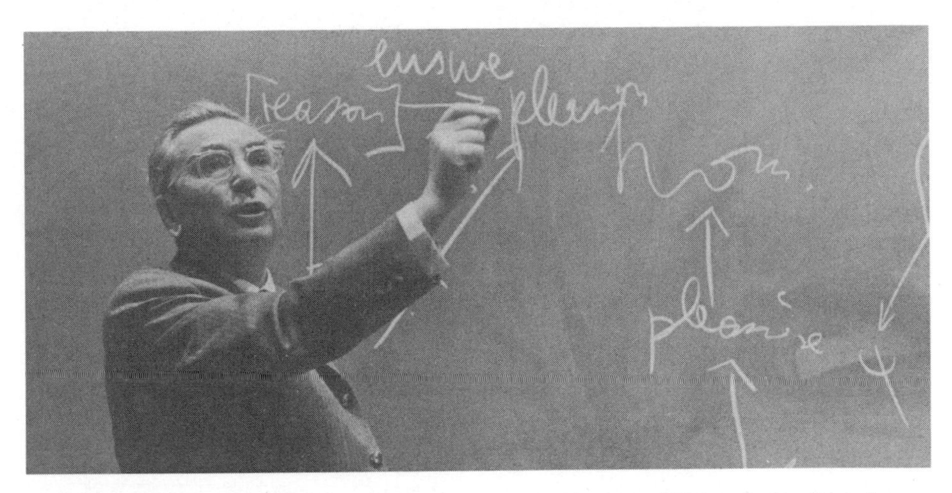

Viktor Frankl lecturing in the United States, 1967. *Credit: Imagno/Hulton Archive/Getty Images*

Today, aspiring to find meaning is now widely considered to be a critical ingredient for flourishing in life.[71] It's not surprising that people who lose meaning in their lives after a cancer diagnosis feel greater distress,[72] or that cocaine addicts who have an increased sense of purpose in life are half as likely to relapse six months after rehab as addicts who do not have that sense of purpose.[73] But what you may find surprising is that increasing evidence suggests that the more meaning and purpose people feel they have, the better health they have.

A two-year study of more than 1,500 adults with heart disease found that every one point increase on a six point "purpose in life" scale resulted in a 27 percent lower risk of suffering a heart attack.[74] Another study that followed 6,000 adults for four years found that every one point increase on a six point purpose scale was correlated with a 22 percent reduction of risk for stroke.[75] Another study that followed more than 900 seniors for seven years to quantify the incidence of Alzheimer's disease found that seniors rated as having a low purpose in life were 2.4 times more likely to develop Alzheimer's than those with a high purpose in life.[76] In a separate study, the same research team also found a slower progression of Alzheimer's among those who had a high purpose in life.[77] There is also accruing evidence that suggests that having meaning and purpose may help you actually live longer.[78]

Researchers are still unravelling the mystery behind why having a strong sense of meaning and purpose has such a significant effect on wellbeing, health, and longevity. The reasons seem to be complex and multifaceted, and may include physiological as well as psychological effects. For example, a 2015 study that tracked people over a ten-year period found that having greater life purpose predicted lower levels of allostatic load.[79] You may recall from Chapter 1 (Stress) that allostatic load refers to the negative effects on the body caused by long-term chronic stress. Purpose in life is also associated with an increase in the immune system's Natural Killer cells that attack viruses and cancer cells.[80] People with a strong sense of purpose sleep better,[81] which we know from Chapter 7 (Sleep) is critical for good health.

In an effort to put this all together, in 2013 a research team reviewed 70 studies that examined the relationship between meaning in life and various indicators of health. They found that overall, "higher levels of meaning are clearly associated with better physical health, as well as with behavioural factors that decrease the probability of negative health outcomes or increase that of positive health outcomes."[82]

The association of meaning in life with healthy behaviour may well be the key to unlocking this health secret. In 2015, researchers found that Hungarian teenagers who reported having greater meaning in their lives were more likely to eat healthily and exercise more.[83] This is supported by a large 2014 study of more than 7,000 Americans that found that the higher people scored on a purpose in life scale, the more likely they were to have various screening tests including cholesterol tests, colonoscopies, mammograms, Pap tests, and prostate exams.[84] At the same time those purpose-driven people spent more time on preventive healthcare, they also spent less time in the hospital.

This idea – that when you have meaning and purpose in your life you are more likely to engage in healthy behaviours – makes total sense. When you feel your existence matters, you have direction and purpose. You feel that what you do every day is important, and you feel driven to behave in ways that allow you to work toward your goals.

Unfortunately there's no tried and tested scientific formula you can apply to finding your life's purpose. But it doesn't have to be a cosmic mission to save the world. While some will find meaning in rallying people to a cause, others will find it in the act of comforting a sick child, or making a nutritious meal to share with others. Some people find meaning in the creation of art or music, others in a neatly prepared spreadsheet. As you move through your life you'll spend time doing mundane and routine things and you'll also spend time doing things that have significance and importance. It's the things that are important to *you* that give you a sense of meaning and purpose. In your search for meaning, in many ways what you're really asking is, "What can I do with my time that is important to me?"

Finding My "Why"

The hard work we put into the making and release of *The Connection* turned out to be worth it. The tour was sold out and people who were inspired to host their own screenings and panel discussions soon began getting in touch. The medical community also responded enthusiastically. Some of the film's biggest advocates are key influencers at hospitals and clinics, and it's uplifting that leaders at some of the most prestigious medical schools in the world continue to screen the film with students and staff. I also hear regularly from people who have seen the film, or read my blog, who tell me about the difference this information has made in their lives. Hearing from them is the fuel to a fire that burns inside me to share what I have learned on my own health journey.

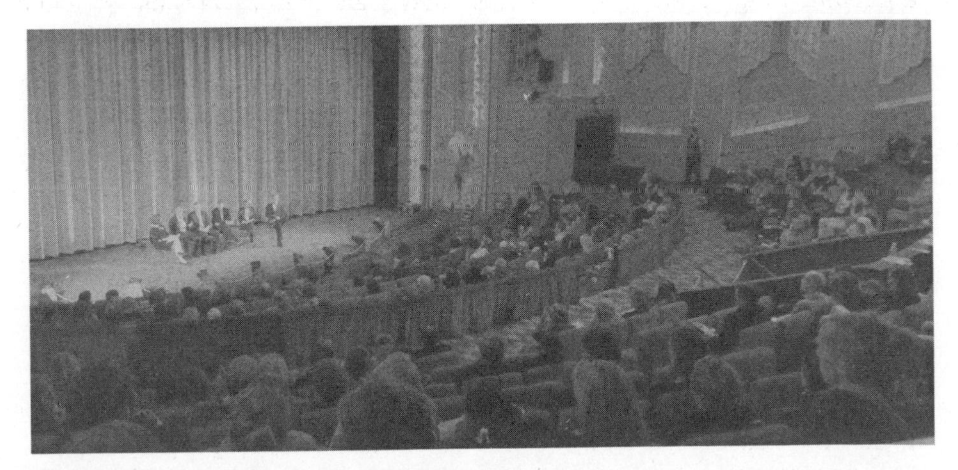

The Sydney premiere of *The Connection* documentary, 2014.

But as important as I feel my work is, when I ask myself, "What really matters in life?" the immediate things that come to mind are my marriage to Jules and my son. In fact, becoming a mother to Theodore brought a whole new meaning to my life which in turn brought my health priorities into razor sharp focus. My love for him, and my desire to be the best mother I possibly can be, drives me to seek health, vitality, and emotional balance.

When I compare the 24-year-old-me who was diagnosed with lupus with the 35-year-old me who writes these words today, I find that I have completely rewritten my list of priorities. In the past, work was always number one. Objectives, targets, and key milestones came unquestioningly before my health and my loved ones. Now, my health is number one, and being a dedicated, present, and reliable wife, mother, and friend is number two. As passionate as I am about my work, it comes in third.

This change in what matters to me most, and in what order those things are on my priority list, has been fundamental to my own journey to better health. It means that during the busy times, like the high-stakes release of the film, moment-to-moment decisions are easy. Write another email, or practice yoga? Yoga. Rush to another meeting, or stop to eat a healthy lunch? Lunch. Take a Saturday morning work call, or hang out in the park with Theodore? Theodore. The small healthy behaviours I do every day have also been transformed from necessary chores to vital allies on my bigger life quest.

Key Takeaways

1 If you're going to make changes in your life as a result of reading this book, then make them sustainable. Think of it as running a marathon, not a sprint. Remember, the healthiest individuals in The Longevity Project were united by a very distinct personality pattern. They were diligent, thorough, hardworking, reliable, responsible, committed, and persevering. In a word, they were *conscientious.*

2 In this busy modern world, having good information and an intention to implement healthy behaviour change doesn't guarantee you'll succeed. (Even if you really, *really* want to change.) You cannot rely on your willpower alone if you want the healthy changes to last. You'll need to put into place a number of strategies to keep yourself on track.

3 Your unthinking routines form the bedrock of what you do in everyday life. The more you repeat a behaviour with a consistent environmental cue, the more automatic the behaviour becomes. With repetition, the mental effort to initiate a new habit gets easier, and over time the action becomes second nature. A simple if-then planning technique can also eliminate the choices you have to make, encourage you to stop and think about the obstacles you'll face in reaching your goal, and makes your behaviour automatic. Combining if-then planning with another exercise called "mental contrasting" encourages you to focus on visualising your goals as well as visualising the obstacles that stand in your way.

4 If you want to give yourself the best chance of success in breaking bad habits and making healthy changes stick, you not only have to plan, but you also need the knowledge, intention, considerable self-regulation, and motivational and volitional strategies. In other words, you have to know *what* you want to do, *how* you are going to do it, and as important, you need to also know *why* you are doing it.

5 The more meaning and purpose you feel you have, the better your health is likely to be. When you feel your existence matters, you have direction and purpose. You feel that what you do every day is important, and you feel driven to behave in ways that allow you to work toward your goals.

Getting Started

FLICK through the chapter headings of this book and choose one aspect of your life in which you'd like to start making healthy changes. For example, you might choose to focus on your sleep and decide that you'd like to start habitually going to bed earlier. Remember, the way to form a new habit is to repeat your chosen behaviour in the same context until it becomes automatic and effortless. I suggest dedicating at least a month to each of the aspects covered in this book that resonate with you in order to make the healthy changes slow and sustainable.

PLACE a visual cue in a prominent part of your home to remind you of your "Why" for wanting to make healthy changes in your life. Remember, finding your "Why" or purpose doesn't necessarily need to involve monumental sacrifice or accomplishing great feats. Finding your "Why" can be as simple as asking: "What do I want to do with my time that is important to me?"

USE the proven if-then planning and mental contrasting techniques to help you stick to your health behaviour goals. You can download instructions from my website. See the following Extra Resources section for details.

USE smart phone apps to help you get started making healthy behaviour changes. Peter Gollwitzer has worked with his New York University psychology colleague Professor Gabrielle Oettingen to develop a free app that combines if-then planning with mental contrasting. The app is called WOOP, short for Wish–Outcome–Obstacle–Plan, and it's free. I keep a list of other recommended apps on my website that I update regularly.

Extra Resources

AVAILABLE AT
www.thewholehealthlife.com/resources

LISTEN to extended audio interviews with the experts including:

- *Peter Gollwitzer (Professor of Psychology in the Psychology Department at New York University)*
- *Stuart Biddle (Professor of Active Living and Public Health at Victoria University's Institute of Sport, Exercise and Active Living). You'll recall Biddle's work on exercise motivation and behaviour change was explored in Chapter 5 (Movement)*

DOWNLOAD instructions for how to get started with your own if-then planning strategies and how to use the mental contrasting techniques used by Gollwitzer and Oettingen in their research.

MY recommended reading list, which I update regularly, is available on my website. Books relevant to this chapter include:

- *The Longevity Project: Surprising Discoveries for Health and Long Life from the Landmark Eight-Decade Study*, Friedman and Martin
- *Man's Search for Meaning*, by Viktor E. Frankl

Epilogue

Beyond

This is the point in the book where I'd love to outline my perfect, healthy life for you. I'd love to tell you that I rise with the sun every morning after a nine hour sleep to perform an hour of yoga, followed by an hour of meditation, before floating through the rest of my day with perfectly balanced emotions, stress levels in "the green zone," and all my relationships in sublime harmony. I'd love to tell you that I have no bad habits, that I only eat foods made from scratch in my "slim by design" kitchen, and that I exercise every day, outside, at exactly the right time to induce the optimum amount of melatonin in a green forest scented with the healing aromas of Japanese cypress and white cedar.

But the reality is, it can be a challenge to always, perfectly, uncompromisingly, live the whole-health life I've outlined in this book. I'm constantly trying to find a balance between my health priorities, and the needs of my small child, my husband, my work, and spending time with my family and friends. Between the cooking and grocery shopping, the errands and appointments, the emails and interviews, the bath time and stories, there's often little time or headspace left to think about my health, let alone to make monumental changes.

I started feeling as if I were getting somewhere when I realised I could turn my attention to just one aspect of my health at a time. For example, once I learned about the importance of sleep and its connection to good health, I spent a month just working on my sleep behaviours – breaking my television habits, changing my bedtime routine, replacing the globes around our house, and getting into bed earlier. When I learned about the new science of movement and exercise that demonstrates it's not only about moving more but also about sitting less, I spent a month finding the right sit-stand work station, and I concentrated on changing the way I moved throughout my work day, using a timer to train myself to get up and move after sitting for an hour. After learning about the mindless eating traps that were set both in my home and out in the wider world, I dedicated a month to doing what I could to counter their power over me. I cleared junk from accessible places in my kitchen, I placed a fruit bowl in the most prominent place, and I started to implement rules for myself, such as never walking down the candy aisle of the supermarket.

This is not to say that during these periods when I focused on specific aspects of a whole-health life that I gave myself free range to let everything else slip. For example, I didn't have an excuse to suddenly binge on junk food just because sleep was my focus that particular month. But while I was concentrating on implementing new behaviours, if I tripped up on something else, I let it go, being careful not to let myself feel like a failure for doing so.

By taking this focussed approach, instead of giving my limited time and energy to a dozen different haphazard ideas that never quite stuck, I started feeling as if I were making progress and I noticed the impact the specific changes I made were having on various aspects of my mental and physical health. I realised, too, that small changes made big differences. This in turn helped create momentum and conviction, and with each successful change came motivation for the next one.

Nowadays, rather than trying to fit everything in, every single day, I look at my health behaviours over the span of a week. One takeaway TV dinner a week isn't a problem. One a day *is*. One night of poor sleep isn't a concern. A week of sleep deprivation gets a big red flag. Not having time to exercise one day isn't a problem. Not having time to exercise for a week is. Some days I take a "just show up" approach too. If I've put an hour of time aside for a walk and it gets derailed by a pressing matter that takes half an hour to resolve, it doesn't mean the walk is pointless. It means I have 30 minutes instead of an hour. Not every meditation I sit down to practice has to lead to blissful stillness. Not every interaction with a friend has to lead to deep and meaningful insights. Not every meal I eat has to be nutritionally optimised. While I'm not a fan of the "everything in moderation" concept – because I think it can sometimes be distorted as an excuse for unhealthy behaviour – my whole-health approach is about what happens on the *whole* that truly matters.

Shortly after *The Connection* was released, I had a routine blood test that showed there was no sign of autoimmune disease in my body. The news truly blew me away. It had been 10 years since a specialist doctor told me he suspected I had lupus, and for a long time I thought the only thing I could do for my illness was diligently take medication that wasn't going to cure me, only suppress my symptoms. Here was yet more evidence that taking the whole-health approach was actually working.

But after following the lead of Professor George Jelinek, who is featured in *The Connection* because of his remarkable recovery from multiple sclerosis, I'm careful that when it comes to describing my health, I use the word *recovery* and not *cure*. The word "cure" implies there's no more work to be done. "Recovery" means an ongoing process. While I may have optimistic blood tests on one day, I'm also aware that how I feel in both the short and the long term is ever-changing based on complex interactions. I also recognise that I have a genetic predisposition toward having an overactive immune system and although there are many things I can do for myself to try to keep those genes from switching on, they will always be part of the blueprint that makes me, me.

Although I did receive that wonderfully encouraging news in late 2014, I've also had setbacks since. The truth is, in 2015 I faced some of the toughest challenges in my journey yet. My first miscarriage happened in February. Two more miscarriages followed in the seven months after that. The worst part was the emotional pain, the hollowness of what could have been but never would be. They took a physical toll on me too. For a couple of weeks afterward I was sore and inflamed with arthritis, exhausted, and drained. But I was never once tempted to go back to my old way of life. I knew that both my mind and body have a remarkable inner capacity for resilience, and that my job was to take care of them. I not only followed the recommendations of the medical experts, I also kept meditating, writing in my diary, and communicating with the people close to me. I went for walks along the sea cliffs near my home. I picked up Theodore early from his preschool so we could just hang out. I went easy on myself, slowed down my work, and booked in for massages. I nourished myself with wholesome foods and allowed myself to sleep as much as I needed to.

Often it wasn't easy to keep up the momentum. Everything I'd learned on my health journey was being put to the test. But I had the evidence I needed to motivate me to keep going. I was able to stick with my whole-health approach and after each set back I bounced back in a matter of weeks, both physically and emotionally.

The idea of going back into "the system" was not something I relished, but despite my previously positive blood test results, we were fearful that my autoimmune disease was at the heart of the problem, so I found an excellent medical team who struck the balance between cutting edge knowledge and compassionate care. Tests were ordered, scans were performed, and blood was drawn. When all the results came in a month later there was nothing to indicate that the miscarriages were autoimmune related. "Just not meant to be" was a non-medical term used by my doctor. The news was wonderfully encouraging, and what we didn't know when we received it last December was that I was already pregnant again. We saw a blob on a screen at six weeks. At eight weeks, a strong heartbeat. At 10 weeks, a blurry hand waving at us. A 12-week blood test told us everything was looking good. At last, we allowed our spirits to soar. In August 2016 I gave birth to a healthy baby brother for Theodore, whom we named Isaac.

As I write these words, I'm the healthiest I have ever been in my life. But my journey isn't over. I continue to delve into the research and find that the science is constantly updating and evolving. While I'm aware that what is considered fact today may be further elucidated tomorrow, I can't see a future where the takeaway message from this book will shift dramatically. Good health is not just about taking our medicine, eating our vegetables, moving regularly, and getting enough sleep. Those things are all essential, but we need to take a whole-health approach. That means reviewing our beliefs and mindsets, tending to our stress levels and emotional wellbeing, surrounding ourselves with healthy people in supportive environments, and of course, nurturing our relationships.

I wrote this book in part for the 24-year-old me who faced a lifetime with a chronic disease and was searching for hope. For many years the question I wanted answered was how to get better. These days, I find myself asking what I can do to stay healthy. And often the answer is the same for both questions.

Wherever you are on your own health journey – whether you're unwell and looking for information you can trust, whether you're well and looking for inspiration to avoid getting sick, or whether you're thinking of the wellbeing of other people in your life, I also wrote this book for you. I hope the information you've read has shown you that there are many straightforward, effective, and inexpensive changes you can do for yourself that will make all the difference and help you live better. I hope this book has shown you that although the changes may sometimes be challenging, they will be unquestionably worth it. There truly is nothing to lose here and everything to gain.

I wish you well.

Shannon

Acknowledgements

If this book were a person, there are some important people that are the body parts that make it whole.

The dedicated and talented team who worked on my film *The Connection* are the legs that kicked the whole thing off. I'd particularly like to mention associate producers Diana Comino and Ellice Mol, director of photography Shing Fung Cheung, editor Mike Connerty, the distribution team including Claire McGinley and Hattie Archibald, and Steve Davis who did the additional cinematography as well as providing boundless support and advice.

The book's stomach are the scientists, researchers and experts who took the time to give me interviews, either on camera for the film, over long email exchanges, or over Skype. Thank you to Fabrizio Benedetti, Herbert Benson, Wendy Berry Mendes, Stuart Biddle, Alice Domar, Damien Finnis, Peter Gollwitzer, Craig Hassed, Hal Hershfield, Sara Lazar, George Jelinek, Jon Kabat-Zinn, David Katz, Rob Knight, Arthur Kramer, Camilla Kring, Dean Ornish, Till Roenneberg, Sarah Pressman, Ken Sheldon, David Spiegel, Esther Sternberg, Brian Wansink, and Andrew Weil. I am deeply grateful for the work that you do, which has changed my health and my life. I hope, as a result of the words in this book, it may do the same for others.

Sarah Hager Johnston is this book's immune system. As a researcher, fact checker and advisor, her expertise in finding, analysing, and communicating complex information have given it the strength and integrity that was so important to me.

Lesley Dahl, who is the editor of this book, forms it's skin. She gave it beauty and elegance, and her constant enthusiasm and encouragement also gave the book its inner glow.

No person is complete without their friends, and when this book was still in its first draft infancy, it made some very special ones, who were kind enough to read it and provide invaluable feedback. Thank you to Jenny Carter, Alice Harvey, Craig Hassed, Keith Mansfield, Simon McNamara, Sarah Moore, Joanie Purcell, Elizabeth Neal, and Justine Taylor.

It has taken 18 months to write this book. My mother- and father-in-law, Max and Alice Harvey, and my parents Kerry and Michael Jones have provided the life support to keep it breathing. Thank you for being the lungs of this book.

The heart and circulatory system of this book, and indeed all the work that I do, is Clark Carter. A friend and co-founder of *The Whole Health Life* project without whom all systems would come to a stop.

My husband Jules Harvey is the Executive Producer of *The Connection* and the managing director of our business, but these titles do not scratch the surface of what he does in order to make a book like *The Whole Health Life* come to life. Jules... thank you doesn't even come close. You are this book's wings.

DID YOU ENJOY THIS BOOK?

Don't forget to leave a review. It only takes a few minutes and I will be very grateful. Your review will help new people discover the book and enable me to continue to research and share this information with you through my books, films, and blog.

Whether it is on Amazon, Goodreads, or any site you prefer they all make a difference. If you are not sure where to start then you can go to my website for some pointers:

www.thewholehealthlife.com/review

If you'd like to keep up to date with the ongoing, latest research on staying healthy in this crazy, busy, modern world, you can read my blog or signup to my newsletter on my website:

www.thewholehealthlife.com

WANT TO LEARN MORE?

You might like to watch my film, *The Connection*.

The Connection is a feature documentary that uncovers the link between your mind, body, and health and proves we have much more to say about our health than we thought possible. It features interviews with many of the world's leading experts in mind-body medicine, as well as people with remarkable stories of healing.

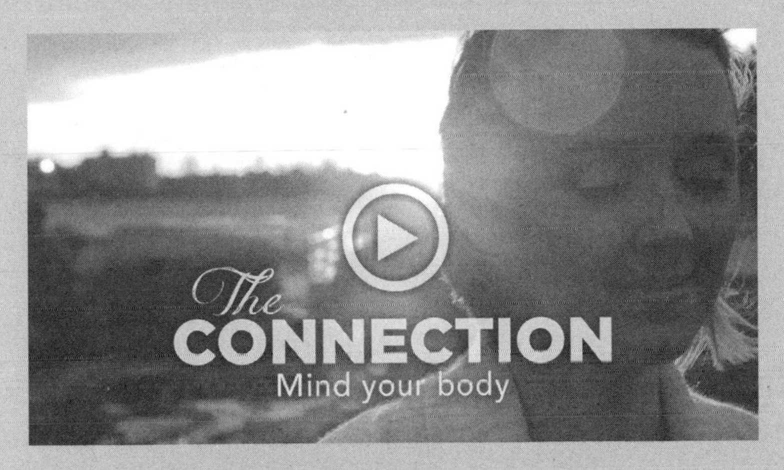

As a special thankyou for reading this book, you can now watch *The Connection* for 10% off at www.thewholehealthlife.com

Simply enter your coupon code at checkout:

10% OFF COUPON CODE: TWHLREADER

End Notes

With the exception of books and a few other cited sources, the resources cited in these notes are available online. If you'd like to explore further or read these studies for yourself, please visit my website www.thewholehealthlife.com/resources, where you will find an expanded version of these citations, complete with links to online sources.

INTRODUCTION

1. World Health Organization, 2014. *Global status report on noncommunicable diseases 2014*. Geneva: World Health Organization. – World Economic Forum, 2011. *The Global economic burden of noncommunicable diseases*. Geneva: World Economic Forum.
2. Bethell CD, Kogan MD, Strickland BB, Schor EL, Robertson J, & Newacheck PW, 2011. A national and state profile of leading health problems and health care quality for us children: key insurance disparities and across-state variations. *Academic Pediatrics,* 11(3), Supplement, Pages S22-S33. doi: 10.1016/j.acap.2010.08.011
3. Patton, M, 2015. Health insurance premiums are rising faster than income, *Forbes*, 30 June.
4. Medibank, n.d. *Helping deliver quality and affordability.* Melbourne: Medibank.
5. World Health Organization, 2014. *Global status report on noncommunicable diseases 2014*. Geneva: World Health Organization.
6. World Economic Forum, 2011. *The Global economic burden of noncommunicable diseases*. Geneva: World Economic Forum.
7. Kelland, K, 2011. WHO warns of enormous burden of chronic disease. Reuters, 27 April.
8. Demaio, Ar, & Lander, F, 2012. Five myths about the global epidemic of chronic diseases. *The Conversation* [online], 29 May. – United Nations, 2011. *Non-communicable diseases deemed development challenge of 'epidemic proportions' in political declaration adopted during landmark general assembly summit.* [news release] 19 September.
9. World Health Organization 2009. *Global health risks: mortality and burden of disease attributable to selected major risks*. Geneva: World Health Organization.
10. Egger G, & Dixon J, 2014. Beyond obesity and lifestyle: a review of 21st century chronic disease determinants. *BioMed Research International*, 2014:731685. doi:10.1155/2014/731685
11. Ward, BW, Schiller, JS, & Goodman, RA, 2014. Multiple chronic conditions among us adults: a 2012 update. *Preventing Chronic Disease* 11:130389, 17 April. – Gerteis J, Izrael D, Deitz D, LeRoy L, Ricciardi R, Miller T, & Basu J., 2014. *Multiple Chronic conditions chartbook: 2010 medical expenditure panel survey data.* (AHRQ Publications No. Q14-0038) Rockville, MD: Agency for Healthcare Research and Quality, April.
12. Dall, T, West, T, Chakrabarti, R, & Iacobucci, W, 2015. *The complexities of physician supply and demand: projections from 2013 to 2025: final report.* Prepared for the Association of American Medical Colleges by HIS, Inc. Washington: Association of American Medical Colleges, March.
13. Brownson, RC, Kreuter, MW, Arrington, BA, & True, WR, 2006. Translating scientific discoveries into public health action: how can schools of public health move us forward? *Public Health Reports*, 121(1), 97-103, January-February. – Schuster, MA, McGlynn, EA, & Brook, RH, 1998. How good is the quality of health care in the United States? *The Milbank Quarterly*, 76(4), 517-563.
14. Shanafelt TD, Boone S, Tan L, Dyrbye, LN, Sotile, W, Satele, D, West, CP, Sloan, J, & Oreskovich, MR, 2012. Burnout and satisfaction with work-life balance among US physicians relative to the general US population. *Archives of Internal Medicine*, 172(18), 1377-1385, 9 October. doi:10.1001/archinternmed.2012.3199
15. Morris, ZS, Wooding, S, & Grant, J, 2011. The answer is 17 years, what is the question: understanding time lags in translational research. *Journal of the Royal Society of Medicine*, 104(12), 510-520, December. doi: 10.1258/jrsm.2011.110180.
16. Hassed, C, [2006 or 2007]. *Mind-body medicine: science, practice and philosophy.* Lifestyle and Culture Lectures [website], Melbourne: School of Philosophy, October 2006 [title page] or 6 July 2007 [interior pages].
17. Kiecolt-Glaser, J, & Glaser, R, 1992. Psychoneuroimmunology: can psychological interventions modulate immunity? *Journal of Consulting and Clinical Psychology,* 60(4), 569-575, August. doi: 10.1037/0022-006X.60.4.569 – Kiecolt-Glaser, JK, Glaser, R, Strain, E, Stout, J, Tarr, K, Holliday, J, & Speicher, CE, 1986. Modulation of cellular immunity in medical students. *Journal of Behavioral Medicine,* 9(1), 5-21, February. doi:10.1007/BF00844640
18. McEwen, BS, 2004. Protection and damage from acute and chronic stress: allostasis and allostatic overload and relevance to the pathophysiology of psychiatric disorders. *Annals of the New York Academy of Sciences*, 1032:1-7, December. doi: 10.1196/annals.1314.001
19. Benhard, JD, Kristeller, J, & Kabat-Zinn, J, 1988. Effectiveness of relaxation and visualization techniques as an adjunct to phototherapy and photochemotherapy of psoriasis. (Letter) *Journal of the American Academy of Dermatology*, 19(3), 572-4, September. doi: http://dx.doi.org/10.1016/S0190-9622(88)80329-3 – Kabat-Zinn J, Wheeler E, Light T, Skillings A, Scharf MJ, Cropley TG, Hosmer D, & Bernhard JD, 1998. Influence of a mindfulness meditation-based stress reduction intervention on rates of skin clearing in patients with moderate to severe psoriasis undergoing phototherapy (UVB) and photochemotherapy (PUVA). *Psychosomatic Medicine*, 60(5), 625-32, September-October.
20. Ornish D, Scherwitz LW, Billings JH, Lance Gould, K, Merritt, TA, Sparler, S, Armstrong, WT, Ports, TA, Kirkeeide, RL, Hogeboom C, & Brand, RJ, 1998. Intensive lifestyle changes for reversal of coronary heart disease. *Journal of the American Medical Association*, 280(23), 2001-2007, 16 December. doi:10.1001/jama.280.23.2001.
21. Ornish D, Brown SE, Scherwitz LW, Billings JH, Armstrong WT, Ports TA, McLanahan SM, Kirkeeide RL, Brand RJ, & Gould KL, 1990. Can lifestyle changes reverse coronary heart disease? The Lifestyle Heart Trial. *Lancet*, 336(8708), 129-33, 21 July. doi: http://dx.doi.org/10.1016/0140-6736(90)91656-U – Ornish D, Scherwitz LW, Billings JH, Brown SE, Gould KL, Merritt TA, Sparler S, Armstrong WT, Ports TA, Kirkeeide RL,

Hogeboom C, & Brand RJ, 1998. Intensive lifestyle changes for reversal of coronary heart disease. *Journal of the American Medical Association*, 280(23), 2001-2007, 16 December. doi:10.1001/jama.280.23.2001. – Gould KL, Ornish D, Scherwitz L, Brown S, Edens RP, Hess MJ, Mullani N, Bolomey L, Dobbs F, Armstrong WT, Merritt, T, Ports, T, Sparler, S, & Billings J, 1995. Changes in myocardial perfusion abnormalities by positron emission tomography after long-term, intense risk factor modification. *Journal of the American Medical Association*, 274(11), 694-701, 20 September. doi:10.1001/jama.1995.03530110056036.

22. Pischke CR, Weidner G, Elliott-Eller M, Scherwitz L, Merritt-Worden TA, Marlin R, Lipsenthal L, Finkel R, Saunders D, McCormac P, Scheer JM, Collins RE, Guarneri EM, & Ornish D, 2006. Comparison of coronary risk factors and quality of life in coronary artery disease patients with versus without diabetes mellitus. *American Journal of Cardiology*, 97(9), 1267-73, 01 May. doi: 10.1016/j.amjcard.2005.11.051 – Ornish D, Weidner G, Fair WR, Marlin R, Pettengill EB, Raisin CJ, Dunn-Emke S, Crutchfield L, Jacobs FN, Barnard RJ, Aronson WJ, McCormac P, McKnight DJ, Fein JD, Dnistrian AM, Weinstein J, Ngo TH, Mendell NR, & Carroll PR, 2005. Intensive lifestyle changes may affect the progression of prostate cancer. *Journal of Urology*, 174(3), 1065-1070, September. doi: 10.1097/01.ju.0000169487.49018.73 – Ornish D, Magbanua MJ, Weidner G, Weinberg V, Kemp C, Green C, Mattie MD, Marlin R, Simko J, Shinohara K, Haqq CM, & Carroll PR, 2008. Changes in prostate gene expression in men undergoing an intensive nutrition and lifestyle intervention. *Proceedings of the National Academy of Sciences of the United States of America*, 105(24), 8369-8374, 17 June. doi: 10.1073/pnas.0803080105
23. Highmark, 2000. *Dean Ornish Program for reversing heart disease: cost effectiveness summary.* Pittsburgh: Highmark, 12 July.
24. Stahl, JE Dossett, ML, LaJoie, AS, Denniger, JW, Mehta, DH, Goldman R, Fricchione GL, & Benson H, 2015. Relaxation response and resiliency training and its effect on healthcare resource utilization. *PLoS ONE* 10(10): e0140212, 13 October. doi: 10.1371/journal.pone.0140212
25. Bhasin MK, Dusek JA, Chang BH, Joseph MG, Denninger JW, Fricchione GL, Benson H, & Libermann TA, 2013. Relaxation response induces temporal transcriptome changes in energy metabolism, insulin secretion and inflammatory pathways. *PLoS ONE*, 8(5): e62817, 01 May. doi: 10.1371/journal.pone.0062817
26. Jelinek, G., 2010. *Overcoming Multiple Sclerosis: An Evidence-Based Guide to Recovery.* Sydney: Allen & Unwin.
27. Jelinek, G. & Law, K., 2013. *Recovering from multiple sclerosis: Real life stories of hope and inspiration.* Sydney: Allen & Unwin.

CHAPTER 1 – STRESS

1. O'Loughlin, T, & Gabbatt, A, 2009. Samoa tsunami: at least 100 feared dead on Pacific islands. *The Guardian*, 30 September.
2. American Psychological Association, 2016. *Discrimination linked to increased stress, poorer health, American Psychological Association survey finds.* [news release] Washington, DC: American Psychological Association, 10 March.
3. Robinson, L, Magee, C, Safadi, M, & Sharma, R, 2014. *Health Profile of Australian Employees.* Prepared by the Centre for Health Initiatives for the Workplace Health Association Australia. Sydney: Workplace Health Association Australia.
4. Health and Safety Executive, 2015. *Work related Stress, Anxiety and Depression Statistics in Great Britain 2015.* London: Health and Safety Executive, October.
5. American Psychological Association, 2016. *Stress in America Press Room* [web site]. Washington, DC: American Psychological Association.
6. Goh, J, Pfeffer, J, & Zenios, SA, 2016. The relationship between workplace stressors and mortality and health costs in the United States. *Management Science* 62(2), 608-628, February. doi: 10.1287/mnsc.2014.2115
7. Oster, S, 2014. In China, 1,600 people die every day from working too hard. *Bloomberg Business*, 03 July.
8. American Psychological Association, 2016. *Stress in America: The impact of discrimination.* (Stress in America™ Survey.) Washington, DC: American Psychological Association, 10 March.
9. Cohen, S, Janicki-Deverts, D, & Miller, GE, 2007. Psychological stress and disease. (Commentary) *Journal of the American Medical Association*, 298(14), 1685-1687, 10 October. doi: 10.1001/jama.298.14.1685 – Gouin, J-P, 2011. Chronic stress, immune dysregulation, and health. *American Journal of Lifestyle Medicine*, 5(6), 476-485, November/December. doi: 10.1177/1559827610395467
10. Ansell, EB, Rando, K, Tuit, K, Guarnaccia, J, & Sinha, R, 2012. Cumulative adversity and smaller gray matter volume in medial prefrontal, anterior cingulate, and insula regions. *Biological Psychiatry*, 2(1), 57-64, 01 July. doi: 10.1016/j.biopsych.2011.11.022.
11. For more information, visit the website of The Stress and Health Research Program in the Institute for Behavioral Medicine Research at the Ohio State University Medical Center (http://pni.osumc.edu/). – American Psychological Association, 2006. *Stress weakens the immune system.* [online] Washington, DC: American Psychological Association, February 23.
12. Epel, ES, Blackburn, EH, Lin, J, Dhabhar, FS, Adler, NE, Morrow, JD, & Cawthon, RM, 2004. Accelerated telomere shortening in response to life stress. *Proceedings of the National Academy of Sciences of the United States of America*, 101(49), 17312-17315, 07 December. doi: 10.1073/pnas.0407162101
13. Dhabhar, FS, 2014. Effects of stress on immune function: the good, the bad, and the beautiful. *Immunologic Research*, 58(2-3), 193-210, May. doi: 10.1007/s12026-014-8517-0.
14. World Surf League, 2015. *Shark attacks Mick Fanning at J-Bay Open.* [video online] Santa Monica, CA: World Surf League, 19 July.
15. Pawle, F, 2015. Great white attacked Mick Fanning, says Andrew Fox, shark expert. *The Australian*, 20 July.
16. ABC News, 2015. *Mick Fanning describes J-Bay shark encounter.* [video online] Sydney: ABC News (Australia), 21 July.
17. Dhabhar, FS, Malarkey, WB, Neri, E, & McEwen, BS, 2012. Stress-induced redistribution of immune cells - from barracks to boulevards to battlefields: a tale of three hormones - Curt Richter Award Winner. *Psychoneuroendocrinology*, 37(9), 1345-1368, September. doi: 10.1016/j.psyneuen.2012.05.008
18. Jansen, AS, Nguyen, XV, Karpitsky, V, Mettenleiter, TC, & Loewy, AD, 1995. Central command neurons of the sympathetic nervous system: basis of the fight-or-flight response. *Science*, 270(5236), 644-646, 27 October. doi: 10.1126/science.270.5236.644
19. Dhabhar, FS, 2014. Effects of stress on immune function: the good, the bad, and the beautiful. *Immunologic Research*, 58(2-3), 193-210, May. doi: 10.1007/s12026-014-8517-0.
20. Cohen, S, Janicki-Deverts, D, Doyle, WJ, Miller, GE, Frank, E, Rabin, BS, & Turner, RB, 2012. Chronic stress, glucocorticoid receptor resistance, inflammation, and disease risk. *Proceedings of the National Academy of Sciences of the United States of America*, 109(16), 5995-5000, 17 April. doi: 10.1073/pnas.1118355109
21. McEwen, BS, 2006. Protective and damaging effects of stress mediators: central role of the brain. *Dialogues in Clinical Neuroscience*, 8(4), 367-381, December.
22. Dhabhar, FS, & Viswanathan, K, 2005. Short-term stress experienced at time of immunization induces a long-lasting increase in immunologic memory. *American Journal of Physiology - Regulatory, Integrative and Comparative Physiology*, 289(3), R738-R744, September. doi: 10.1152/ajpregu.00145.2005 – TEDTalentSearch, 2012. Firdaus Dhabhar: *The positive effects of stress.* [video online]. New York: TED, 25 June.
23. Rosenberger, PH, Ickovics, JR, Epel, E, Nadler, E, Jokl, P, Fulkerson, JP, Tillie, JM & Dhabhar, FS, 2009. Surgical stress-induced immune cell

redistribution profiles predict short-term and long-term postsurgical recovery. *The Journal of Bone and Joint Surgery (American volume)*, 91(12), 2783-2794, 01 December. doi: 10.2106/JBJS.H.00989
24. Sainani, K, 2014. What, me worry? *Stanford Magazine*, May/June.
25. Dhabhar, FS 2009. A hassle a day may keep the pathogens away: the fight-or-flight stress response and the augmentation of immune function. *Integrative and Comparative Biology*, 49(3), 215-236, September. doi: 10.1093/icb/icp045.
26. MologhWNews, 2015. *Julian Wilson in tears as he recounts...* [video online] s.l.: MologhWNews, 19 July.
27. Taylor, SE, Klein, LC, Lewis, BP, Gruenewald, TL, Gurung, RAR, & Updegraff, JA, 2000. Biobehavioral responses to stress in females: tend-and-befriend, not fight-or-flight. *Psychological Review*, 107(3), 411-429, July. http://dx.doi.org/10.1037/0033-295X.107.3.411
28. Hidenobu, S, Nakae, A, Kanai, R, & Ishiguro, H, 2013. Huggable communication medium decreases cortisol levels. *Scientific Reports* 3:3034, 23 October. doi: 10.1038/srep03034 – Cohen, S, Janicki-Deverts, D, Turner, RB, & Doyle, WJ, 2015. Does hugging provide stress-buffering social support? a study of susceptibility to upper respiratory infection and illness. *Psychological Science* 26(2), 135-147, February. doi: 10.1177/0956797614559284.
29. Selye, H, 1975. Implications of stress concept, *New York State Journal of Medicine*, 75: 2139-2145, October.
30. Le Fevre, M, Kolt, GS, & Matheny, J, 2006. Eustress, distress and their interpretation in primary and secondary occupational stress management interventions: which way first? *Journal of Managerial Psychology*, 21(6), pp.547-565, July. doi: 10.1108/02683940610684391
31. Szabo, S, Tache, Y, & Somogyi, A, 2012. The legacy of Hans Selye and the origins of stress research: a retrospective 75 years after his landmark brief "Letter" to the Editor of *Nature*. *Stress* 15(5), 472-478, September. doi: 10.3109/10253890.2012.710919.
32. Le Fevre, M, Kolt, GS, & Matheny, J, 2006. Eustress, distress and their interpretation in primary and secondary occupational stress management interventions: which way first? *Journal of Managerial Psychology*, 21(6), pp.547-565, July. doi: 10.1108/02683940610684391
33. Petticrew, MP, & Lee, K, 2011. The "Father of Stress" meets "Big Tobacco": Hans Selye and the tobacco industry. *American Journal of Public Health*, 101(3), 411-418, March. doi: 10.2105/AJPH.2009.177634.
34. Trotter, RJ, 1975, Stress: confusion & controversy, *Science News*, 107(22), 356-357, 359. – Lazarus, RS, 1993. From psychological stress to the emotions: a history of changing outlooks. *Annual review of psychology*, 44: 1-21, February. doi: 10.1146/annurev.ps.44.020193.000245 – Mason, JW, 1975. A historical view of the stress field. *Journal of Human Stress*, 1(1), 6-12, March. doi:10.1080/0097840X.1975.9940399.
35. Jeremy, JP, Mendes, WB, Blackstock, E, & Schmader, T, 2010. Turning the knots in your stomach into bows: reappraising arousal improves performance on the GRE. *Journal of Experimental Social Psychology*, 46(1), 208-212. doi:10.1016/j.jesp.2009.08.015 – Vine, SJ, Freeman, P, Moore, LJ, Chandra-Ramanan, R & Wilson, MR, 2013. Evaluating stress as a challenge is associated with superior attentional control and motor skill performance: testing the predictions of the biopsychosocial model of challenge and threat, *Journal of Experimental Psychology: Applied*, 19(3), 185-194, September. doi: 10.1037/a0034106. – Jamieson JP, Nock MK, & Mendes WB, 2012. Mind over matter: reappraising arousal improves cardiovascular and cognitive responses to stress, *Journal of Experimental Psychology: General*, 141(3), 417-422, August. doi: 10.1037/a0025719.
36. Epel, ES, Blackburn, EH, Lin, J, Dhabhar, FS, Adler, NE, Morrow, JD & Cawthon, RM, 2004. Accelerated telomere shortening in response to life stress. *Proceedings of the National Academy of Sciences of the United States of America*, 101(49), 17312-17315, 07 December. doi: 10.1073/pnas.0407162101.
37. Keller, A, Litzelman, K, Wisk, LE, Maddox, T, Cheng, ER, Creswell, PD, & Witt, WP, 2012. Does the perception that stress affects health matter? the association with health and mortality. *Health Psychology*, 31(5), 677-684, September. http://doi.org/10.1037/a0026743.
38. Benson, H, 1975. *The Relaxation response*. New York: HarperCollins.
39. Wallace, RK, Benson, H, & Wilson, AF, 1971. A wakeful hypometabolic physiologic state. *American Journal of Physiology*, 221(3), 795-799, September. – Benson, H, Beary, JF, & Carol, MP, 1974. The relaxation response. *Psychiatry*, 37(1), 37-46, February. – Beary JF & Benson H, 1974. A simple psychophysiologic technique which elicits the hypometabolic changes of the relaxation response. Psychosomatic Medicine, 36(2), 115-120, March-April. – Wallace, RK, & Benson, H, 1972. The physiology of meditation. *Scientific American* 226(2), 84-90, February. – Benson, H, 1975. *The Relaxation response*. New York: HarperCollins.
40. Bhasin, MK, Dusek, JA, Chang, BH, Joseph, MG, Denninger, JW, Fricchione, GL, Benson, H, & Libermann, TA, 2013. Relaxation response induces temporal transcriptome changes in energy metabolism, insulin secretion and inflammatory pathways. *PLoS ONE*, 8(5), 01 May. doi: 10.1371/journal.pone.0062817.
41. Mcgreevey, S, 2013. Mind-body genomics. *Harvard Medical School News*, 01 May.
42. Mccubbin, T, Dimidjian, S, Kempe, K, Glassey, MS, Ross, C, & Beck, A, 2014. Mindfulness-based stress reduction in an integrated care delivery system: one-year impacts on patient-centered outcomes and health care utilization. *Permanente Journal*, 18(4), 4-9, Fall. doi: 10.7812/TPP/14-014. – Khoury, B, Sharma, M, Rush, SE, & Fournier, C, 2015. Mindfulness-based stress reduction for healthy individuals: A meta-analysis. *Journal of Psychosomatic Research*, 78(6), 519-528, June. doi: 10.1016/j.jpsychores.2015.03.009. – Crowe, M, Jordan, J, Burrell, B, Jones, V, Gillon, D, & Harris, S, 2016. Mindfulness-based stress reduction for long-term physical conditions: A systematic review. The Australian and New Zealand Journal of Psychiatry, 50(1), 21-32, January. doi: 10.1177/0004867415607984.
43. Kabat-Zinn, J, Wheeler, E, Light, T, Skillings, A, Scharf, MJ, Cropley, TG, Hosmer, D & Bernhard, JD, 1998. Influence of a mindfulness meditation-based stress reduction intervention on rates of skin clearing in patients with moderate to severe psoriasis undergoing phototherapy (UVB) and photochemotherapy (PUVA). *Psychosomatic Medicine*, 60(5), 625-632, September-October.
44. Kabat-Zinn, J, 2014. Interview in *Conversation Series* (Episode 5). Interviewed by Shannon Harvey. [video online] The Connection & Elemental Media, 2014.
45. Pickert, K, 2014. The mindful revolution, *TIME Magazine*, 03 February.
46. Essig, T, 2012. Google teaches employees to 'search inside yourself.' *Forbes*, 30 April.
47. Gregoire, C, 2013. The daily habit of these outrageously successful people. *The Huffington Post*, 05 July.
48. Huffington, A, 2013. Mindfulness, meditation, wellness and their connection to corporate America's bottom line. *The Huffington Post*, 18 March.
49. Davidson, RJ, Kabat-Zinn, J, Schumacher, J, Rosenkranz, M, Muller, D, Santorelli, SF, Urbanowski, F, Harrington, A, Bonus, K, & Sheridan, JF, 2003. Alterations in brain and immune function produced by mindfulness meditation. *Psychosomatic Medicine*, 65(4), 564-570, July-August. doi: 10.1097/01.PSY.0000077505.67574.E3
50. Grossman, P, Niemann, L, Schmidt, S, & Walach, H, 2003. Mindfulness-based stress reduction and health benefits. *The Journal of Psychosomatic Research*, 57(1), 35-43. doi: http://dx.doi.org/10.1016/S0022-3999(03)00573-7
51. Goyal, M, Singh, S, Sibinga, EM, Gould, NF, Rowland-Seymour, A, Sharma, R, Berger, Z, Sleicher, D, Maron, DD, Shihab, HM, Ranasinghe, PD, Linn, S, Saha, S, Bass, EB, & Haythornthwaite, JA, 2014. Meditation programs for psychological stress and well-being: a systematic review and meta-analysis. JAMA Internal Medicine, 174(3), 357-368, March. doi: 10.1001/jamainternmed.2013.13018.
52. Slagter, HA, Lutz, A, Greischar, LL, Francis, AD, Nieuwenhuis, S, Davis, JM, & Davidson, RJ, 2007. Mental training affects distribution of limited brain resources, *PLOS Biology*, 5(6), e138, June. doi:10.1371/journal.pbio.0050138
53. Tang, YY, Ma, Y, Wang, J, Fan, Y, Feng, S, Lu, Q, Yu, Q, Sui, D, Rothbart, MK, Fan, M, & Posner, MI, 2007. Short-term meditation training improves attention and self-regulation *Proceedings of the National Academy of Sciences of the United States of America*, 104(43), 17152-17156, 23 October. doi: 10.1073/pnas.0707678104
54. Hölzel, BK, Carmody, J, Evans, KC, Hoge, E.A, Dusek, JA, Morgan, L, Pitman, RK, & Lazar, SW, 2010. Stress reduction correlates with structural changes in the amygdala. *Social Cognitive and Affective Neuroscience*, 5(1), 11-17, March. . doi: 10.1093/scan/nsp034
55. Cervellin, G, & Lippi, G, 2011. From music-beat to heart-beat: A journey in the complex interactions between music, brain, and heart. *European Journal of Internal Medicine*, 22(4), 371-374, August. doi: 10.1016/j.ejim.2011.02.019. – Bernatzky, G, Presch, M, Anderson, M, & Panksepp, J, 2011. Emotional foundations of music as a non-pharmacological pain management tool in modern medicine, *Neuroscience and Biobehavioral Reviews*, 35(9), 1989-1999, October. doi: 10.1016/j.neubiorev.2011.06.005.

56. Lindgren, L, Rundgren, S, Winsö, O, Lehtipalo, S, Wiklund, U, Karlsson, M, Stenlund, H, Jacobsson, C, & Brulin, C, 2010. Physiological responses to touch massage in healthy volunteers. *Autonomic Neuroscience: Basic & Clinical*, 158(1-2), 105-110, December. doi: 10.1016/j.autneu.2010.06.011.
57. Sloan, DM, Feinstein, BA, & Marx, BP, 2009. The durability of beneficial health effects associated with expressive writing. *Anxiety, Stress, and Coping*, 22(5), 509-523, October. doi: 10.1080/10615800902785608.
58. Mimica, N, & Kalinić, D, 2011. Art therapy may be benefitial [sic] for reducing stress-related behaviours in people with dementia – case report. *Psychiatria Danubina*, 23(1), 125-128, March.
59. Morita, E, Fukuda, S, Nagano, J, Hamajima, N, Yamamoto, H, Iwai, Y, Nakashima, T, Ohira, H, & Shirakawa, T, 2007. Psychological effects of forest environments on healthy adults: Shinrin-yoku (forest-air bathing, walking) as a possible method of stress reduction. *Public Health*, 121(1), 54-63, January. doi: http://dx.doi.org/10.1016/j.puhe.2006.05.024
60. Faraut, B, Boudjeltia, KZ, Dyzma, M, Rousseau, A, David, E, Stenuit, P, Franck, T, Van Antwerpen, P, Vanhaeverbeek, M, & Kerkhofs, M, 2011. Benefits of napping and an extended duration of recovery sleep on alertness and immune cells after acute sleep restriction. *Brain, Behavior, and Immunity*, 25(1), 16-24, January. doi: 10.1016/j.bbi.2010.08.001.
61. Light, KC, Grewen, KM, & Amico, JA, 2005. More frequent partner hugs and higher oxytocin levels are linked to lower blood pressure and heart rate in premenopausal women, *Biological Psychology*, 69(1), 5-21, April. doi:10.1016/j.biopsycho.2004.11.002
62. Steptoe, A, Gibson, EL, Vuononvirta, R, Williams, ED, Hamer, M, Rycroft, JA, Erusalimsky, JD, & Wardle, J, 2007. The effects of tea on psychophysiological stress responsivity and post-stress recovery: a randomised double-blind trial, *Psychopharmacology*, 190(1), 81-89, January. doi 10.1007/s00213-006-0573-2.
63. Scholey, A, Haskell, C, Robertson, B, Kennedy, D, Milne, A, & Wetherell, M, 2009. Chewing gum alleviates negative mood and reduces cortisol during acute laboratory psychological stress, *Physiology and Behaviour*, 97(3-4), 304-312, 22 June. doi: 10.1016/j.physbeh.2009.02.028.
64. American Psychological Association, 2008. *Stress in America*. [news release] Washington, DC: American Psychological Association, October 7.
65. van Leeuwen, S, Singer, W, & Melloni, L, 2012. Meditation increases the depth of information processing and improves the allocation of attention in space. *Frontiers in Human Neuroscience*, volume 6, article 133, 1-16, 15 May. doi: 10.3389/fnhum.2012.00133
66. Lazar, SW, Kerr, CE, Wasserman, RH, Gray, JR, Greve, DN, Treadway, MT, McGarvey, M, Quinn, BT, Dusek, JA, Benson, H, Rauch, SL, Moore, CI, & Fischl, B, 2005. Meditation experience is associated with increased cortical thickness. *Neuroreport*, 16(17), 1893-1897, 28 November. doi: 10.1097/01.wnr.0000186598.66243.19
67. Moore, A, Gruber, T, Derose, J, & Malinowski, P, 2012. Regular, brief mindfulness meditation practice improves electrophysiological markers of attentional control. *Frontiers in Human Neuroscience*, volume 6, article 18, 1-5, 10 February. doi: 10.3389/fnhum.2012.00018.
68. Hölzel, BK, Carmody, J, Vangel, M, Congleton, C, Yerramsetti, SM, Gard, T, & Lazar, SW, 2011. Mindfulness practice leads to increases in regional brain gray matter density, *Psychiatry Research*, 191(1), 36-43, 30 January. doi: 10.1016/j.pscychresns.2010.08.006.
69. Zeidan, F, Johnson, SK, Diamondc, BJ, David, Z, & Goolkasian, P, 2010. Mindfulness meditation improves cognition: evidence of brief mental training. *Consciousness and Cognition*, 19(2), 597-605, June. doi: 10.1016/j.concog.2010.03.014.
70. Zeidan, F, Gordon, NS, Merchant, J, & Goolkasian, P, 2009. The Effects of brief mindfulness meditation training on experimentally induced pain. *The Journal of Pain*, 11(3), 199-209, March. doi: 10.1016/j.jpain.2009.07.015.
71. Moore, A, Gruber, T, Derose, J, & Malinowski, P, 2012. Regular, brief mindfulness meditation practice improves electrophysiological markers of attentional control. *Frontiers in Human Neuroscience*, volume 6, article 18, 1-15, February. doi: 10.3389/fnhum.2012.00018.

CHAPTER 2 – EMOTIONS

1. Harrington, A, 2008. *The cure within: A history of mind-body medicine*. New York: W.W. Norton.
2. Gottman, J, 2012. Interview: Paul Ekman. *The Milton H. Erickson Foundation Newsletter* 32(2), 1, 26-28, Summer/Fall. – Sample, I, 2003. Can you guess how I'm feeling? *The Guardian*, July 9.
3. Ekman, P, 2003. *Emotions revealed: Recognizing faces and feelings to improve communication and emotional life*. New York: Times Books.
4. Darwin, C, 1886. *The Expression of the emotions in man and animals*. London: Appleton.
5. Davidson, RJ, Ekman, P, Saron, CD, Senulis, JA, & Friesen, WV, 1990. Approach-withdrawal and cerebral asymmetry: emotional expression and brain physiology. I. *Journal of personality and social psychology*, 58(2), 330-341, February. doi: 10.1037/0022-3514.58.2.330 – Ekman, P, Davidson, RJ, & Friesen, WV, 1990. The Duchenne smile: emotional expression and brain physiology. II. *Journal of personality and social psychology*, 58(2), 342-353, February. doi: 10.1037/0022-3514.58.2.342
6. Kang, DH, Davidson, RJ, Coe, CL, Wheeler, RE, Tomarken, AJ, & Ershler WB, 1991. Frontal brain asymmetry and immune function. *Behavioral Neuroscience*, 105(6), 860-869, December. doi: 10.1037/0735-7044.105.6.860
7. Davidson, RJ, & Begley, S, 2012. *The Emotional life of your brain: how its unique patterns affect the way you think, feel, and live–and how you can change them*. New York: Hudson Street Press, page 133.
8. Davidson, RJ, Coe, CC, Dolski, I, & Donzella, B, 1999. Individual differences in prefrontal activation asymmetry predict natural killer cell activity at rest and in response to challenge. *Brain, Behavior, and Immunity*, 13(2), 93-108, June. doi:10.1006/brbi.1999.0557
9. Pressman, SD, & Cohen, S, 2005. Does positive affect influence health? *Psychological Bulletin*, 131(6), 925-971, November. doi: 10.1037/0033-2909.131.6.925
10. Brummett, BH, Helms, MJ, Dahlstrom, WG, & Siegler, IC, 2006. Prediction of all-cause mortality by the Minnesota Multiphasic Personality Inventory Optimism-Pessimism Scale scores: Study of a college sample during a 40-year follow-up period. *Mayo Clinic Proceedings*, 81(12), 1541-1544, December. doi: http://dx.doi.org/10.4065/81.12.1541
11. Diener, E, & Chan, MY, 2011. Happy people live longer: Subjective well-being contributes to health and longevity. *Applied Psychology: Health and Well-Being*, 3(1), 1-43, January. doi:10.1111/j.1758-0854.2010.01045.x
12. Carver, CS, Scheier, MF, & Segerstrom, SC, 2010. Optimism. *Clinical Psychology Review*, 30(7), 879-889, November. http://doi.org/10.1016/j.cpr.2010.01.006
13. Lench, HHG, 2011. Personality and health outcomes. Making positive expectations a reality. *Journal of Happiness Studies*, 12(3), 493-507. http://doi.org/10.1007/s10902-010-9212-z
14. Robles, TF, Brooks, KP, & Pressman, SD, 2009. Trait positive affect buffers the effects of acute stress on skin barrier recovery. Health Psychology, 28(3), 373-378, May. doi: 10.1037/a0014662
15. Cohen, S, Doyle, WJ, Turner, RB, Alper, CM, & Skoner, DP. 2003. Emotional style and susceptibility to the common cold. *Psychosomatic Medicine*, 65(4), 652-657, July-August. doi: 10.1097/01.PSY.0000077508.57784.DA
16. Cohen, S, Alper, CM, Doyle, WJ, Treanor, JJ, & Turner, RB, 2006. Positive emotional style predicts resistance to illness after experimental exposure to rhinovirus or influenza A virus. *Psychosomatic Medicine*, 68, 809-815, November-December doi: 10.1097/01.psy.0000245867.92364.3c
17. Ein-Dor, T, Mikulincer, M, & Shaver, PR, 2011. Effective reaction to danger: attachment insecurities predict behavioral reactions to an experimentally induced threat above and beyond general personality traits. *Social Psychological and Personality Science*, 2(5), 467-473, August. doi: 10.1177/1948550610397843
18. Ein-Dor, T, 2012. Social defense theory: How a mixture of personality traits in group contexts may promote our survival. In: M. Mikulincer & PR Shaver, eds., 2014. *Mechanisms of social connection: From brain to group*. (The Herzliya series on personality and social psychology.) Washington, DC: American Psychological Association, 357-372.
19. Forgas, JP, 1998. On being happy and mistaken: mood effects on the fundamental attribution error. *Journal of Personality and Social Psychology*, 75(2), 318-331, August. doi: 10.1037/0022-3514.75.2.318
20. Forgas, JP, Goldenberg, L, & Unkelbach, C, 2009. Can bad weather

improve your memory? An unobtrusive field study of natural mood effects on real-life memory. *Journal of Experimental Social Psychology*, 45(1), 254-257, January. doi: 10.1016/j.jesp.2008.08.014

21. Forgas, JP, 2011. The upside of feeling down: The benefits of negative mood for social cognition and social behaviour. In: *14th Sydney Symposium of Social Psychology, 2011: Social Thinking and Interpersonal Behaviour.* Sydney: University of New South Wales, 15-17 March 2011.
22. Forgas, JP, 2007. When sad is better than happy: negative affect can improve the quality and effectiveness of persuasive messages and social influence strategies. *Journal of Experimental Social Psychology*, 43(4), 513-528, July. doi: 10.1016/j.jesp.2006.05.006
23. Friedman, HS, 2000. Long-term relations of personality and health: dynamisms, mechanisms, tropisms. *Journal of Personality*, 68(6), 1089-1107, December. doi: 10.1111/1467-6494.00127
24. Veenhoven, R, 2008. Healthy happiness: effects of happiness on physical health and the consequences for preventive health care. *Journal of Happiness Studies*, 9(3), 449-469, September. doi: 10.1007/s10902-006-9042-1 – Friedman, HS, & Kern, ML, 2014. Personality, well-being, and health. *Annual Review of Psychology*, 65, 719-742. doi: 10.1146/annurev-psych-010213-115123
25. Coyne, JC, Pajak, TF, Harris, J, Konski, A, Movsas, B, Ang, K, & Watkins Bruner D, 2007. Emotional well-being does not predict survival in head and neck cancer patients: a Radiation Therapy Oncology Group study. *Cancer*, 110(11), 2568-2575, December. doi: 10.1002/cncr.23080
26. Spiegel, D, & Kraemer, HC, 2008. Emotional well-being does not predict survival in head and neck cancer patients: a Radiation Therapy Oncology Group study (Correspondence). *Cancer*, 112(10), 2326-2327, 15 May. doi : 10.1002/cncr.23435
27. Coyne, JC & Tennen, H, 2010. Positive psychology in cancer care: bad science, exaggerated claims, and unproven medicine. *Annals of Behavioral Medicine*, 39(1), 16-26, February. doi: 10.1007/s12160-009-9154-z
28. Pressman, SD, & Cohen, S, 2005. Does positive affect influence health? *Psychological Bulletin*, 131(6), 925-971, November. doi: 10.1037/0033-2909.131.6.925.
29. World Health Organization, 2015. *Depression.* (Fact Sheet). Geneva: World Health Organization, April.
30. Marcus, M, Yasamy, MT, van Ommeren, M, Chisholm, D, & Saxena S, 2012. Depression: a global public health concern. In: World Federation for Mental Health, *Depression: A Global Crisis; World Mental Health Day, October 10 2012.* Occoquan, VA: World Federation for Mental Health, October 10, pp.6-8.
31. Kessler, RC, McGonagle, KA, Zhao, S, Nelson, CB, Hughes, M, Eshleman, S, Wittchen, HU, & Kendler, KS, 1994. Lifetime and 12-month prevalence of DSM-III-R psychiatric disorders in the United States: Results from the National Comorbidity Survey. *Archives of General Psychiatry*, 5(1), 8-19, January. doi: 10.1001/archpsyc.1994.03950010008002
32. Marcus, M, Yasamy, MT, van Ommeren, M, Chisholm, D, & Saxena S, 2012. Depression: a global public health concern. In: World Federation for Mental Health, *Depression: A Global Crisis; World Mental Health Day, October 10 2012.* Occoquan, VA: World Federation for Mental Health, October 10, pp.6-8.
33. American Psychiatric Association, 1994. *Diagnostic and statistical manual of mental disorders.* 4th ed. Arlington, VA: American Psychiatric Association.
34. Chapman, DP, Perry, GS, & Strine, TW, 2005. The vital link between chronic disease and depressive disorders. *Preventing Chronic Disease: Public Health Research, Practice, and Policy*, 2(1), 1-10, January.
35. Ali, S, Stone, MA, Peters, JL, Davies, MJ, & Khunti, K, 2006. The prevalence of co-morbid depression in adults with Type 2 diabetes: a systematic review and meta-analysis. *Diabetic Medicine*, 23(11), 1165-1173, November. doi: 10.1111/j.1464-5491.2006.01943.x – Spijkerman, T, de Jonge, P, van den Brink, RH, Jansen, JH, May, JF, Crijns, HJ, & Ormel, J, 2005. Depression following myocardial infarction: first-ever versus ongoing and recurrent episodes. *General Hospital Psychiatry*, 27(6), 411-417, December. doi: http://dx.doi.org/10.1016/j.genhosppsych.2005.05.007
36. Patten, SB, 2001. Long-term medical conditions and major depression in a Canadian population study at waves 1 and 2. *Journal of Affective Disorders*, 63(1-3), 35-41, March. doi: http://dx.doi.org/10.1016/S0165-0327(00)00186-5
37. Reddy, MS, 2010. Depression: The disorder and the burden. *Indian Journal of Psychological Medicine*, 32(1), 1-2, January. doi: 10.4103/0253-7176.70510
38. Murray, CJL & Lopez, AD, eds., 1996. *The global burden of disease: A comprehensive assessment of mortality and disability from diseases, injuries, and risk factors in 1990 and projected to 2020.* (Global burden of disease and injury series, volume 1) [Cambridge, MA]: Published by the Harvard School of Public Health on behalf of the World Health Organization and the World Bank.
39. Reddy, MS, 2010. Depression: the disorder and the burden. *Indian Journal of Psychological Medicine*, 32(1), 1-2, January. doi: 10.4103/0253-7176.70510
40. DiMatteo, MR, Lepper, HS, & Croghan, TW, 2000. Depression is a risk factor for noncompliance with medical treatment: meta-analysis of the effects of anxiety and depression on patient adherence. *Archives of Internal Medicine*, 160(14), 2101-2107, July. doi: 10.1001/archinte.160.14.2101.
41. Cuijpers, P, Berking, M, Andersson, G, Quigley, L, Kleiboer, A, & Dobson, KS, 2013. A meta-analysis of cognitive-behavioural therapy for adult depression, alone and in comparison with other treatments. *Canadian Journal of Psychiatry*, 58(7), 376-385, July. doi: 10.1177/070674371305800702
42. Barnhofer, T, Crane, C, Hargus, E, Amarasinghe, M, Winder, R, & Williams, JM, 2009. Mindfulness-based cognitive therapy as a treatment for chronic depression: A preliminary study. Behavior Research and Therapy, 47(5), 366-373, May. doi: 10.1016/j.brat.2009.01.019. – Britton, WB, Shahar, B, Szepsenwol, O, & Jacobs, WJ, 2012. Mindfulness-based cognitive therapy improves emotional reactivity to social stress: Results from a randomized controlled trial. *Behavior Therapy*, 43(2), 365-380, June. doi: 10.1016/j.beth.2011.08.006
43. Sin, NL, & Lyubomirsky, S, 2009. Enhancing well-being and alleviating depressive symptoms with positive psychology interventions: a practice-friendly meta-analysis. *Journal of Clinical Psychology*, 65(5), 467-487, May. doi: 10.1002/jclp.20593 – Sin, NL, Della Porta, MD, & Lyubomirsky, S, 2011. Tailoring positive psychology interventions to treat depressed individuals. In SI Donaldson, M Csikszentmihalyi, & J Nakamura, eds., 2011. *Applied positive psychology: Improving everyday life, health, schools, work, and society* (Applied Psychology Series). New York: Routledge, 79-96.
44. Britton, WB, Shahar, B, Szepsenwol, O, & Jacobs, WJ, 2012. Mindfulness-based cognitive therapy improves emotional reactivity to social stress: Results from a randomized controlled trial. *Behavior Therapy*, 43(2), 365-380, June. doi: 10.1016/j.beth.2011.08.006
45. Wang, PS, Berglund, PA, Olfson, M, & Kessler, RC, 2004. Delays in Initial Treatment Contact after First Onset of a Mental Disorder. *HSR: Health Services Research*, 39(2), 393-416, April. doi: 10.1111/j.1475-6773.2004.00234.x
46. Fredrickson, BL, 2009. *Positivity: Top-notch research reveals the upward spiral that will change your life.* New York: Harmony Books.
47. Ehrenreich, BB, 2010. *Bright-sided: How positive thinking is undermining America.* New York: Picador.
48. Hershfield, HE, Scheibe, S, Sims, TL, & Carstensen, LL, 2013. When feeling bad can be good: mixed emotions benefit physical health across adulthood. *Social Psychological and Personality Science*, 4(1), 54-61, January. doi: 10.1177/1948550612444616
49. Folkman, S, & Moskowitz, JT, 2000. Stress, positive emotion, and coping. *Current Directions in Psychological Science*, 9(4), 115-118, August. doi: 10.1111/1467-8721.00073
50. Tully, SM, Hershfield, HE, & Meyvis, T, 2015. Seeking lasting enjoyment with limited money: financial constraints increase preference for material goods over experiences. *Journal of Consumer Research*, Vol. 42, 59-75. doi: 10.1093/jcr/ucv007.
51. Adler, JM, & Hershfield, HE, 2012. Mixed emotional experience is associated with and precedes improvements in psychological well-being. *PLoS ONE*, 7(4), e35633. doi: 10.1371/journal.pone.0035633
52. Hershfield, HE, Scheibe, S, Sims, TL, & Carstensen, LL, 2013. When feeling bad can be good: mixed emotions benefit physical health across adulthood. *Social Psychological and Personality Science*, 4(1), 54-61, January. doi: 10.1177/1948550612444616
53. Kashdan, TB, & Biswas-Diener, R, 2014. *The upside of your dark side: why being your whole self–not just your "good" self–drives success and fulfillment.* New York: Hudson Street Press.
54. Chapman, BP, Fiscella, K, Kawachi, I, Duberstein, P, & Muennig P, 2013. Emotion suppression and mortality risk over a 12-year follow-up. *Journal of Psychosomatic Research*, 75(4), 381-385, October. doi: 10.1016/j.jpsychores.2013.07.014.
55. Evers, C, Marijn Stok, F, & de Ridder, DT, 2010. Feeding your feelings: emotion regulation strategies and emotional eating. *Personality and Social Psychology Bulletin*, 36(6), 792-804, June. doi: 10.1177/0146167210371383.

56. Mund, M, & Mitte K, 2012. The costs of repression: a meta-analysis on the relation between repressive coping and somatic diseases. *Health Psychology*, 31(5), 640-649, September. doi: 10.1037/a0026257.
57. Gleiberman, L, 2007. Repressive/defensive coping, blood pressure, and cardiovascular rehabilitation. *Current Hypertension Reports*, 9(1), 7-12, March. doi: 10.1007/s11906-007-0003-9
58. Harburg, E, Julius, M, Kaciroti, N, Gleiberman, L, & Schork, MA, 2003. Expressive/suppressive anger-coping responses, gender, and types of mortality: a 17-year follow-up (Tecumseh, Michigan, 1971-1988). *Psychosomatic Medicine*, 65(4), 588-597, July-August. doi: 10.1097/01.PSY.0000075974.19706.3B – Denollet, J, Gidron, Y, Vrints, CJ, & Conraads, VM, 2010. Anger, suppressed anger, and risk of adverse events in patients with coronary artery disease. *American Journal of Cardiology*, 105(110, 1555-1560, June. doi: 10.1016/j.amjcard.2010.01.015. – Stürmer, T, Hasselbach, P, & Amelang, M, 2006. Personality, lifestyle, and risk of cardiovascular disease and cancer: follow-up of population based cohort. *BMJ*, 332(7554), 1359, 10 June. doi: 10.1136/bmj.38833.479560.80.
59. Frattaroli, J, 2006. Experimental disclosure and its moderators: A meta-analysis. *Psychological Bulletin*, 132(6), 823-865, November. doi: 10.1037/0033-2909.132.6.823
60. Pennebaker, JW, & Francis, ME, 1996. Cognitive, emotional, and language processes in disclosure. *Cognition and Emotion*, 10(6), 601-626, September. doi: 10.1080/026999396380079
61. Pennebaker, JW, Kiecolt-Glaser, JK, & Glaser, R, 1988. Disclosure of traumas and immune function: health implications for psychotherapy. *Journal of Consulting and Clinical Psychology*, 56(2), 239-245, April. doi: 10.1037/0022-006X.56.2.239
62. Petrie, KJ, Booth, RJ, Pennebaker, JW, Davison, KP, & Thomas, MG, 1995. Disclosure of trauma and immune response to a hepatitis B vaccination program. *Journal of Consulting and Clinical Psychology*, 63(5), 787-792, October. doi: 10.1037/0022-006X.63.5.787
63. Lepore, SJ, 1997. Expressive writing moderates the relation between intrusive thoughts and depressive symptoms. *Journal of Personality and Social Psychology*, 73(5), 1030-1037, November. doi: 10.1037/0022-3514.73.5.1030 – Murray, EJ, & Segal, DJ, 1994. Emotional processing in vocal and written expression of feelings about traumatic experiences. *Journal of Traumatic Stress*, 7(3), 391-405, July. doi: 10.1002/jts.2490070305
64. Sloan, DM, Marx, BP, & Epstein, EM, 2005. Further examination of the exposure model underlying the efficacy of written emotional disclosure. *Journal of Consulting and Clinical Psychology*, 73(3), 549-554, June. doi: 10.1037/0022-006X.73.3.549
65. Pennebaker, JW, & Chung, CK, 2011. Expressive writing: Connections to physical and mental health. In: H. S. Friedman, ed., 2011. *The Oxford handbook of health psychology*. Oxford; New York: Oxford University Press, Chapter 18. doi: 10.1093/oxfordhb/9780195342819.013.0018 – Krpan, KM, Kross, E, Berman, MG, Deldin, PJ, Askren, MK, & Jonides, J, 2013. An everyday activity as a treatment for depression: The benefits of expressive writing for people diagnosed with major depressive disorder. *Journal of Affective Disorders*, 150(3), 1148-1151, 25 September. doi: 10.1016/j.jad.2013.05.065
66. Pennebaker, JW, & Chung, CK, 2011. Expressive writing: Connections to physical and mental health. In: H. S. Friedman, ed., 2011. *The Oxford handbook of health psychology*. Oxford; New York: Oxford University Press, Chapter 18. doi: 10.1093/oxfordhb/9780195342819.013.0018
67. Brickman, P, Coates, D, & Janoff-Bulman, R, 1978. Lottery winners and accident victims: Is happiness relative? *Journal of Personality and Social Psychology*, 36(8), 917-927, August.
68. Headey, B, & Wearing, A, 1989. Personality, life events, and subjective well-being: Toward a dynamic equilibrium model. *Journal of Personality and Social Psychology*, 57(4), 731-739, September. doi: 10.1037/0022-3514.57.4.731
69. Davidson, RJ and Begley, S, 2012. *The Emotional life of your brain: how its unique patterns affect the way you think, feel, and live–and how you can change them*. New York: Hudson Street Press.
70. Bartels, M, & Boomsma, DI, 2009. Born to be happy? The etiology of subjective well-being. *Behavior Genetics*, 39(6), 605-615, November. doi: 10.1007/s10519-009-9294-8 – Lykken, D, & Tellegen, A, 1996. Happiness is a stochastic phenomenon. *Psychological Science*, 7(3), 186-189, May. doi: 10.1111/j.1467-9280.1996.tb00355.x – Røysamb, E, Harris, JR, Magnus, P, Vittersø, J, & Tambs, K, 2002. Subjective well-being: sex-specific effects of genetic and environmental factors. *Personality and Individual Differences*, 32(2), 211-223, January. doi: 10.1016/S0191-8869(01)00019-8 – Stubbe, JH, Posthuma, D, Boomsma, DI, & De Geus, EJC, 2005. Heritability of life satisfaction in adults: a twin-family study. *Psychological Medicine*, 35(11), 1581-1588, November. doi: 10.1017/S0033291705005374 – Nes, RB, Røysamb, E, Tambs, K, Harris, JR, & Reichborn-Kjennerud, T, 2006. Subjective well-being: genetic and environmental contributions to stability and change. *Psychological Medicine*, 36(7), 1033-1042, July. doi: 10.1017/S0033291706007409
71. Lykken, D, & Tellegen, A, 1996. Happiness is a stochastic phenomenon. *Psychological Science*, 7(3), 186-189, May. doi: 10.1111/j.1467-9280.1996.tb00355.x
72. Sheldon, KM, & Lyubomirsky, S, 2007. Is it possible to become happier? (And if so, how?). *Social and Personality Psychology Compass*, 1(1), 129-145, November. doi: 10.1111/j.1751-9004.2007.00002.x
73. Sheldon, KM, & Lyubomirsky, S, 2012. The challenge of staying happier: testing the hedonic adaptation prevention model. *Personality and Social Psychology Bulletin*, 38(5), 670-680, May. doi: 10.1177/0146167212436400
74. Wood AM, Froh JJ, & Geraghty AW, 2010. Gratitude and well-being: a review and theoretical integration. *Clinical Psychology Review*, 30(7), 890-905, November. doi: 10.1016/j.cpr.2010.03.005. – Jose, PE, Lim, BT, & Bryant, FB, 2012. Does savoring increase happiness? A daily diary study, *The Journal of Positive Psychology*, 7(3), 176-187, April. doi: 10.1080/17439760.2012.671345 – Musick, MA, Herzog, AR, & House, JS, 1999. Volunteering and mortality among older adults: findings from a national sample. *The Journals of Gerontology Series B: Psychological Sciences and Social Sciences*, 54(3), S173-S180. – Poulin, MJ, Brown, SL, Dillard, AJ, & Smith, DM, 2013. Giving to others and the association between stress and mortality. *American Journal of Public Health*, 103(9), 1649-1655, September. doi: 10.2105/AJPH.2012.300876
75. Sin, NL, & Lyubomirsky, S, 2009. Enhancing well-being and alleviating depressive symptoms with positive psychology interventions: a practice-friendly meta-analysis. *Journal of Clinical Psychology*, 65(5), 467-487, May. doi: 10.1002/jclp.20593
76. Bolier, L, Haverman, M, Westerhof, GJ, Riper, H, Smit, F, & Bohlmeijer, E, 2013. Positive psychology interventions: a meta-analysis of randomized controlled studies. *BMC Public Health*, 13:119, 08 February. doi: 10.1186/1471-2458-13-119.
77. Sheldon, KM, Boehm, J, & Lyubomirsky, S, 2013. Variety is the spice of happiness: the hedonic adaptation prevention model. In S. David, I. Boniwell, & A.C. Ayers (eds.), *Oxford handbook of happiness*. Oxford: Oxford University Press, pp. 901-914. doi: 10.1093/oxfordhb/9780199557257.013.0067
78. Lyubomirsky, S, Dickerhoof, R, Boehm, JK, & Sheldon, KM, 2011. Becoming happier takes both a will and a proper way: an experimental longitudinal intervention to boost well-being. *Emotion*, 11(2), 391-402, April. doi:10.1037/a0022575.
79. Coyne, JC and Tennen, H, 2010. Positive psychology in cancer care: bad science, exaggerated claims, and unproven medicine. *Annals of Behavioral Medicine*, 39(1), 16-26, February. doi: 10.1007/s12160-009-9154-z – Thombs, BD, Roseman, M, Coyne, JC, de Jonge, P, Delisle, VC, Arthurs, E, Levis, B, & Ziegelstein, RC, 2013. Does evidence support the American Heart Association's recommendation to screen patients for depression in cardiovascular care? An updated systematic review. *PLoS ONE*, 8(1), e52654. doi: 10.1371/journal.pone.0052654.
80. Friedman, HS, & Kern, ML, 2014. Personality, well-being, and health. *Annual Review of Psychology*, 65, 719-742. doi: 10.1146/annurev-psych-010213-115123

CHAPTER 3 – BELIEF

1. Ozkan, S, Murk, W, & Arici, A, 2008. Endometriosis and infertility: epidemiology and evidence-based treatments. *Annals of the New York Academy of Sciences*, 1127:92-100, April. doi: 10.1196/annals.1434.007. – Viganò, P, Parazzini, F, Somigliana, E, Vercellini, P, 2004. Endometriosis: epidemiology and aetiological factors. *Best practice & research. Clinical obstetrics & gynaecology*, 18(2), 177-200, April. doi: 10.1016/j.bpobgyn.2004.01.007
2. Abbott, J, Hawe, J, Hunter, D, Holmes, M, Finn, P, & Garry, R, 2004. Laparoscopic excision of endometriosis: a randomized, placebo-controlled trial. *Fertility and Sterility*, 82(4), 878-884, October. doi: 10.1016/j.fertnstert.2004.03.046

3. Abbott, JA, Jarvis, SK, Lyons, SD, Thomson, A, & Vancaille, TG, 2006. Botulinum toxin type A for chronic pain and pelvic floor spasm in women: A randomized controlled trial. *Obstetrics and Gynecology*, 108(4), 915-923, October. doi: 10.1097/01.AOG.0000237100.29870.cc – Levine, JD, Gordon, NC, & Fields, HL, 1978. The mechanism of placebo analgesia. *Lancet*, 312(8091), 654-657, 23 September. doi: 10.1016/S0140-6736(78)92762-9 – Price, DD, Milling, LS, Kirsch, I, Duff, A, Montgomery, GH, & Nicholls, SS, 1999. An analysis of factors that contribute to the magnitude of placebo analgesia in an experimental paradigm. *Pain*, 83:2), 147-156, November. doi: 10.1016/S0304-3959(99)00081-0 – Amanzio, M, Pollo, A, Maggi, G, & Benedetti, F, 2001. Response variability to analgesics: a role for non-specific activation of endogenous opioids. *Pain*, 90(3), 205-215, February. doi: 10.1016/S0304-3959(00)00486-3 – Moerman, DE, 2002. Explanatory mechanisms for placebo effects: cultural influences and the meaning response. In HA Guess, A Kleinman, JW Kusek, & LW Engel (eds.), *The science of the placebo: toward an interdisciplinary research agenda*. London: BMJ Books, pages 77-107. – Flaten, MA, Simonsen, T, & Olsen, H, 1999. Drug-related information generates placebo and nocebo responses that modify the drug response. *Psychosomatic Medicine*, 61(2), 250-255, March-April.
4. Beecher, HK, 1946. Pain in men wounded in battle. *Annals of Surgery*, 123(1), 96-105, January. – Beecher, HK, 1955. The control of pain in men wounded in battle. In Hays, SB, Surgery in World War II, Part I, Chapter II. In JB Coates, ME Debakey, WP Giddings, & EM Mcfetridge (eds.), Volume II, *General Surgery*. Washington, DC: Office of the Surgeon General, Department of the Army, 1955.
5. Beecher, HK, 1946. Pain in men wounded in battle. *Annals of Surgery*, 123(1), 96-105, January.
6. Beecher, HK, 1955. The powerful placebo. *Journal of the American Medical Association*, 159(17), 1602-1606, December 24. doi:10.1001/jama.1955.02960340022006.
7. Kienle, GS, & Kiene, H, 1997. The powerful placebo effect: fact or fiction? *Journal of Clinical Epidemiology*, 50(12), 1311-1318, December. doi: http://dx.doi.org/10.1016/S0895-4356(97)00203-5
8. Roberts, AH, Kewman, DG, Mercier, L, & Hovell, M, 1993. The power of nonspecific effects in healing: implications for psychosocial and biological treatments. *Clinical Psychology Review*, 13(5), 375-391. doi:10.1016/0272-7358(93)90010-J
9. De Craen, AJ, Moerman, DE, Heisterkamp, SH, Tytgat, GN, Tijssen, JG, & Kleijnen, J, 1999. Placebo effect in the treatment of duodenal ulcer. *British Journal of Clinical Pharmacology*, 48(6), 853-860, December. doi: 10.1046/j.1365-2125.1999.00094.x
10. Wilson IB, 2010. Adherence, placebo effects, and mortality. Comment on Avins, AL, et al, 2010. Placebo adherence and its association with morbidity and mortality in the studies of left ventricular dysfunction. [*Journal of General Internal Medicine*, 25(12), 1275-1281, December, doi: 10.1007/s11606-010-1477-8]. *Journal of General Internal Medicine*, 25(12), 1270-1272, December doi: 10.1007/s11606-010-1530-7. – Hartz, A, & He, T, 2013. Why is greater medication adherence associated with better outcomes. *Emerging Themes in Epidemiology* 10(1). doi: 10.1186/1742-7622-10-1
11. Egerton-Warburton, D, Meek, R, Mee, MJ, & Braitberg, G, 2014. Antiemetic use for nausea and vomiting in adult emergency department patients: randomized controlled trial comparing ondansetron, metoclopramide, and placebo. *Annals of Emergency Medicine*, 64(5), 526-532, November. doi: 10.1016/j.annemergmed.2014.03.017
12. de Craen, AJM, Tijssen, JGP, de Gans, J, & Kleijnen, J 2000. Placebo effect in the acute treatment of migraine: subcutaneous placebos are better than oral placebos. *Journal of Neurology*, 247(3), 183-188, March. doi: 10.1007/s004150050560
13. Kam-Hansen, S, Jakubowski, M, Kelley, JM, Kirsch, I, Hoaglin, DC, Kaptchuk, TJ, & Burstein, R, 2014. Altered placebo and drug labeling changes the outcome of episodic migraine attacks. *Science Translational Medicine*, 6(218), 218ra5, January. doi: 10.1126/scitranslmed.3006175.
14. Waber, RL, Shiv, B, Carmon, Z, & Ariely, D, 2008. Commercial features of placebo and therapeutic efficacy. (Research Letter) *The Journal of the American Medical Association*, 299(9), 1016-1017, 05 March. doi: 10.1001/jama.299.9.1016.
15. de Craen, AJM, Roos, PJ, de Vries, AL, Kleijnen, J, 1996. Effect of colour of drugs: systematic review of perceived effect of drugs and of their effectiveness. *British Medical Journal*, 313, 1624-1626, 21 December.
16. Cattaneo, AD, Lucchelli, PE, & Filippucci, G, 1970. Sedative effects of placebo treatment. *European Journal of Clinical Pharmacology*, 3(1), 43-45, December.
17. Holtedahl, R, Brox, JI, & Tjomsland, O, 2015. Placebo effects in trials evaluating 12 selected minimally invasive interventions: a systematic review and meta-analysis. *BMJ Open*, 5(1). doi:10.1136/bmjopen-2014-007331
18. Ader, R, & Cohen, N, 1975. Behaviorally conditioned immunosuppression. *Psychosomatic Medicine*, 37(4), 333-340, July-August.
19. Goebel, MU, Trebst, AE, Steiner, J, Xie, YF, Exton, MS, Frede, S, Canbay, AE, Michel, MC, Heemann, U, Schedlowski, M, 2002. Behavioral conditioning of immunosuppression is possible in humans. *FASEB Journal*, 16(14), 1869-1873, December. doi: 10.1096/fj.02-0389com
20. Benedetti, F, Pollo, A, & Colloca, L, 2007. Opioid-mediated placebo responses boost pain endurance and physical performance: is it doping in sport competitions? *Journal of Neuroscience*, 27(44), 11934-11939. doi:10.1523/JNEUROSCI.3330-07.2007
21. Ader, R, Mercurio, MG, Walton, J, James, D, Davis, M, Ojha, V, Kimball, AB, Fiorentino, D, 2010. Conditioned pharmacotherapeutic effects: a preliminary study. *Psychosomatic Medicine*, 72(2), 192-197, February. doi:/10.1097/PSY.0b013e3181cbd38b
22. University of Rochester Medical Center, 2009. *Study redefines placebo effect as part of effective treatment: It's not drug or placebo; it's drug and placebo*. [news release] Rochester, NY: University of Rochester Medical Center, 22 December.
23. Arnold, MH, Finniss, DG, & Kerridge, I, 2014. Medicine's inconvenient truth: the placebo and nocebo effect. *Internal Medicine Journal*, 44(4), 398-405, April. doi: 10.1111/imj.12380.
24. Benedetti, F, Frisaldi, E, Carlino, E, Giudetti, L, Pampallona, A, Zibetti, M, Lanotte, M, & Lopiano, L, 2016. Teaching neurons to respond to placebos. *Journal of Physiology*, 24 February. doi:10.1113/JP271322
25. Benedetti, F, 2014. *Placebo effect* (2nd ed.) Oxford: Oxford University Press.
26. Amanzio, M, & Benedetti, F, 1999. Neuropharmacological dissection of placebo analgesia: expectation-activated opioid systems versus conditioning activated specific subsystems. *Journal of Neuroscience*, 19(1), 484-494, January.
27. de la Fuente-Fernández, R, Ruth, TJ, Sossi, V, Schulzer, M, Calne, DB, & Stoessl, AJ, 2001. Expectation and dopamine release: mechanism of the placebo effect in Parkinson's disease. *Science*, 293(5532), 1164-1166, 10 August. – de la Fuente-Fernández, R, Phillips, AG, Zamburlini, M, Sossi, V, Calne, DB, Ruth, TJ, & Stoessl AJ, 2002. Dopamine release in human ventral striatum and expectation of reward. *Behavioural Brain Research*, 136(2), 359-363, 15 November. doi:10.1016/S0166-4328(02)00130-4
28. Benedetti, F, Carlino, E, & Pollo, A, 2011. How placebos change the patient's brain. *Neuropsychopharmacology*, 36(1), 339-354, January. doi: 10.1038/npp.2010.81.
29. Benedetti, F, Carlino, E, & Pollo, A, 2011. How placebos change the patient's brain. *Neuropsychopharmacology*, 36(1), 339-354, January. doi: 10.1038/npp.2010.81.
30. Benedetti, F, Durando, J, & Vighetti, S, 2014. Nocebo and placebo modulation of hypobaric hypoxia headache involves the cyclooxygenase-prostaglandins pathway. *Pain*, 155(5), 921-928, May. doi: 10.1016/j.pain.2014.01.016.
31. Mendes, WB, 2013. Inspired by the question, not the measure: exploiting neurobiological responses in the service of intergroup research. In B Derks, D Scheepers, & N Ellemers (eds.), 2013, *Neuroscience of Prejudice and Intergroup Relations*. New York: Psychology Press, 2013. Chapter 16.
32. Kirschbaum, C, Pirke, KM, & Hellhammer, DH, 1993. The 'Trier Social Stress Test': a tool for investigating psychobiological stress responses in a laboratory setting. *Neuropsychobiology*, 28(1-2), 76-81. doi: 10.1159/000119004 – Birkett, MA, 2011. The Trier Social Stress Test protocol for inducing psychological stress. *Journal of Visualized Experiments*, 56, 3238, 19 October. doi: 10.3791/3238 – Frisch, JU, Häusser, JA, Mojzisch, A, 2015. The Trier Social Stress Test as a paradigm to study how people respond to threat in social interactions. *Frontiers in Psychology*, 6(14), 1-15, 02 February. doi: 10.3389/fpsyg.2015.00014.
33. Emotions, thoughts, and health: what all aging bodies should know; Emotions, decisions, and behavior across the life span: surprises from social psychology, 2012. Presented by Wendy Berry Mendes. UCSF Osher Mini Medical School for the Public [Show ID: 23207] [video] La Jolla, CA: University of California Television (UCTV), April 19. – Jamieson, JP, Nock, MK, & Mendes, WB, 2012. Mind over matter: reappraising arousal improves cardiovascular and cognitive responses to stress. *Journal of Experimental Psychology*, 141(3), 417-422, August. doi: 10.1037/a0025719.
34. Mendes, WB, Blascovich, J, Hunter, SB, Lickel, B, & Jost, JT, 2007. Threatened by the unexpected: physiological responses during social interac-

tions with expectancy-violating partners. *Journal of Personality and Social Psychology* 92(4), 698-716, April. doi: 10.1037/0022-3514.92.4.698

35. UBS, 2009. Restatement of UBS's annual report 2008: Important notice. Zurich: UBS, May 20; modified on 22 May 2013.
36. Crum, AJ, Salovey, P, & Achor, S, 2013. Rethinking stress: The role of mindsets in determining the stress response. *Journal of Personality and Social Psychology*, 104(4), 716-733, April. doi: 10.1037/a0031201
37. Change your mindset, change the game. 2014. [video] Presented by A Crum. Traverse City, MI: TEDx.
38. Crum, AJ, Salovey, P, & Achor, S, 2013. Rethinking stress: The role of mindsets in determining the stress response. *Journal of Personality and Social Psychology*, 104(4), 716-733, April. doi: 10.1037/a0031201
39. Levy, BR, & Myers, LM, 2004. Preventive health behaviors influenced by self-perceptions of aging. *Preventive Medicine*, 39(3), 625-629, September. doi:10.1016/j.ypmed.2004.02.029
40. Coyne, J, 2014. Eminent Harvard psychologist, mother of positive psychology, New Age quack? *Science-Based Medicine*, November 16.
41. Feinberg, C, 2010. The mindfulness chronicles: on "the psychology of possibility." *Harvard Magazine*, September-October.
42. Rippon, I, & Steptoe, A, 2014. Feeling old vs being old: Associations between self-perceived age and mortality. *JAMA Internal Medicine*, 175(2), 307-309, December. doi: 10.1001/jamainternmed.2014.6580 – Kotter-Grühn, D, Kleinspehn-Ammerlahn, A, Gerstorf, D, & Smith, J, 2009. Self-perceptions of aging predict mortality and change with approaching death: 16-year longitudinal results from the Berlin Aging Study. *Psychology and Aging*, 24(3), 654-667, September. doi: 10.1037/a0016510. – Uotinen, V, Rantanen, T, & Suutama, T, 2005. Perceived age as a predictor of old age mortality: A 13-year prospective study. *Age and Ageing*, 34(4), 368-372, July. doi: 10.1093/ageing/afi091 – Levy, BR, Slade, MD, Kunkel, SR, & Kasl, SV, 2002. Longevity increased by positive self-perceptions of aging. *Journal of Personality and Social Psychology*, 83(2), 261-270, August. doi: 10.1037/0022-3514.83.2.261
43. Langer, EJ, 2009. *Counter clockwise: mindful health and the power of possibility*. New York: Ballantine Books.
44. Chvetzoff, G, & Tannock, IF, 2003. Placebo effects in oncology. *Journal of the National Cancer Institute*, 95(1), 19-29, January. doi: 10.1093/jnci/95.1.19
45. Zhang, W, Robertson, J, Jones, AC, Dieppe, PA, & Doherty, M, 2008. The placebo effect and its determinants in osteoarthritis: Meta analysis of randomised controlled trials. *Annals of the Rheumatic Diseases*, 67(12), 1716-1723, December. doi: 10.1136/ard.2008.092015
46. Furmark, T, Appel, L, Henningsson, S, Åhs, F, Faria, V, Linnman, C, Pissiota, A, Frans, O, Bani, M, Bettica, P, Pich, EM, Jacobsson, E, Wahlstedt, K, Oreland, L, Långström, B, Eriksson, E, & Fredrikson, M, 2008. A link between serotonin-related gene polymorphisms, amygdala activity, and placebo-induced relief from social anxiety. *Journal of Neuroscience*, 28(49), 13066-13074, 03 December. doi: 10.1523/JNEUROSCI.2534-08.2008
47. Hall, KT, Lembo, AJ, Kirsch, I, Ziogas, DC, Douaiher, J, Jensen, KB, Conboy, LA, Kelley, JM, Kokkotou, E, Kaptchuk, TJ, 2012. Catechol-O-methyltransferase val158met polymorphism predicts placebo effect in irritable bowel syndrome. *PLoS ONE*, 7(10), e48135. doi: 10.1371/journal.pone.0048135
48. Hall, KT, Loscalzo, J, & Kaptchuk, TJ, 2015. Genetics and the placebo effect: the placebome. *Trends in Molecular Medicine*, 21(5), 285-294, May. doi: 10.1016/j.molmed.2015.02.009
49. Kavoussi B, & Ross, BE, 2007. The neuroimmune basis of anti-inflammatory acupuncture. *Integrative Cancer Therapies*, 6(3), 251-7, September. DOI: 10.1177/1534735407305892

CHAPTER 4 – FOOD

1. Australian Competition and Consumer Commission, 2009. *Allergy treatment declared misleading*. (Media release no. NR 210/09) [news release] Canberra: Australian Competition and Consumer Commission, 27 August. – Australian Competition and Consumer Commission v Allergy Pathway Pty Ltd [2009] FCA 960. Melbourne: Federal Court of Australia, 27 August.
2. Sofi, F, Abbate, R, Gensini, GF, & Casini, A, 2013. Importance of diet on disease prevention. International *Journal of Medicine and Medical Sciences*, 5(2), 55-59, February. doi: 10.5897/IJMMS12.107
3. World Health Organization, 2002. *The world health report 2002: reducing risks, promoting healthy life*. Geneva: World Health Organization, page 230. – World Health Organization, [2004, updated 2015]. *Promoting fruit and vegetable consumption around the world*. Geneva: World Health Organization.
4. World Health Organization, 2015. *Increasing fruit and vegetable consumption to reduce the risk of noncommunicable diseases*. Geneva: World Health Organization, 08 October.
5. World Health Organization, [2004, updated 2015]. *Promoting fruit and vegetable consumption around the world*. Geneva: World Health Organization.
6. Blot, WJ, & Tarone, RE, 2015. Doll and Peto's quantitative estimates of cancer risks: holding generally true for 35 years. *Journal of the National Cancer Institute*, 107(4), djv044, March. doi: 10.1093/jnci/djv044
7. International Food Information Council Foundation, 2012. *Americans find doing their own taxes simpler than improving diet and health*. (Executive Summary, 2012 Food & Health Survey). Washington, DC: International Food Information Council Foundation.
8. Katz, DL, & Meller, S, 2014. Can we say what diet is best for health? *Annual Review of Public Health*, 35, 83-103. doi: 10.1146/annurev-publhealth-032013-182351
9. Zeevi, D, Korem, T, Zmora, N, Israeli, D, Rothschild, D, Weinberger, A, Ben-Yacov, O, Lador, D, Avnit-Sagi, T, Lotan-Pompan, M, Suez, J, Mahdi, JA, Matot, E, Malka, G, Kosower, N, Rein, M, Zilberman-Schapira, G, Dohnalová, L, Pevsner-Fischer, M, Bikovsky, R, Halpern, Z, Elinav, E, & Segal, E, 2015. Personalized nutrition by prediction of glycemic responses. *Cell*, 163(5), 1079-1094, 19 November. doi: 10.1016/j.cell.2015.11.001. doi: 10.1016/j.cell.2015.11.001
10. Lock, K, Pomerleau, J, Causer, L, & McKee, M, 2004. Low fruit and vegetable consumption. In M Ezzati, AD Lopez, A Rodgers, & CJL Murray (eds.), *Comparative quantification of health risks: global and regional burden of diseases attributable to selected major risk factors*. Geneva: World Health Organization, volume 1, pages 597-728.
11. Springmann, M, Godfray, HCJ, Rayner, M, & Scarborough, P, 2016. Analysis and valuation of the health and climate change cobenefits of dietary change. *Proceedings of the National Academy of Sciences of the United States of America*, 113 (15), 4146-4151, 12 April. doi:10.1073/pnas.1523119113
12. Pollan, M, 2007. Unhappy meals. *The New York Times Magazine*, 28 January.
13. Aristotle, 1998. *Aristotle's Metaphysics*, trans. H Lawson-Tancred. London: Penguin. – Beresford, MJ, 2010. Medical reductionism: lessons from the great philosophers. *QJM*, 103(9), 721-724, September. doi: 10.1093/qjmed/hcq057
14. The 'Law of the intestine.' 1928. *Journal of the American Medical Association*, 90(3), 208. doi: 10.1001/jama.1928.02690300048019 – Bayliss, WM, & Starling, EH, 1899. The movements and innervation of the small intestine. *Journal of Physiology*, 24(2), 99-143, 11 May.
15. Van Oudenhove, L, McKie, S, Lassman, D, Uddin, B, Paine, P, Coen, S, Gregory, L, Tack, J, & Aziz, Q, 2011. Fatty acid-induced gut-brain signaling attenuates neural and behavioral effects of sad emotion in humans. *Journal of Clinical Investigation*, 121(8), 3094-3099, August. doi: 10.1172/JCI46380. – Cizza, G, & Rother KI, 2011. Was Feuerbach right: are we what we eat? (Commentary) *Journal of Clinical Investigation*, 121(8), 2969-2971, August. doi: 10.1172/JCI58595.
16. Powley, TL, & Phillips, RJ, 2002. Musings on the wanderer: what's new in our understanding of vago-vagal reflexes? I. Morphology and topography of vagal afferents innervating the GI tract. *American Journal of Physiology. Gastrointestinal and Liver Physiology*, 283(6), G1217-G1225, December. doi: 10.1152/ajpgi.00249.2002
17. Nahas, Z, Marangell, LB, Husain, MM, Rush, AJ, Sackeim, HA, Lisanby, SH, Martinez, JM, & George, MS, 2005. Two-year outcome of vagus nerve stimulation (VNS) for treatment of major depressive episodes. *Journal of Clinical Psychiatry*, 66(9), 1097-1104, September.
18. Food and Drug Administration, 2013. VNS Therapy System - P970003s050. Washington, DC: Food and Drug Administration, 04 September.
19. Lyte, M, 2014. Microbial endocrinology: host-microbiota neuroendocrine interactions influencing brain and behavior. *Gut Microbes*, 5(3), 381-389, May-June. doi: 10.4161/gmic.28682 – Carabotti, M, Scirocco, A, Maselli, MA, & Severi, C, 2015. The gut-brain axis: interactions between enteric microbiota, central and enteric nervous systems. *Annals of Gastroenterology*, 28(2), 203-209, April-June. – Norris, V, Molina, F, & Gewirtz, AT, 2013. Hypothesis: bacteria control host appetites. *Journal of Bacteriology*, 195(3), 411-416, February. doi: 10.1128/JB.01384-12

20. Dominguez-Bello, MG, Costello, EK, Contreras, M, Magris, M, Hidalgo, G, Fierer, N, & Knight, R, 2010. Delivery mode shapes the acquisition and structure of the initial microbiota across multiple body habitats in newborns. *Proceedings of the National Academy of Sciences of the United States of America*, 107(26), 11971-11975, 29 June. doi: 10.1073/pnas.1002601107.
21. Kero, J, Gissler, M, Grönlund, M-M, Kero, P, Koskinen, P, Hemminki, E, & Isolauri, E. 2002. Mode of delivery and asthma – is there a connection? *Pediatric Research*, 52(1), 6-11, July. doi: 10.1203/00006450-200207000-00004 – Couzin-Frankel, J, 2010. Bacteria and asthma: untangling the links. *Science*, 330(6008), 1168-1169, 26 November. doi: 10.1126/science.330.6008.1168. – Ege, MJ, Mayer, M, Normand, AC, Genuneit, J, Cookson, WO, Braun-Fahrländer, C, Heederik, D, Piarroux, R, von Mutius, E, & GABRIELA Transregio 22 Study Group, 2011. Exposure to environmental microorganisms and childhood asthma. Exposure to environmental microorganisms and childhood asthma. *New England Journal of Medicine*, 364(8), 701-709, 24 February. doi: 10.1056/NEJMoa1007302. – Algert, CS, McElduff, A, Morris, JM, & Roberts, CL, 2009. Perinatal risk factors for early onset of Type 1 diabetes in a 2000-2005 birth cohort. *Diabetic Medicine*, 26(12), 1193-1197, December. doi: 10.1111/j.1464-5491.2009.02878.x. – Ajslev, TA, Andersen, CS, Gamborg, M, Sørensen, TI, & Jess, T, 2011. Childhood overweight after establishment of the gut microbiota: the role of delivery mode, pre-pregnancy weight and early administration of antibiotics. *International Journal of Obesity*, 35(4), 522-529, April. doi: 10.1038/ijo.2011.27. – Mueller, NT, Whyatt, R, Hoepner, L, Oberfield, S, Dominguez-Bello, MG, Widen, EM, Hassoun, A, Perera, F, & Rundle, A, 2015. Prenatal exposure to antibiotics, cesarean section and risk of childhood obesity. *International Journal of Obesity*, 39(4), 665-670, April. doi: 10.1038/ijo.2014.180. – Castanys-Muñoz, E, Martin, MJ, & Vazquez, E, 2016. Building a beneficial microbiome from birth. *Advances in Nutrition*, 7(2), 323-330, 15 March. doi: 10.3945/an.115.010694. – Renz, H, Brandtzaeg, P, & Hornef, M, 2011. The impact of perinatal immune development on mucosal homeostasis and chronic inflammation. *Nature Reviews. Immunology*, 12(1), 9-23, 09 December. doi: 10.1038/nri3112.
22. Sender, R, Fuchs, S, & Milo, R, 2016. Revised estimates for the number of human and bacteria cells in the body. *bioRxiv*, 06 January. doi: 10.1101/036103
23. May, KT, 2014. How microbes could cure disease: Rob Knight at TED2014. *TEDBlog*, 19 March. – Lozupone, CA, Stombaugh, JI, Gordon, JI, Jansson, JK, & Knight, R, 2012. Diversity, stability and resilience of the human gut microbiota. *Nature*, 489(7415), 220-230, 13 September. doi: 10.1038/nature11550.
24. Chow, J, Lee, SM, Shen, Y, Khosravi, A, & Mazmanian, SK, 2010. Host-bacterial symbiosis in health and disease. *Advances in Immunology*, 107, 243-274. doi: 10.1016/B978-0-12-381300-8.00008-3. – Fukuda, S, Toh, H, Hase, K, Oshima, K, Nakanishi, Y, Yoshimura, K, Tobe, T, Clarke, JM, Topping, DL, Suzuki, T, Taylor, TD, Itoh, K, Kikuchi, J, Morita, H, Hattori, M, & Ohno, H, 2010. Bifidobacteria can protect from enteropathogenic infection through production of acetate. *Nature*, 469(7331), 543-547, 27 January. doi: 10.1038/nature09646. – Sonnenburg, JL, Xu, J, Leip, DD, Chen, CH, Westover, BP, Weatherford, J, Buhler, JD, & Gordon, JI, 2005. Glycan foraging in vivo by an intestine-adapted bacterial symbiont. *Science*, 307(5717), 1955-1959, 25 March. – Turnbaugh, PJ, Ley, RE, Mahowald, MA, Magrini, V, Mardis, ER, & Gordon JI, 2006. An obesity-associated gut microbiome with increased capacity for energy harvest. *Nature*, 444(7122), 1027-1031, 21 December. – Collins, SM, Surette, M, & Bercik, P, 2012. The interplay between the intestinal microbiota and the brain. *Nature Reviews. Microbiology*, 10(11), 735-742, November. doi: 10.1038/nrmicro2876.
25. Turnbaugh, PJ, Ley, RE, Mahowald, MA, Magrini, V, Mardis, ER, & Gordon JI, 2006. An obesity-associated gut microbiome with increased capacity for energy harvest. *Nature*, 444(7122), 1027-1031, 21 December. – Kallus, SJ, & Brandt, LJ, 2012. The intestinal microbiota and obesity. *Journal of Clinical Gastroenterology*, 46(1), 16-24, January. doi: 10.1097/MCG.0b013e31823711fd – Ley, RE, Turnbaugh, PJ, Klein, S, & Gordon, JI, 2006. Microbial ecology: human gut microbes associated with obesity. *Nature*, 444(7122), 1022-1023, 21 December. doi: 10.1038/4441022a – Koeth, RA, Wang, Z, Levison, BS, Buffa, JA, Org, E, Sheehy, BT, Britt, EB, Fu, X, Wu, Y, Li, L, Smith, JD, DiDonato, JA, Chen, J, Li, H, Wu, GD, Lewis, JD, Warrier, M, Brown, JM, Krauss, RM, Tang, WH, Bushman, FD, Lusis, AJ, & Hazen, SL, 2013. Intestinal microbiota metabolism of L-carnitine, a nutrient in red meat, promotes atherosclerosis. *Nature Medicine*, 19(5), 576-585, 19 May. doi: 10.1038/nm.3145. – Gao, Z, Guo, B, Gao, R, Zhu, Q, & Qin, H, 2015. Microbiota disbiosis is associated with colorectal cancer. *Frontiers in Microbiology*, 6, 20, 109, February. doi: 10.3389/fmicb.2015.00020. – Qin, J, Li, Y, Cai, Z, Li, S, Zhu, J, Zhang, F, Liang, S, Zhang, W, Guan, Y, Shen, D, Peng, Y, Zhang, D, Jie, Z, Wu, W, Qin, Y, Xue, W, Li, J, Han, L, Lu, D, Wu, P, Dai, Y, Sun, X, Li, Z, Tang, A, Zhong, S, Li, X, Chen, W, Xu, R, Wang, M, Feng, Q, Gong, M, Yu, J, Zhang, Y, Zhang, M, Hansen, T, Sanchez, G, Raes, J, Falony, G, Okuda, S, Almeida, M, Le Chatelier, E, Renault, P, Pons, N, Batto, JM, Zhang, Z, Chen, H, Yang, R, Zheng, W, Li, S, Yang, H, Wang, J, Ehrlich, SD, Nielsen, R, Pedersen, O, Kristiansen, K, & Wang, J, 2012. A metagenome-wide association study of gut microbiota in type 2 diabetes. *Nature*, 490(7418), 55-60, 04 October. doi: 10.1038/nature11450. – Gevers, D, Kugathasan, S, Denson, LA, Vázquez-Baeza, Y, Van Treuren, W, Ren, B, Schwager, E, Knights, D, Song, SJ, Yassour, M, Morgan, XC, Kostic, AD, Luo, C, González, A, McDonald, D, Haberman, Y, Walters, T, Baker, S, Rosh, J, Stephens, M, Heyman, M, Markowitz, J, Baldassano, R, Griffiths, A, Sylvester, F, Mack, D, Kim, S, Crandall, W, Hyams, J, Huttenhower, C, Knight, R, & Xavier, RJ, 2014. The treatment-naive microbiome in new-onset Crohn's disease. *Cell Host & Microbe*, 15(3), 382-392, 12 March. doi: 10.1016/j.chom.2014.02.005. – Morgan, XC, Tickle, TL, Sokol, H, Gevers, D, Devaney, KL, Ward, DV, Reyes, JA, Shah, SA, LeLeiko, N, Snapper, SB, Bousvaros, A, Korzenik, J, Sands, BE, Xavier, RJ, & Huttenhower, C, 2012. Dysfunction of the intestinal microbiome in inflammatory bowel disease and treatment. *Genome Biology* 13(9), R79, 16 April. doi: 10.1186/gb-2012-13-9-r79. – Proal, AD, Albert, PJ, & Marshall, TG, 2013. The human microbiome and autoimmunity. *Current Opinion in Rheumatology*, 25(2), 234-240, March. doi: 10.1097/BOR.0b013e32835cedbf. – Mielcarz, DW, & Kasper, LH, 2015. The gut microbiome in multiple sclerosis. *Current Treatment Options in Neurology*, 17(4), 344, April. doi: 10.1007/s11940-015-0344-7. – Hsiao, EY, McBride, SW, Hsien, S, Sharon, G, Hyde, ER, McCue, T, Codelli, JA, Chow, J, Reisman, SE, Petrosino, JF, Patterson, PH, & Mazmanian, SK, 2013. Microbiota modulate behavioral and physiological abnormalities associated with neurodevelopmental disorders. *Cell*, 155(7), 1451-1463, 19 December. doi: 10.1016/j.cell.2013.11.024. – Mielcarz, DW, & Kasper, LH, 2015. The gut microbiome in multiple sclerosis. *Current Treatment Options in Neurology*, 17(4), 344, April. doi: 10.1007/s11940-015-0344-7.
26. Prince, BT, Mandel, MJ, Nadeau, K, & Singh, AM, 2015. Gut microbiome and the development of food allergy and allergic disease. *Pediatric Clinics of North America*, 62(6), 1479-1492, December. doi: 10.1016/j.pcl.2015.07.007.
27. Baquero, F, & Nombela, C, 2012. The microbiome as a human organ. *Clinical Microbiology and Infection*, 18(Supplement 4), 2-4, July. doi: 10.1111/j.1469-0691.2012.03916.x.
28. Chandler, J, 2015. Gut feelings: the mysteries of the microbiome. *The Monthly: Australian politics, society, and culture*, May.
29. Spector, T, 2015. *The diet myth: the real science behind what we eat*. London: Orion.
30. Spector, T, 2015. Your gut bacteria don't like junk food - even if you do. *The Conversation*, May 10.
31. David, LA, Maurice, CF, Carmody, RN, Gootenberg, DB, Button, JE, Wolfe, BE, Ling, AV, Devlin, AS, Varma, Y, Fischbach, MA, Biddinger, SB, Dutton, RJ, & Turnbaugh, PJ. Diet rapidly and reproducibly alters the human gut microbiome. *Nature*, 505(7484), 559-563, 23 January. doi: 10.1038/nature12820.
32. O'Keefe, SJ, Li, JV, Lahti, L, Ou, J, Carbonero, F, Mohammed, K, Posma, JM, Kinross, J, Wahl, E, Ruder, E, Vipperla, K, Naidoo, V, Mtshali, L, Tims, S, Puylaert, PG, DeLany, J, Krasinskas, A, Benefiel, AC, Kaseb, HO, Newton, K, Nicholson, JK, de Vos, WM, Gaskins, HR, & Zoetendal, EG, 2015. Fat, fibre and cancer risk in African Americans and rural Africans. *Nature Communications*, 6:6342, 28 April. doi: 10.1038/ncomms7342.
33. Myles, IA, 2014. Fast food fever: reviewing the impacts of the Western diet on immunity. *Nutrition Journal*, 13, 61, 17 June. doi: 10.1186/1475-2891-13-61.
34. Chassaing, B, Koren, O, Goodrich, JK, Poole, AC, Srinivasan, S, Ley, RE, & Gewirtz, AT, 2015. Dietary emulsifiers impact the mouse gut microbiota promoting colitis and metabolic syndrome. *Nature*, 519(7541), 92-96, 05 March. doi: 10.1038/nature14232 – Cani, PD, & Everard, A, 2015. Keeping gut lining at bay: Impact of emulsifiers. *Trends in Endocrinology & Metabolism*, 26(6), 273-274, June. doi: 10.1016/j.tem.2015.03.009. – Suez, J, Korem, T, Zeevi, D, Zilberman-Schapira, G, Thaiss, CA, Maza, O, Israeli, D, Zmora, N, Gilad, S, Weinberger, A, Kuperman, Y, Harmelin, A, Kolodkin-Gal, I, Shapiro, H, Halpern, Z, Segal, E, & Elinav, E, 2014.

Artificial sweeteners induce glucose intolerance by altering the gut microbiota. *Nature*, 514(7521), 181-186, 09 October. doi: 10.1038/nature13793. – Suez, J, Korem, T, Zilberman-Schapira, G, Segal, E, & Elinav, E, 2015. Non-caloric artificial sweeteners and the microbiome: findings and challenges. *Gut Microbes*, 6(2), 149-155, 01 April. doi: 10.1080/19490976.2015.1017700.

35. Chassaing, B, Koren, O, Goodrich, JK, Poole, AC, Srinivasan, S, Ley, RE, & Gewirtz, AT, 2015. Dietary emulsifiers impact the mouse gut microbiota promoting colitis and metabolic syndrome. *Nature*, 519(7541), 92-96, 05 March. doi: 10.1038/nature14232
36. Cani, PD, Amar, J, Iglesias, MA, Poggi, M, Knauf, C, Bastelica, D, Neyrinck, AM, Fava, F, Tuohy, KM, Chabo, C, Waget, A, Delmée, E, Cousin, B, Sulpice, T, Chamontin, B, Ferrières, J, Tanti, JF, Gibson, GR, Casteilla, L, Delzenne, NM, Alessi, MC, & Burcelin, R, 2007. Metabolic endotoxemia initiates obesity and insulin resistance. *Diabetes*, 56(7), 1761-1772, July. doi: 10.2337/db06-1491
37. Office of Disease Prevention and Health Promotion, [2015]. Food and nutrient intakes, and health: Current status and trends. In *Scientific Report of the 2015 Dietary Guidelines Advisory Committee*, Part D, Chapter 1. Washington, DC. Office of Disease Prevention and Health Promotion, [28 January].
38. Vikraman, S, Fryar, CD, & Ogden, CL, 2015. *Caloric Intake from Fast Food among Children and Adolescents in the United States, 2011-2012*. (NCHS Data Brief No. 213). Hyattsville, MD: Centers for Disease Control and Prevention, September.
39. Kaakoush, NO, Martire, SI, Raipuria, M, Mitchell, HM, Nielsen, S, Westbrook, RF, & Morris, MJ, 2016. Alternating or continuous exposure to cafeteria diet leads to similar shifts in gut microbiota compared to chow diet. *Molecular Nutrition & Food Research*, 14 January. doi: 10.1002/mnfr.201500815
40. Greenwood, C, Morrow, AL, Lagomarcino, AJ, Altaye, M, Taft, DH, Yu, Z, Newburg, DS, Ward, DV, & Schibler, KR, 2014. Early empiric antibiotic use in preterm infants is associated with lower bacterial diversity and higher relative abundance of Enterobacter. *Journal of Pediatrics*, 165(1), 23-29, July. doi: 10.1016/j.jpeds.2014.01.010. – Blaser, M, 2011. Antibiotic overuse: Stop the killing of beneficial bacteria. *Nature*, 476(7361), 393-394, 24 August. doi: 10.1038/476393a. – Willing, BP, Russell, SL, & Finlay, BB, 2011. Shifting the balance: antibiotic effects on host-microbiota mutualism. *Nature Reviews. Microbiology*, 9(4), 233-243, April. doi: 10.1038/nrmicro2536. – Jakobsson, HE, Jernberg, C, Andersson, AF, Sjölund-Karlsson, M, Jansson, JK, Engstrand, L, 2010. Short-term antibiotic treatment has differing long-term impacts on the human throat and gut microbiome. *PLoS ONE*, 5(3), e9836, 24 March. doi: 10.1371/journal.pone.0009836.
41. Zaura, E, Brandt, BW, Teixeira de Mattos, MJ, Buijs, MJ, Caspers, MP, Rashid, MU, Weintraub, A, Nord, CE, Savell, A, Hu, Y, Coates, AR, Hubank, M, Spratt, DA, Wilson, M, Keijser, BJ, & Crielaard, W, 2015. Same exposure but two radically different responses to antibiotics: resilience of the salivary microbiome versus long-term microbial shifts in feces. *MBio*, 6(6), e01693-15, 10 November. doi: 10.1128/mBio.01693-15.
42. Lynch, SV, 2016. Gut microbiota and allergic disease: new insights. *Annals of the American Thoracic Society*, 13(Supplement 1), S51-S54., March. doi: 10.1513/AnnalsATS.201507-451MG – Gupta, RS, Springston, EE, Warrier, MR, Smith, B, Kumar, R, Pongracic, J, & Holl JL, 2011. The prevalence, severity, and distribution of childhood food allergy in the United States. *Pediatrics*, 128(1), e9-18, July. doi: 10.1542/peds.2011-0204. – Gupta, R, Sheikh, A, Strachan, DP, & Anderson, HR, 2007. Time trends in allergic disorders in the UK. *Thorax*, 62(1), 91-96, January. doi: 10.1136/thx.2004.038844 – Foliaki, S, Pearce, N, Björkstén, B, Mallol, J, Montefort, S, von Mutius, E, & International Study of Asthma and Allergies in Childhood Phase III Study Group, 2009. Antibiotic use in infancy and symptoms of asthma, rhinoconjunctivitis, and eczema in children 6 and 7 years old: International Study of Asthma and Allergies in Childhood Phase III. *Journal of Allergy and Clinical Immunology*, 124(5), 982-989, November. doi: 10.1016/j.jaci.2009.08.017. – Feehley, T, Stefka, AT, Cao, S, & Nagler, CR, 2012. Microbial regulation of allergic responses to food. *Seminars in Immunopathology*, 34(5), 671-688, September. doi: 10.1007/s00281-012-0337-5. – Lange, K, Buerger, M, Stallmach, A, Bruns, T, 2016. Effects of Antibiotics on Gut Microbiota. *Digestive Diseases*, 34(3), 260-268. doi: 10.1159/000443360.
43. Johnson, CC, Ownby, DR, Alford, SH, Havstad, SL, Williams, LK, Zoratti, EM, Peterson, EL, & Joseph, CL, 2005. Antibiotic exposure in early infancy and risk for childhood atopy. *Journal of Allergy and Clinical Immunology*, 115(6), 1218-1224, June. doi: 10.1016/j.jaci.2005.04.020.
44. Abrahamsson, TR, Jakobsson, HE, Andersson, AF, Björkstén, B, Engstrand, L, & Jenmalm, MC, 2012. Low diversity of the gut microbiota in infants with atopic eczema. *Journal of Allergy and Clinical Immunology*, 129(2), 434-440.e12, February. doi: 10.1016/j.jaci.2011.10.025.
45. Gould, IM, & Bal, AM, 2013. New antibiotic agents in the pipeline and how they can help overcome microbial resistance. *Virulence*, 4(2), 185-191, February. doi: 10.4161/viru.22507.
46. Tackett KL, & Atkins A, 2012. Evidence-based acute bronchitis therapy. *Journal of Pharmacy Practice*, 25(6), 586-590, December. doi: 10.1177/0897190012460826. – Albert, RH, 2010. Diagnosis and treatment of acute bronchitis. *American Family Physician*, 82(11), 1345-1350, December.
47. Ventola, CL, 2015. The antibiotic resistance crisis: part 1: causes and threats. *Pharmacy and Therapeutics*, 40(4), 277-283, April. – Centers for Disease Control and Prevention, 2013. *Antibiotic resistance threats in the United States, 2013*. (Report CS239559-B) Atlanta, GA: Centers for Disease Control and Prevention, page 113.
48. Ventola, CL, 2015. The antibiotic resistance crisis: part 1: causes and threats. *Pharmacy and Therapeutics*, 40(4), 277-283, April.
49. McFarland, LV, 2014. Use of probiotics to correct dysbiosis of normal microbiota following disease or disruptive events: a systematic review. *BMJ Open*, 4(8), e005047, 23 August. doi: 10.1136/bmjopen-2014-005047
50. Zhang, YJ, Li, S, Gan, RY, Zhou, T, Xu, DP, & Li, HB, 2015. Impacts of gut bacteria on human health and diseases. *International Journal of Molecular Sciences*, 16(4), 7493-7519, 02 April. doi: 10.3390/ijms16047493.
51. Goodrich, JK, Waters, JL, Poole, AC, Sutter, JL, Koren, O, Blekhman, R, Beaumont, M, Van Treuren, W, Knight, R, Bell, JT, Spector, TD, Clark, AG, & Ley, RE, 2014. Human genetics shape the gut microbiome. *Cell*, 159(4), 789-799, 06 November. doi: 10.1016/j.cell.2014.09.053.
52. Walters, WA, Xu, Z, & Knight, R, 2014. Meta-analyses of human gut microbes associated with obesity and IBD. *FEBS Letters*, 588(22), 4223-4233, 17 November. doi: 10.1016/j.febslet.2014.09.039. – Knights, D, Parfrey, LW, Zaneveld, J, Lozupone, C, & Knight, R, 2011. Human-associated microbial signatures: examining their predictive value. *Cell Host & Microbe*, 10(4), 292-296, 20 October. doi: 10.1016/j.chom.2011.09.003. – Le Chatelier, E, Nielsen, T, Qin, J, Prifti, E, Hildebrand, F, Falony, G, Almeida, M, Arumugam, M, Batto, JM, Kennedy, S, Leonard, P, Li, J, Burgdorf, K, Grarup, N, Jørgensen, T, Brandslund, I, Nielsen, HB, Juncker, AS, Bertalan, M, Levenez, F, Pons, N, Rasmussen, S, Sunagawa, S, Tap, J, Tims, S, Zoetendal, EG, Brunak, S, Clément, K, Doré, J, Kleerebezem, M, Kristiansen, K, Renault, P, Sicheritz-Ponten, T, de Vos, WM, Zucker, JD, Raes, J, Hansen, T, MetaHIT Consortium, Bork, P, Wang, J, Ehrlich, SD, & Pedersen, O, 2013. Richness of human gut microbiome correlates with metabolic markers. *Nature*, 500(7464), 541-546, 29 August. doi:10.1038/nature12506 – Speliotes, EK, Willer, CJ, Berndt, SI, et al., 2010. Association analyses of 249,796 individuals reveal eighteen new loci associated with body mass index. *Nature Genetics*, 42(11), 937-948, November. Published online 2010 Oct 10. doi: 10.1038/ng.686
53. Ohland, CL, Kish, L, Bell, H, Thiesen, A, Hotte, N, Pankiv, E, & Madsen, KL, 2013. Effects of *Lactobacillus helveticus* on murine behavior are dependent on diet and genotype and correlate with alterations in the gut microbiome. *Psychoneuroendocrinology*, 38(9), 1738-1747, September. doi: 10.1016/j.psyneuen.2013.02.008.
54. Mackos, AR, Eubank, TD, Parry, NM, & Bailey, MT, 2013. Probiotic *Lactobacillus reuteri* attenuates the stressor-enhanced severity of *Citrobacter rodentium* infection. *Infection and Immunity*, 81(9), 3253-3263, September. doi: 10.1128/IAI.00278-13.
55. Carasi, P, Racedo, SM, Jacquot, C, Romanin, DE, Serradell, MA, & Urdaci, MC, 2015. Impact of kefir derived *Lactobacillus kefiri* on the mucosal immune response and gut microbiota. *Journal of Immunology Research*, 2015:361604. doi: 10.1155/2015/361604.
56. Dapoigny, M, Piche, T, Ducrotte, P, Lunaud, B, Cardot, JM, & Bernalier-Donadille, A, 2012. Efficacy and safety profile of LCR35 complete freeze-dried culture in irritable bowel syndrome: a randomized, double-blind study. *World Journal of Gastroenterology*, 18(17), 2067-2075, 07 May. doi: 10.3748/wjg.v18.i17.2067.
57. Messaoudi, M, Lalonde, R, Violle, N, Javelot, H, Desor, D, Nejdi, A, Bisson, JF, Rougeot, C, Pichelin, M, Cazaubiel, M, & Cazaubiel, JM, 2011. Assessment of psychotropic-like properties of a probiotic formulation (*Lactobacillus helveticus* R0052 and *Bifidobacterium longum* R0175) in rats and human subjects. *British Journal of Nutrition*, 105(5), 755-764, March. doi: 10.1017/S0007114510004319.

58. Scher, JU, Sczesnak, A, Longman, RS, Segata, N, Ubeda, C, Bielski, C, Rostron, T, Cerundolo, V, Pamer, EG, Abramson, SB, Huttenhower, C, & Littman, DR, 2013. Expansion of intestinal *Prevotella copri* correlates with enhanced susceptibility to arthritis. *eLife*, 2, e01202, 05 November. doi: 10.7554/eLife.01202.
59. Scher, JU, Ubeda, C, Artacho, A, Attur, M, Isaac, S, Reddy, SM, Marmon, S, Neimann, A, Brusca, S, Patel, T, Manasson, J, Pamer, EG, Littman, DR, & Abramson, SB, 2015. Decreased bacterial diversity characterizes the altered gut microbiota in patients with psoriatic arthritis, resembling dysbiosis in inflammatory bowel disease. *Arthritis & Rheumatology*, 67(1), 128-139, January. doi: 10.1002/art.38892.
60. Tillisch, K, Labus, J, Kilpatrick, L, Jiang, Z, Stains, J, Ebrat, B, Guyonnet, D, Legrain-Raspaud, S, Trotin, B, Naliboff, B, & Mayer, EA, 2013. Consumption of fermented milk product with probiotic modulates brain activity. *Gastroenterology*, 144(7), 1394-401, 1401.e1-4, June. doi: 10.1053/j.gastro.2013.02.043.
61. Sonnenburg, JL, 2015. Engineering the human microbiome shows promise for treating disease. *Scientific American*, March 01.
62. Transparency Market Research, 2016. *Global probiotics market to expand at 7.40% CAGR from 2014 to 2020.* [news release] Albany, NY: Transparency Market Research, January 15.
63. Hungin, AP, Mulligan, C, Pot, B, Whorwell, P, Agréus, L, Fracasso, P, Lionis, C, Mendive, J, Philippart, de Foy, JM, Rubin, G, Winchester, C, de Wit, N, & European Society for Primary Care Gastroenterology, 2013. Systematic review: probiotics in the management of lower gastrointestinal symptoms in clinical practice -- an evidence-based international guide. *Alimentary Pharmacology & Therapeutics*, 38(8), 864-86, October. doi: 10.1111/apt.12460.
64. Kechagia, M, Basoulis, D, Konstantopoulou, S, Dimitriadi, D, Gyftopoulou, K, Skarmoutsou, N, & Fakiri, EM, 2013. Health benefits of probiotics: a review. *ISRN Nutrition*, 2013:481651, 02 January. doi: 10.5402/2013/481651.
65. Fuller, R, 1991. Probiotics in human medicine. *Gut*, 32(4), 439-442, April. – Govender, M, Choonara, YE, Kumar, P, du Toit, LC, van Vuuren, S, & Pillay, V, 2014. A review of the advancements in probiotic delivery: conventional vs. non-conventional formulations for intestinal flora supplementation. *AAPS PharmSciTech*, 15(1), 29-43, February. doi: 10.1208/s12249-013-0027-1.
66. Marcobal, A, Underwood, MA, & Mills, DA, 2008. Rapid determination of the bacterial composition of commercial probiotic products by terminal restriction fragment length polymorphism analysis. *Journal of Pediatric Gastroenterology & Nutrition*, 46(5), 608-611, May. doi: 10.1097/MPG.0b013e3181660694.
67. Weese, JS, & Martin, H, 2008. Assessment of commercial probiotic bacterial contents and label accuracy. *Canadian Veterinary Journal*, 52(1), 43-46, January. doi: 10.1097/MPG.0b013e3181660694
68. Alang, N, & Kelly, CR, 2015. Weight gain after fecal microbiota transplantation. *Open Forum Infectious Diseases*, 2(1), ofv004, 04 February. doi: 10.1093/ofid/ofv004
69. Lozupone, CA, Stombaugh, JI, Gordon, JI, Jansson, JK, & Knight, R, 2012. Diversity, stability and resilience of the human gut microbiota. *Nature*, 489(7415), 220-230, 13 September. doi: 10.1038/nature11550. – Cotillard, A, Kennedy, SP, Kong, LC, Prifti, E, Pons, N, Le Chatelier, E, Almeida, M, Quinquis, B, Levenez, F, Galleron, N, Gougis, S, Rizkalla, S, Batto, JM, Renault, P, ANR MicroObes consortium, Doré, J, Zucker, JD, Clément, K, & Ehrlich, SD, 2013. Dietary intervention impact on gut microbial gene richness. *Nature*, 500(7464), 585-588, 29 August. doi: 10.1038/nature12480. – Le Chatelier, E, Nielsen, T, Qin, J, Prifti, E, Hildebrand, F, Falony, G, Almeida, M, Arumugam, M, Batto, JM, Kennedy, S, Leonard, P, Li, J, Burgdorf, K, Grarup, N, Jørgensen, T, Brandslund, I, Nielsen, HB, Juncker, AS, Bertalan, M, Levenez, F, Pons, N, Rasmussen, S, Sunagawa, S, Tap, J, Tims, S, Zoetendal, EG, Brunak, S, Clément, K, Doré, J, Kleerebezem, M, Kristiansen, K, Renault, P, Sicheritz-Ponten, T, de Vos, WM, Zucker, JD, Raes, J, Hansen, T, MetaHIT Consortium, Bork, P, Wang, J, Ehrlich, SD, & Pedersen, O, 2013. Richness of human gut microbiome correlates with metabolic markers. *Nature*, 500(7464), 541-546, 29 August. doi:10.1038/nature12506
70. Chang, JY, Antonopoulos, DA, Kalra, A, Tonelli, A, Khalife, WT, Schmidt, TM, & Young, VB, 2008. Decreased diversity of the fecal microbiome in recurrent Clostridium difficile-associated diarrhea. Journal of Infectious Diseases, 197(3), 435-438, 01 February. doi: 10.1086/525047. – Rook, GA, Raison, CL, & Lowry, CA, 2014. Microbial 'old friends', immunoregulation and socioeconomic status. *Clinical & Experimental Immunology*, 177(1), 1-12, July. doi: 10.1111/cei.12269. – Andoh, A, 2016. Physiological role of gut microbiota for maintaining human health. *Digestion*, 93(3), 176-181, June. doi: 10.1159/000444066
71. Scher, JU, Sczesnak, A, Longman, RS, Segata, N, Ubeda, C, Bielski, C, Rostron, T, Cerundolo, V, Pamer, EG, Abramson, SB, Huttenhower, C, & Littman, DR, 2013. Expansion of intestinal *Prevotella copri* correlates with enhanced susceptibility to arthritis. *eLife*, 2, e01202, 05 November. doi: 10.7554/eLife.01202. – Frank, DN, St Amand, AL, Feldman, RA, Boedeker, EC, Harpaz, N, & Pace, NR, 2007. Molecular-phylogenetic characterization of microbial community imbalances in human inflammatory bowel diseases. *Proceedings of the National Academy of Sciences of the United States of America*, 104(34), 13780-13785, 21 August. 10.1073/pnas.0706625104. – Turnbaugh, PJ, Hamady, M, Yatsunenko, T, Cantarel, BL, Duncan, A, Ley, RE, Sogin, ML, Jones, WJ, Roe, BA, Affourtit, JP, Egholm, M, Henrissat, B, Heath, AC, Knight, R, & Gordon, JI, 2009. A core gut microbiome in obese and lean twins. *Nature*, 457(7228), 480-484, 22 January. doi: 10.1038/nature07540.
72. Xu, Z, & Knight, R, 2015. Dietary effects on human gut microbiome diversity. *British Journal of Nutrition*, 113, Supplement S1, S1-S5, January. doi: 10.1017/S0007114514004127. – Wu, GD, Chen, J, Hoffmann, C, Bittinger, K, Chen, YY, Keilbaugh, SA, Bewtra, M, Knights, D, Walters, WA, Knight, R, Sinha, R, Gilroy, E, Gupta, K, Baldassano, R, Nessel, L, Li, H, Bushman, FD, & Lewis, JD, 2011. Linking long-term dietary patterns with gut microbial enterotypes. *Science*, 334(6052), 105-108, 07 October. doi: 10.1126/science.1208344.
73. Pollan, M, 2007. Unhappy meals. *The New York Times Magazine*, 28 January.
74. Cotillard, A, Kennedy, SP, Kong, LC, Prifti, E, Pons, N, Le Chatelier, E, Almeida, M, Quinquis, B, Levenez, F, Galleron, N, Gougis, S, Rizkalla, S, Batto, JM, Renault, P, ANR MicroObes consortium, Doré, J, Zucker, JD, Clément, K, & Ehrlich, SD, 2013. Dietary intervention impact on gut microbial gene richness. *Nature*, 500(7464), 585-588, 29 August. doi: 10.1038/nature12480. – Le Chatelier, E, Nielsen, T, Qin, J, Prifti, E, Hildebrand, F, Falony, G, Almeida, M, Arumugam, M, Batto, JM, Kennedy, S, Leonard, P, Li, J, Burgdorf, K, Grarup, N, Jørgensen, T, Brandslund, I, Nielsen, HB, Juncker, AS, Bertalan, M, Levenez, F, Pons, N, Rasmussen, S, Sunagawa, S, Tap, J, Tims, S, Zoetendal, EG, Brunak, S, Clément, K, Doré, J, Kleerebezem, M, Kristiansen, K, Renault, P, Sicheritz-Ponten, T, de Vos, WM, Zucker, JD, Raes, J, Hansen, T, MetaHIT Consortium, Bork, P, Wang, J, Ehrlich, SD, & Pedersen, O, 2013. Richness of human gut microbiome correlates with metabolic markers. *Nature*, 500(7464), 541-546, 29 August. doi:10.1038/nature12506
75. David, LA, Maurice, CF, Carmody, RN, Gootenberg, DB, Button, JE, Wolfe, BE, Ling, AV, Devlin, AS, Varma, Y, Fischbach, MA, Biddinger, SB, Dutton, RJ, & Turnbaugh, PJ. Diet rapidly and reproducibly alters the human gut microbiome. *Nature*, 505(7484), 559-563, 23 January. doi: 10.1038/nature12820. – Walker, AW, Ince, J, Duncan, SH, Webster, LM, Holtrop, G, Ze, X, Brown, D, Stares, MD, Scott, P, Bergerat, A, Louis, P, McIntosh, F, Johnstone, AM, Lobley, GE, Parkhill, J, & Flint, HJ, 2011. Dominant and diet-responsive groups of bacteria within the human colonic microbiota. *ISME Journal*, 5(2), 220-230, February. doi: 10.1038/ismej.2010.118. – Wu, GD, Chen, J, Hoffmann, C, Bittinger, K, Chen, YY, Keilbaugh, SA, Bewtra, M, Knights, D, Walters, WA, Knight, R, Sinha, R, Gilroy, E, Gupta, K, Baldassano, R, Nessel, L, Li, H, Bushman, FD, & Lewis, JD, 2011. Linking long-term dietary patterns with gut microbial enterotypes. *Science*, 334(6052), 105-108, 07 October. doi: 10.1126/science.1208344.
76. Sonnenburg, ED, & Sonnenburg, JL, 2014. Starving our microbial self: the deleterious consequences of a diet deficient in microbiota-accessible carbohydrates. *Cell Metabolism*, 20(5), 779-786, 04 November. doi: 10.1016/j.cmet.2014.07.003.
77. Sonnenburg, JL, & Sonnenburg, ED, 2015 *The good gut: Taking control of your weight, your mood, and your long-term health.* New York, NY: Penguin Press.
78. Hoy MK, & Goldman JD, 2014. *Fiber intake of the U.S. population: what we eat in America*, NHANES 2009-2010. (Food Surveys Research Group Dietary Data Brief No. 12) Beltsville, MD: United States Department of Agriculture, September. – Bliss, RM, 2015. Shifting out of high-calorie habits. *AgResearch Magazine*, 63(3), March.
79. Schnorr, SL, Candela, M, Rampelli, S, Centanni, M, Consolandi, C, Basaglia, G, Turroni, S, Biagi, E, Peano, C, Severgnini, M, Fiori, J, Gotti, R, De Bellis, G, Luiselli, D, Brigidi, P, Mabulla, A, Marlowe, F, Henry, AG, & Crittenden, AN, 2014. Gut microbiome of the Hadza hunter-gatherers. *Nature Communications*, 5(3654), 15 April. doi: 10.1038/ncomms4654. –

Bliss, RM, 2015. Shifting out of high-calorie habits. *AgResearch Magazine*, 63(3), March. – Calorie Control Council, 2014. *Closing the dietary fiber gap: aligning dietary fiber policy, research, and communication.* Washington, DC: Calorie Control Council.

CHAPTER 5 – MOVEMENT

1. National Center for Complementary and Integrative Health, 2005, updated 2015. *Ayurvedic medicine: in depth.* (Publication D287) Bethesda, MD: National Center for Complementary and Integrative Health.
2. Burzynska, AZ, Wong, CN, Chaddock-Heyman, L, Olson, EA, Gothe, NP, Knecht, A, Voss, MW, McAuley, E, & Kramer AF, 2016. White matter integrity, hippocampal volume, and cognitive performance of a world-famous nonagenarian track-and-field athlete. *Neurocase*, 22(2), 135-144. 03 August. doi: 10.1080/13554794.2015.1074709.
3. Erickson, KI, Voss, MW, Prakash, RS, Basak, C, Szabo, A, Chaddock, L, Kim, JS, Heo, S, Alves, H, White, SM, Wojcicki, TR, Mailey, E, Vieira, VJ, Martin, SA, Pence, BD, Woods, JA, McAuley, E, & Kramer, AF, 2011. Exercise training increases size of hippocampus and improves memory. *Proceedings of the National Academy of Sciences of the United States of America*, 108(7), 3017-3022, 15 February. doi: 10.1073/pnas.1015950108.
4. Szuhany, KL, Bugatti, M, & Otto, MW, 2015. A meta-analytic review of the effects of exercise on brain-derived neurotrophic factor. *Journal of Psychiatric Research*, 60, 56-64, January. doi: 10.1016/j.jpsychires.2014.10.003.
5. Cohen Cory, S, Kidane, AH, Shirkey, NJ, & Marshak, S, 2010. Brain-derived neurotrophic factor and the development of structural neuronal connectivity. *Developmental Neurobiology*, 70(5), 271-288, April. doi: 10.1002/dneu.20774.
6. Blair, SN, Goodyear, NN, Gibbons, LW, & Cooper, KH, 1984. Physical fitness and incidence of hypertension in healthy normotensive men and women. *Journal of the American Medical Association*, 252(4), 487-490, 27 July. doi:10.1001/jama.1984.03350040017014. – Adamopoulos, S, Parissis, J, Kroupis, C, Georgiadis, M, Karatzas, D, Karavolias, G, Koniavitou, K, Coats, AJ, & Kremastinos, DT, 2001. Physical training reduces peripheral markers of inflammation in patients with chronic heart failure. *European Heart Journal*, 22(9), 791-797, May. doi:10.1053/euhj.2000.2285 – McGavock, J, Mandic, S, Lewanczuk, R, Koller, M, Muhll, IV, Quinney, A, Taylor, D, Welsh, R, & Haykowsky, M, 2004. *Cardiovascular Diabetology*, 3(3), 15 March. doi: 10.1186/1475-2840-3-3
7. Warburton, DE, Glendhill, N, & Quinney, A, 2001. The effects of changes in musculoskeletal fitness on health. *Canadian Journal of Applied Physiology*, 26(2), 161-216, April. 10.1139/h01-012. – Wilmore JH, & Knuttgen H, 2003. Aerobic exercise and endurance improving fitness for health benefits. *Physician and Sportsmedicine* 31 (5), 45-51, May. doi: 10.3810/psm.2003.05.367. – Seidell, JC, Cigolini, M, Deslypere, JP, Charzewska, J, Ellsinger, BM, & Cruz, A, 1991. Body fat distribution in relation to physical activity and smoking habits in 38-year-old European men: The European Fat Distribution Study. *American Journal of Epidemiology*, 133(3), 257-265, 01 February. – Tremblay, A, Després, JP, Leblanc, C, Craig, CL, Ferris, B, Stephens, T, & Bouchard, C, 1990. Effect of intensity of physical activity on body fatness and fat distribution. *American Journal of Clinical Nutrition*, 51(2), 153-157, February.
8. Chapman, SB, Aslan, S, Spence, JS, Defina, LF, Keebler, MW, Didehbani, N, & Lu, H, 2013. Shorter term aerobic exercise improves brain, cognition, and cardiovascular fitness in aging. *Frontiers in Aging Neuroscience*, 5, 75, 12 November. doi: 10.3389/fnagi.2013.00075.
9. Pennington, R, & Hanna, S, 2013. The acute effects of exercise on cognitive performances of older adults. *Journal of the Arkansas Academy of Science*, 67, 109-114.
10. Bjørnebekk, A, Mathé, AA, & Brené, S, 2005. The antidepressant effect of running is associated with increased hippocampal cell proliferation. *International Journal of Neuropsychopharmacology*, 8(3), 357-368, September. doi :10.1017/S1461145705005122. – Callaghan, P, 2004. Exercise: A neglected intervention in mental health care? *Journal of Psychiatric and Mental Health Nursing*, 11(4), 476-483, August. doi: 10.1111/j.1365-2850.2004.00751.x – Guszkowska, M, 2004. [Effects of exercise on anxiety, depression and mood.] [article in Polish] *Psychiatria Polska*, 38(4), 611-620, July-August.
11. Warburton, DE, Nicol, CW, & Bredin, SS, 2006. Health benefits of physical activity: the evidence. *Canadian Medical Association Journal*, 174(6), 801-809, March. doi: 10.1503/cmaj.051351
12. Franco, OH, de Laet, C, Peeters, A, Jonker, J, Mackenbach, J, & Nusselder, W, 2005. Effects of physical activity on life expectancy with cardiovascular disease. *Archives of Internal Medicine*, 165(20), 2355-2360, 14 November. doi:10.1001/archinte.165.20.2355. – Paffenbarger, RS Jr, Hyde, RT, Wing, AL, & Hsieh, CC, 1986. Physical activity, all-cause mortality, and longevity of college alumni. *New England Journal of Medicine*, 314(10, 605-613, 06 March. doi: 10.1056/NEJM198603063141003.
13. Pimlott, N, 2010. The miracle drug. [editorial] *Canadian Family Physician*, 56(5), 407, 409, May.
14. World Health Organization, 2010. *Global recommendations on physical activity for health.* Geneva: World Health Organization.
15. American Heart Association, 2014, 2016. *American Heart Association Recommendations for Physical Activity in Adults.* Dallas, TX: American Heart Association.
16. Garber, CE, Blissmer, B, Deschenes, MR, Franklin, BA, Lamonte, MJ, Lee, IM, Nieman, DC, & Swain, DP, 2011. American College of Sports Medicine position stand: Quantity and quality of exercise for developing and maintaining cardiorespiratory, musculoskeletal, and neuromotor fitness in apparently healthy adults: guidance for prescribing exercise. *Medicine and science in sports and exercise*, 43(7), 1334-1359, July. doi: 10.1249/MSS.0b013e318213fefb.
17. Harris, CD, Watson, KB, Carlson, SA, Fulton, JE, Dorn, JM, & Elam-Evans, L, 2013. Adult participation in aerobic and muscle-strengthening physical activities – United States, 2011. *Morbidity and Mortality Weekly Report*, 62(17), 326-330, 03 May. – Farrell, F, Hollingsworth, B, Propper, C, & Shields, MA, 2013. *The Socioeconomic Gradient in physical inactivity in England.* (CMPO Working Paper Series No. 13/311) Bristol, England: University of Bristol, The Centre for Market and Public Organisation, July. – Colley, RC, Garriguet, D, Janssen, I, Craig, CL, Clarke, J, & Tremblay, MS, 2011. Physical activity of Canadian adults: accelerometer results from the 2007 to 2009 Canadian Health Measures Survey. *Health Reports*, 22(1), 7-14, March.
18. World Health Organization, [n.d.]. *Physical Inactivity: A global public health problem.* Geneva: World Health Organization.
19. Mansoubi, M, Pearson, N, Biddle, SJ, & Clemes, S, 2014. The relationship between sedentary behaviour and physical activity in adults: a systematic review. *Preventive Medicine*, 69:28-35.December. doi: 10.1016/j.ypmed.2014.08.028.
20. Church, TS, Thomas, DM, Tudor-Locke, C, Katzmarzyk, PT, Earnest, CP, Rodarte, RQ, Martin, CK, Blair, SN, & Bouchard, C, 2011. Trends over 5 decades in U.S. occupation related physical activity and their associations with obesity. *PLoS One*, 6(5), e19657, 25 May. doi: 10.1371/journal.pone.0019657.
21. Kuper, S, 2009. The man who invented exercise. *Financial Times*, 11 September.
22. Morris, JN, Heady, JA, Raffle, PA, Roberts, CG, & Parks JW, 1953. Coronary heart disease and physical activity of work. *Lancet*, 265(6796), 1111-1120, 28 November. DOI: 10.1016/S0140-6736(53)91495-0 – Heady, JA, Morris, JN, Kagan, A, & Raffle, PA, 1961. Coronary heart disease in London busmen: a progress report with particular reference to physique. *British Journal of Preventive & Social Medicine*, 15(4), 143-153, October. – Morris, JN, & Raffle, PA, 1954. Coronary heart disease in transport workers: a progress report. *British Journal of Industrial Medicine*, 11(4), 260-264, October. – Paffenbarger, RS, Blair, SN, & Lee, IM, 2001. A history of physical activity, cardiovascular health and longevity: the scientific contributions of Jeremy N Morris, DSc, DPH, FRCP. *International Journal of Epidemiology*, 30(5), 1184-1192, October. doi: 10.1093/ije/30.5.1184
23. Hevesi, D, 2009. Jeremy Morris, who proved exercise is heart-healthy, dies at 99½. *The New York Times*, 07 November.
24. National Health Service, 2014. *Why sitting too much is bad for your health.* National Health Service, October 14. – Wilmot, EG, Edwardson, CL, Achana, FA, Davies, MJ, Gorely, T, Gray, LJ, Khunti, K, Yates, T, & Biddle, SJ, 2012. Sedentary time in adults and the association with diabetes, cardiovascular disease and death: systematic review and meta-analysis. *Diabetologia*, 55(11), 2895-2905, November. doi: 10.1007/s00125-012-2677-z.
25. Matthews, CE, Chen, KY, Freedson, PS, Buchowski, MS, Beech, BM, Pate, RR, & Troiano, RP, 2008. Amount of time spent in sedentary behaviors in the United States, 2003-2004. *American Journal of Epidemiology*, 167(7), 875-881, 01 April. doi: 10.1093/aje/kwm390
26. Australian Bureau of Statistics, 2013. *Australian health survey: Physical activity, 2011-12.* Canberra: Australian Bureau of Statistics, 19 July.
27. Hu, FB, Li, TY, Colditz, GA, Willett, WC, & Manson, JE, 2003. Television watching and other sedentary behaviors in relation to risk of obesity and

type 2 diabetes mellitus in women. *Journal of the American Medical Association*, 289(14), 1785-1791, 09 April. doi:10.1001/jama.289.14.1785. – Jakes, RW, Day, NE, Khaw, KT, Luben, R, Oakes, S, Welch, A, Bingham, S, & Wareham, NJ, 2003. Television viewing and low participation in vigorous recreation are independently associated with obesity and markers of cardiovascular disease risk: EPIC-Norfolk population-based study. *European Journal of Clinical Nutrition*, 57(9), 1089-1096, September. doi:10.1038/sj.ejcn.1601648. – Healy, GN, Dunstan, DW, Salmon, J, Cerin, E, Shaw, JE, Zimmet, PZ, & Owen, N, 2007. Objectively measured light-intensity physical activity is independently associated with 2-h plasma glucose. *Diabetes Care*, 30(6), 1384-1389, June. doi: 10.2337/dc07-0114 – Hu, FB, Leitzmann, MF, Stampfer, MJ, Colditz, GA, Willett, WC, & Rimm, EB, 2001. Physical activity and television watching in relation to risk for type 2 diabetes mellitus in men. *Archives of Internal Medicine*, 161(12), 1542-1548, 25 June. doi:10.1001/archinte.161.12.1542. – Beunza, JJ, Martínez-González, MA, Ebrahim, S, Bes-Rastrollo, M, Núñez, J, Martínez, JA, & Alonso, A, 2007. Sedentary behaviors and the risk of incident hypertension: the SUN Cohort. *American Journal of Hypertension*, 20(11), 1156-1162, November. doi: 10.1016/j.amjhyper.2007.06.007 – Hamilton, MT, Hamilton, DG, & Zderic, TW, 2007. Role of low energy expenditure and sitting in obesity, metabolic syndrome, type 2 diabetes, and cardiovascular disease. *Diabetes*, 56(11), 2655-2667, November. doi: 10.2337/db07-0882. – Warburton, DE, Nicol, CW, & Bredin, SSD, 2006. Health benefits of physical activity: the evidence. *Canadian Medical Association Journal*, 174(6), 801-809, March. doi: 10.1503/cmaj.051351 – Albanes, D, Blair, A, & Taylor, PR, 1989. Physical activity and risk of cancer in the NHANES I population. *American Journal of Public Health*, 79(6), 744-750, June. doi: 10.2105/AJPH.79.6.744

28. Veerman, JL, Healy, GN, Cobiac, LJ, Vos, T, Winkler, EA, Owen, N, & Dunstan, DW, 2012. Television viewing time and reduced life expectancy: a life table analysis. *British Journal of Sports Medicine*, 46(13), 927-930, October. doi 10.1136/bjsm.2011.085662.
29. Shaw, M, Mitchell, R, & Dorling, D, 2000. Time for a smoke? One cigarette reduces your life by 11 minutes. *British Medical Journal*, 320(7226), 53, 01 January. doi: 10.1136/bmj.320.7226.53
30. Ravn, K, 2013. Don't just sit there: Really. *Los Angeles Times*, May 23.
31. Ezzati, M, & Lopez, AD, 2003. Estimates of global mortality attributable to smoking in 2000. *Lancet*, 362(9387), 847-852, 13 September. doi: 10.1016/S0140-6736(03)14338-3
32. Lee, IM, Shiroma, EJ, Lobelo, F, Puska, P, Blair, SN, Katzmarzyk, PT, & Lancet Physical Activity Series Working Group, 2012. Effect of physical inactivity on major non-communicable diseases worldwide: an analysis of burden of disease and life expectancy. *Lancet*, 380(9839), 219-229, 21 July. doi: 10.1016/S0140-6736(12)61031-9. – Wen, CP, & Wu, X, 2012. Stressing harms of physical inactivity to promote exercise. *Lancet*, 380(9838), 192-193, 21 July. doi: 10.1016/S0140-6736(12)60954-4.
33. Schmid, D, & Leitzmann, MF, 2014. Television viewing and time spent sedentary in relation to cancer risk: a meta-analysis. *Journal of the National Cancer Institute*, 106(7), dju098, 09 July. doi:10.1093/jnci/dju098
34. Dunstan, DW, Salmon, J, Owen, N, Armstrong, T, Zimmet, PZ, Welborn, TA, Cameron, AJ, Dwyer, T, Jolley, D, Shaw, JE; & AusDiab Steering Committee, 2005. Associations of TV viewing and physical activity with the metabolic syndrome in Australian adults. *Diabetologia*, 48(11), 2254-2261, November. doi: 10.1007/s00125-005-1963-4 – Healy, GN, Dunstan, DW, Salmon, J, Shaw, JE, Zimmet, PZ, & Owen, N, 2008. Television time and continuous metabolic risk in physically active adults. *Medicine and Science in Sports and Exercise*, 40(4), 639-645, April. doi: 10.1249/MSS.0b013e3181607421
35. Bey, L, & Hamilton, MT, 2003. Suppression of skeletal muscle lipoprotein lipase activity during physical inactivity: a molecular reason to maintain daily low-intensity activity. *Journal of Physiology*, 551(part 2), 673-682, 01 September. doi: 10.1113/jphysiol.2003.045591
36. Zderic, TW, & Hamilton MT, 2012. Identification of hemostatic genes expressed in human and rat leg muscles and a novel gene (LPP1/PAP2A) suppressed during prolonged physical inactivity (sitting). *Lipids in Health and Disease*, 11: 137, 12 October. doi: 10.1186/1476-511X-11-137.
37. Boller, PF, 1996. *Presidential Anecdotes*. 2nd ed. New York: Oxford University Press USA, page 195.
38. Marx, R, [n.d.] The Health of the President: Theodore Roosevelt. Healthguidance.org. – Koepp, S, 2014. *The Roosevelts: the American family that changed the world*. New York: TIME Books.
39. Pedersen, BK, & Saltin, B, 2015. Exercise as medicine: Evidence for prescribing exercise as therapy in 26 different chronic diseases. *Scandinavian Journal of Medicine & Science in Sports*, 25(Suppl. 3), 1-72. doi: 10.1111/sms.12581.
40. Cooke, GE, Wetter, NC, Banducci, SE, Mackenzie, MJ, Zuniga, KE, Awick, EA, Roberts, SA, Sutton, BP, McAuley, E, & Kramer, AF, 2016. Moderate physical activity mediates the association between white matter lesion volume and memory recall in breast cancer survivors. *PLoS One*, 11(2), e0149552, 25 February. doi: 10.1371/journal.pone.0149552.
41. Widener, WM, as quoted in *Roosevelt, Theodore. An Autobiography, with Illustrations*. New York: Macmillan, 1913, 1916, page 350.
42. Rhodes, RE, & Plotnikoff, RC, 2006. Understanding action control: Predicting physical activity intention-behavior profiles across 6 months in a Canadian sample. *Health Psychology*, 25(3), 292-299, May. doi: 10.1037/0278-6133.25.3.292
43. Rhodes, RE, & de Bruijn, GJ, 2013.How big is the physical activity intention-behaviour gap? a meta-analysis using the action control framework. *British Journal of Health Psychology*, 18(2), 296-309, May. doi: 10.1111/bjhp.12032.
44. Webb, TL, & Sheeran, P, 2006. Does changing behavioral intentions engender behavior change? a meta-analysis of the experimental evidence. *Psychological Bulletin*, 132(2), 249-268, March. doi: 10.1037/0033-2909.132.2.249
45. Rhodes, RE, & de Bruijn, GJ, 2013.How big is the physical activity intention-behaviour gap? a meta-analysis using the action control framework. *British Journal of Health Psychology*, 18(2), 296-309, May. doi: 10.1111/bjhp.12032.
46. Gardner, B, Smith, L, Lorencatto, F, Hamer, M, & Biddle, SJ, 2016. How to reduce sitting time? A review of behaviour change strategies used in sedentary behaviour reduction interventions among adults. *Health Psychology Review*, 10(1), 89-112. doi:10.1080/17437199.2015.1082146.
47. Torbeyns, T, Bailey, S, Bos, I, & Meeusen, R, 2014. Active workstations to fight sedentary behaviour. *Sports Medicine*, 44(9), 1261-1273, September. doi: 10.1007/s40279-014-0202-x
48. Dunstan, DW, Kingwell, BA, Larsen, R, Healy, GN, Cerin, E, Hamilton, MT, Shaw, JE, Bertovic, DA, Zimmet, PZ, Salmon, J, & Owen, N, 2012. Breaking up prolonged sitting reduces postprandial glucose and insulin responses. *Diabetes Care*, 35(5), 976-983, May. doi: 10.2337/dc11-1931.
49. Biddle, SJ, Mutrie, N, & Gorely, T, 2015. *Psychology of physical activity: Determinants, well-being, and interventions*. 3rd ed. London: Routledge.
50. Williams, DM, 2008. Exercise, affect, and adherence: an integrated model and a case for self-paced exercise. *Journal of Sport & Exercise Psychology*. 30(5), 471-496, October. doi: 10.1123/jsep.30.5.471
51. Kwan, BM, & Bryan, AD, 2010. Affective response to exercise as a component of exercise motivation: Attitudes, norms, self-efficacy, and temporal stability of intentions. *Psychology of Sport and Exercise*, 11(1), 71-79, 01 January. doi: 10.1016/j.psychsport.2009.05.010
52. Williams, DM, Dunsiger, S, Ciccolo, JT, Lewis, BA, Albrecht, AE, & Marcus, BH, 2008. Acute affective response to a moderate-intensity exercise stimulus predicts physical activity participation 6 and 12 months later. *Psychology of Sport and Exercise*, 9(3), 231-245, May. doi: 10.1016/j.psychsport.2007.04.002
53. Annesi, J, 2005. Relations of self-motivation, perceived physical condition, and exercise-induced changes in revitalization and exhaustion with attendance in women initiating a moderate cardiovascular exercise regimen. *Women and Health*, 42(3), 77-93. doi: 10.1300/J013v42n03_05
54. Biondolillo, MJ, & Pillemer, DB, 2015. Using memories to motivate future behaviour: an experimental exercise intervention. *Memory*, 23(3), 390-402. doi: 10.1080/09658211.2014.889709
55. Thompson, CE, & Wankel, LM, 1980. The effects of perceived activity choice upon frequency of exercise behavior. *Journal of Applied Social Psychology*, 10(5), 436-443, July. doi: 10.1111/j.1559-1816.1980.tb00722.x
56. Rodgers, WM, & Brawley, LM, 1993. Using both self-efficacy theory and the theory of planned behavior to discriminate adherers and dropouts from structured programs. *Journal of Applied Sport Psychology*, 5(2), 195-206, September. doi:10.1080/10413209308411314
57. Kwasnicka, D, Presseau, J, White, M, & Sniehotta, FF, 2013. Does planning how to cope with anticipated barriers facilitate health-related behaviour change? a systematic review. *Health Psychology Review*, 7(2), 129-145. doi :10.1080/17437199.2013.766832
58. Luszczynska, A, 2006. An implementation intentions intervention, the use of a planning strategy, and physical activity after myocardial infarction. *Social Science & Medicine*, 62(4), 900-908, February. doi:10.1016/j.socscimed.2005.06.043
59. Gollwitzer, PM, & Sheeran, P, 2006. Implementation intentions and goal achievement: A meta�analysis of effects and processes. *Advances*

in Experimental Social Psychology, 38, 69-119, December. doi:10.1016/S0065-2601(06)38002-1
60. Lavigne, GL, Vallerand, RJ, & Crevier-Braud, L, 2011. The fundamental need to belong: on the distinction between growth and deficit-reduction orientations. *Personality & Social Psychology Bulletin*, 37(9), 1185-1201, September. doi: 10.1177/0146167211405995.
61. Baumeister, RF, & Leary, MR, 1995. The need to belong: desire for interpersonal attachments as a fundamental human motivation. *Psychological Bulletin*, 117(3), 497-529, May. doi: 10.1037/0033-2909.117.3.497
62. Viljoen, JE, & Christie, CJ, 2015. The change in motivating factors influencing commencement, adherence and retention to a supervised resistance training programme in previously sedentary post-menopausal women: a prospective cohort study. *BMC Public Health*, 15:236, 12 March. doi: 10.1186/s12889-015-1543-6.

CHAPTER 6 – ENVIRONMENT

1. Hoersten, G, 2015. Reunited after 39 years: A look back at the 'Jim Twins.' *Lima News*, 28 July.
2. Goleman, D, 1986. Major personality study finds that traits are mostly inherited. *The New York Times*, 02 December.
3. Tellegen, A, Lykken, DT, Bouchard, TJ, Wilcox, KJ, Segal, NL, & Rich, S, 1988. Personality similarity in twins reared apart and together. *Journal of Personality and Social Psychology*, 54(6), 1031-1039.
4. Joseph, J, 2001. Separated twins and the genetics of personality differences: a critique. *The American Journal of Psychology*, 114(1), 1-30, Spring. – Segal, NL, Cortez, FA, Zettel-Watson, L, Cherry, BJ, Mechanic, M, Munson, JE, Velázquez, JM, & Reed B, 2015. Genetic and experiential influences on behavior: twins reunited at seventy-eight years. *Personality and Individual Differences*, 73:110-117, January 1. – Turkheimer, E, Pettersson, E, & Horn EE, 2014. A phenotypic null hypothesis for the genetics of personality. *Annual Review of Psychology*, 65: 515-540, January. doi: 10.1146/annurev-psych-113011-143752.
5. Galetzka, D, Hansmann, T, El Hajj, N, Weis, E, Irmscher, B, Ludwig, M, Schneider-Rätzke, B, Kohlschmidt, N, Beyer, V, Bartsch, O, Zechner, U, Spix, C, & Haaf, T, 2012. Monozygotic twins discordant for constitutive BRCA1 promoter methylation, childhood cancer and secondary cancer. *Epigenetics*, 7(1), 47-54, January. doi: 10.4161/epi.7.1.18814
6. O'connor, T, 2014. Sins of the fathers and the mothers: how day-to-day choices can affect your DNA. *Sydney Morning Herald*, 20 January. – Spector, TD, 2012. *Identically different: Why you can change your genes.* London: George Weidenfeld & Nicholson.
7. Bell, JT, & Spector, TD, 2011. A twin approach to unraveling epigenetics. *Trends in Genetics*, 27(3), 116-125, March. doi: 10.1016/j.tig.2010.12.005. – Svendsen, AJ, Kyvik, KO, Houen, G, Junker, P, Christensen, K, Christiansen, L, Nielsen, C, Skytthe, A, & Hjelmborg, JV, 2013. On the origin of rheumatoid arthritis: The impact of environment and genes – A population based twin study. *PLoS One*, 8(2), e57304, February. doi: 10.1371/journal.pone.0057304.
8. Fraga, MF, Ballestar, E, Paz, MF, Ropero, S, Setien, F, Ballestar, ML, Heine-Suñer, D, Cigudosa, JC, Urioste, M, Benitez, J, Boix-Chornet, M, Sanchez-Aguilera, A, Ling, C, Carlsson, E, Poulsen, P, Vaag, A, Stephan, Z, Spector, TD, Wu, YZ, Plass, C, & Esteller, M, 2005. Epigenetic differences arise during the lifetime of monozygotic twins. *Proceedings of the National Academy of Sciences of the United States of America*, 102(30), 10604-10609, 26 July. doi: 10.1073/pnas.0500398102 – Kaminsky, ZA, Tang, T, Wang, SC, Ptak, C, Oh, GH, Wong, AH, Feldcamp, LA, Virtanen, C, Halfvarson, J, Tysk, C, McRae, AF, Visscher, PM, Montgomery, GW, Gottesman, II, Martin, NG, & Petronis, A, 2009. DNA methylation profiles in monozygotic and dizygotic twins. *Nature Genetics*, 41(2), 240-245, February. doi: 10.1038/ng.286. – Haque, FN, Gottesman, II, & Wong, AH, 2009. Not really identical: epigenetic differences in monozygotic twins and implications for twin studies in psychiatry. *American Journal of Medical Genetics. Part C, Seminars in Medical Genetics*, 151C(2), 136-141, 15 May. doi: 10.1002/ajmg.c.30206. – Silva, S, Martins, Y, Matias, A, & Blickstein I, 2011. Why are monozygotic twins different? *Journal of Perinatal Medicine*, 39(2), 195-202, March. doi: 10.1515/JPM.2010.140.
9. Bouchard, TJ, 1997. Whenever the Twain shall meet. *The Sciences*, 37(5), 52-57, September-October. doi: 10.1002/j.2326-1951.1997.tb03343.
10. Wansink, B, & Park, SB, 2001. At the movies: How external cues and perceived taste impact consumption volume. *Food Quality and Preference*, 12(1), 69-74. doi: 10.1016/S0950-3293(00)00031-8.
11. Wansink, B, 2006. *Mindless eating: Why we eat more than we think.* New York: Bantam Books. – Wansink, B, & Kim, J, 2005 Bad popcorn in big buckets: portion size can influence intake as much as taste. *Journal of Nutrition Education and Behavior*, 37(5), 242-245, September-October. doi:10.1016/S1499-4046(06)60278-9 – Kral, TV, 2006. Effects on hunger and satiety, perceived portion size and pleasantness of taste of varying the portion size of foods: a brief review of selected studies. *Appetite* 46(1), 103-105, January. doi:10.1016/j.appet.2005.05.006
12. Wansink, B, & Sobal, J, 2007. Mindless eating: the 200 daily food decisions we overlook. *Environment and Behavior*, 39(1), 106-123, January. doi: 10.1177/0013916506295573.
13. Wansink, B, & Cheney, MM, 2005. Super bowls: serving bowl size and food consumption. *Journal of the American Medical Association*, 293(14), 1723-1728, 13 April. doi: 10.1001/jama.293.14.1727 – Wansink, B, & van Ittersum, K, 2007. Portion size me: downsizing our consumption norms. *Journal of the American Dietetic Association*, 107(7), 1103-1106, July. doi: 10.1016/j.jada.2007.05.019
14. Wansink, B, & Chandon, P, 2014. Slim by design: redirecting the accidental drivers of mindless overeating. *Journal of Consumer Psychology*, 24(3), 413-431. doi: 10.1016/j.jcps.2014.03.006
15. Wansink, B, 2015. Change their choice! changing behavior using the CAN approach and activism research. *Psychology and Marketing*, 32(5), 486-500. doi: 10.1002/mar.20794
16. Li, Q, Morimoto, K, Nakadai, A, Inagaki, H, Katsumata, M, Shimizu, T, Hirata, Y, Hirata, K, Suzuki, H, Miyazaki, Y, Kagawa, T, Koyama, Y, Ohira, T, Takayama, N, Krensky, AM, & Kawada, T, 2007. Forest bathing enhances human natural killer activity and expression of anti-cancer proteins. *International Journal of Immunopathology and Pharmacology*, 20(Suppl 2), 3-8, April-June. doi: 10.1177/03946320070200S202
17. Li, Q, 2010. Effect of forest bathing trips on human immune function. *Environmental Health and Preventive Medicine*, 15(1), 9-17, January. doi: 10.1007/s12199-008-0068-3
18. James, P, Banay, RF, Hart, JE, & Laden, F, 2015. A review of the health benefits of greenness. *Current Epidemiology Reports*, 2(2), 131-142, June. doi: 10.1007/s40471-015-0043-7
19. Miyazaki, Y, Ikei, H, & Song, C, 2014. Forest medicine research in Japan. *Nippon Eiseigaku Zasshi. Japanese Journal of Hygiene*, 69(2), 122-135. doi: 10.1265/jjh.69.122
20. Williams, F, 2012. Take two hours of pine forest and call me in the morning. *Outside Magazine*, December.
21. Williams, F, 2012. Take two hours of pine forest and call me in the morning. *Outside Magazine*, December.
22. United Nations Department of Economic and Social Affairs, 2014. World's population increasingly urban with more than half living in urban areas. New York: United Nations, 10 July.
23. Gleave, J, & Cole-Hamilton, I, 2012. *A world without play: a literature review.* Barnet, England: Play England. – Playday, 2007. Our streets too! Street play opinion poll summary. London: Playday.
24. Medibank, 2014. Health Check #1 – Community views on the health impact of screen time. Melbourne: Medibank.
25. Pretty, JN, 2004. How nature contributes to mental and physical health. *Spirituality and Health*, 5(2), 68-78. doi:10.1002/shi.220
26. Whiteford, HA, Degenhardt, L, Rehm, J, Baxter, AJ, Ferrari, AJ, Erskine, HE, Charlson, FJ, Norman, RE, Flaxman, AD, Johns, N, Burstein, R, Murray, CJ, & Vos, T, 2013. Global burden of disease attributable to mental and substance use disorders. *The Lancet*, 382(9904), 1575-1586, 9 November. doi: 10.1016/S0140-6736(13)61611-6.
27. Lederbogen, F, Kirsch, P, Haddad, L, Streit, F, Tost, H, Schuch, P, Wüst, S, Pruessner, JC, Rietschel, M, Deuschle, M, & Meyer-Lindenberg, A, 2011. City living and urban upbringing affect neural social stress processing in humans. *Nature*, 474(7352), 498-501, 22 June. doi: 10.1038/nature10190.
28. Bratman, GN, Hamilton, JP, Hahn, KS, Daily, GC, & Gross, JJ, 2015. Nature experience reduces rumination and subgenual prefrontal cortex activation. *Proceedings of the National Academy of Sciences of the United States of America*, 112(28), 8567-8572, 14 July. doi: 10.1073/pnas.1510459112
29. Aspinall, P, Mavros, P, Coyne, R, & Roe, J, 2015. The urban brain: Analysing outdoor physical activity with mobile EEG. *British Journal of Sports Medicine*, 49(4), 272-276, February. doi: 10.1136/bjsports-2012-091877
30. National Recreation and Parks Association, 2014. *Prescribing parks for better health: success stories.* Ashburn, VA: National Recreation and Parks Association. – Zarr, R, 2013. "Why I prescribe nature": In D.C., pioneering pediatricians offer new hope and health through park Rx. Minneapolis: Children and Nature Network, 05 November.

31. Association of Nature and Forest Therapy Guides and Programs.
32. Williams, F, 2016. This is your brain on nature. *National Geographic*, January.
33. Li, Q, & Kawada T, 2010. Healthy forest parks make healthy people: forest environments enhance human immune function. (Unpublished manuscript)
34. Li, Q, Kobayashi, M, Wakayama, Y, Inagaki, H, Katsumata, M, Hirata, Y, Hirata, K, Shimizu, T, Kawada, T, Park, BJ, Ohira, T, Kagawa, T, & Miyazaki, Y, 2009. Effect of phytoncide from trees on human natural killer cell function. *International Journal of Immunopathology and Pharmacology*, 22(4), 951-959, October-December. doi: 10.1177/039463200902200410
35. Li, Q, Nakadai, A, Matsushima, H, Miyazaki, Y, Krensky, AM, Kawada, T, & Morimoto, K, 2006. Phytoncides (wood essential oils) induce human natural killer cell activity. *Immunopharmacology and Immunotoxicology*, 28(2), 319-333. doi: 10.1080/08923970600809439
36. Matsubara, E, & Kawai, S, 2014. VOCs emitted from Japanese cedar (Cryptomeria japonica) interior walls induce physiological relaxation. *Building and Environment*, 72, 125-130, February. doi:10.1016/j.buildenv.2013.10.023
37. da Silva, SL, Figueiredo, PM, & Yano, T, 2007. Chemotherapeutic potential of the volatile oils from Zanthoxylum rhoifolium Lam leaves. *European Journal of Pharmacology*, 576(1-3), 180-188, December. doi:10.1016/j.ejphar.2007.07.065
38. Grassmann, J, Hippeli, S, Vollmann, R, & Elstner, EF, 2003. Antioxidative properties of the essential oil from Pinus mugo. *Journal of Agricultural and Food Chemistry*, 51(26), 7576-7582, 17 December.
39. Baggoley, C, 2015. *Review of the Australian government rebate on natural therapies for private health insurance*. Canberra: Department of Health.
40. Beute, F, & de Kort, Y, 2013. Let the sun shine! measuring explicit and implicit preference for environments differing in naturalness, weather type and brightness. *Journal of Environmental Psychology*, 36, 162-178, July. doi: 10.1016/j.jenvp.2013.07.016
41. Boubekri, M, Cheung, IN, Reid, KJ, Wang, CH, & Zee, PC, 2014. Impact of windows and daylight exposure on overall health and sleep quality of office workers: a case-control pilot study. *Journal of Clinical Sleep Medicine*, 10(6), 603-611, 15 June. doi: 10.5664/jcsm.3780.
42. Harb, F, Hidalgo, MP, & Martau, B, 2015. Lack of exposure to natural light in the workspace is associated with physiological, sleep and depressive symptoms. *Chronobiology International*, 32(3), 368-375, April. doi: 10.3109/07420528.2014.982757
43. Roenneberg, T, Kantermann, T, Juda, M, Vetter, C, & Allebrandt, KV, 2013. Light and the human circadian clock. In: A Kramer & M Merrow, eds., *Circadian Clocks*. (Series: *Handbook of Experimental Pharmacology*, volume 217) Berlin: Springer-Verlag, pages 311-331. doi: 10.1007/978-3-642-25950-0_13.
44. Kauffman, JM, 2009. Benefits of vitamin D supplementation. *Journal of American Physicians and Surgeons*, 14(2), 38-45, Summer.
45. Lansdowne, AT, & Provost, SC, 1988. Vitamin D3 enhances mood in healthy subjects during winter. *Psychopharmacology*, 135(4), 319-323, February.
46. Berwick, M, Buller, DB, Cust, A, Gallagher, R, Lee, TK, Meyskens, F, Pandey, S, Thomas, NE, Veierød, MB, & Ward, S, 2016. Melanoma epidemiology and prevention. In: HL Kaufman and JM Megner, eds., *Melanoma*. (Series: Cancer Treatment and Research, volume 167) Cham, Switzerland: Springer International, pages 17-49. doi: 10.1007/978-3-319-22539-5_2.
47. Wolpowitz, D, & Gilchrest, BA, 2006. The vitamin D questions: How much do you need and how should you get it? *Journal of the American Academy of Dermatology*, 54(2), 301-317, February. doi: http://dx.doi.org/10.1016/j.jaad.2005.11.1057 – American Cancer Society, 2016. *Cancer Facts & Figures, 2016*. Atlanta: American Cancer Society.
48. Graedel, L, Merker, M, Felder, S, Kutz, A, Haubitz, S, Faessler, L, Kaeslin, M, Huber, A, Mueller, B, & Schuetz, P, 2016. Vitamin D deficiency strongly predicts adverse medical outcome across different medical inpatient populations: results from a prospective study. *Medicine*, 95(19), e3533, May. doi: 10.1097/MD.0000000000003533.
49. Holick, MF, & Chen, TC, 2008. Vitamin D deficiency: A worldwide problem with health consequences. *American Journal of Clinical Nutrition*, 87(4), 1080S-1086S, April.
50. Kriegel, MA, Manson, JE, & Costenbader, KH, 2011. Does vitamin D affect risk of developing autoimmune disease? a systematic review. *Seminars in Arthritis and Rheumatism*, 40(6), 512-531, e8. June. doi: 10.1016/j.semarthrit.2010.07.009. – Baeke, F, van Etten, E, Gysemans, C, Overbergh, L, & Mathieu, C, 2008. Vitamin D signaling in immune-mediated disorders: Evolving insights and therapeutic opportunities. *Molecular Aspects of Medicine*, 29(6), 376-387, December. doi: 10.1016/j.mam.2008.05.004. – Wagner, CL, Taylor, SN, Johnson, DD, & Hollis, BW, 2012. The role of vitamin D in pregnancy and lactation: emerging concepts. *Women's Health*, 8(3), 323-340, May. doi: 10.2217/whe.12.17. – Chiang, M, Natarajan, R, & Fan, X, 2016. Vitamin D in schizophrenia: a clinical review. *Evidence-Based Mental Health*, 19(1), 6-9, February. doi: 10.1136/eb-2015-102117 – Muscogiuri, G, Nuzzo, V, Gatti, A, Zuccoli, A, Savastano, S, Di Somma, C, Pivonello, R, Orio, F, & Colao, A, 2016. Hypovitaminosis D: a novel risk factor for coronary heart disease in type 2 diabetes? *Endocrine*, 51(2), 268-273, February. doi: 10.1007/s12020-015-0609-7.
51. Tagliabue, E, Raimondi, S, & Gandini, S, 2015. Meta-analysis of vitamin D-binding protein and cancer risk. *Cancer Epidemiology, Biomarkers & Prevention*, 24(11), 1758-1765, November. doi: 10.1158/1055-9965.EPI-15-0262. – Holick, MF, 2004. Vitamin D: Importance in the prevention of cancers, type 1 diabetes, heart disease, and osteoporosis. *American Journal of Clinical Nutrition*, 79(3), 362-371, March. – Garland, CF, 2003. More on preventing skin cancer: Sun avoidance will increase incidence of cancers overall. (Letter) *British Medical Journal*, 327(7425), 1228, 22 November. doi: 10.1136/bmj.327.7425.1228-a.
52. Theodoratou, E, Tzoulaki I, Zgaga, L, & Ioannidis, JPA, 2014. Vitamin D and multiple health outcomes: umbrella review of systematic reviews and meta-analyses of observational studies and randomised trials. *British Medical Journal*, 348, g2035, 01 April. doi: 10.1136/bmj.g2035.
53. Holick, MF, & Chen, TC, 2008. Vitamin D deficiency: A worldwide problem with health consequences. *American Journal of Clinical Nutrition*, 87(4), 1080S-1086S, April.
54. Frandsen, TB, Pareek, M, Hansen, JP, & Nielsen, CT, 2014. Vitamin D supplementation for treatment of seasonal affective symptoms in healthcare professionals: A double-blind randomised placebo-controlled trial. *BMC Research Notes*, 7, 528, August. doi: 10.1186/1756-0500-7-528. – Dumville, JC, Miles, JN, Porthouse, J, Cockayne, S, Saxon, L, & King, C, 2006. Can vitamin D supplementation prevent winter-time blues? a randomised trial among older women. *Journal of Nutrition, Health, and Aging*, 10(2), 151-153, March-April. – Theodoratou, E, Tzoulaki I, Zgaga, L, & Ioannidis, JPA, 2014. Vitamin D and multiple health outcomes: umbrella review of systematic reviews and meta-analyses of observational studies and randomised trials. *British Medical Journal*, 348, g2035, 01 April. doi: 10.1136/bmj.g2035. – Reid, IR, 2016. What diseases are causally linked to vitamin D deficiency? *Archives of Disease in Childhood*, 101(2), 185-189, February. doi: 10.1136/archdischild-2014-307961. – Sperati, F, Vici, P, Maugeri-Saccà, M, Stranges, S, Santesso, N, Mariani, L, Giordano, A, Sergi, D, Pizzuti, L, Di, Lauro, L, Montella, M, Crispo, A, Mottolese, M, & Barba, M, 2013. Vitamin D supplementation and breast cancer prevention: a systematic review and meta-analysis of randomized clinical trials. *PLoS One*, 22, 8(7), e69269, July. doi: 10.1371/journal.pone.0069269.
55. Sanders, KM, Stuart, AL, Williamson, EJ, Simpson, JA, Kotowicz, MA, Young, D, & Nicholson, GC, 2010. Annual high-dose oral vitamin D and falls and fractures in older women: A randomized controlled trial. *Journal of the American Medical Association*, 303(18), 1815-1822, 12 May. doi: 10.1001/jama.2010.594.
56. Wolpowitz, D, & Gilchrest, BA, 2006. The vitamin D questions: How much do you need and how should you get it? *Journal of the American Academy of Dermatology*, 54(2), 301-317, February. doi: http://dx.doi.org/10.1016/j.jaad.2005.11.1057 – Norval, M, & Wulf, HC, 2009. Does chronic sunscreen use reduce vitamin D production to insufficient levels? *British Journal of Dermatology*, 161(4), 732-736, October. doi: 10.1111/j.1365-2133.2009.09332.x
57. Münzel, T, Gori, T, Babisch, W, & Basner, M, 2014. Cardiovascular effects of environmental noise exposure. *European Heart Journal*, 35(13), 829-836, April. doi: 10.1093/eurheartj/ehu030.
58. Hammer, MS, Swinburn, TK, Neitzel, RL, 2014. Environmental noise pollution in the United States: developing an effective public health response. *Environmental Health Perspectives*, 122(2), 115-119, February. doi: 10.1289/ehp.1307272.
59. World Health Organization, 2015. *1 billion people at risk of hearing loss: WHO highlights serious threat posed by exposure to recreational noise.* [news release] Geneva: World Health Organization, 27 February.
60. Bronzaft, AL, 1981. The effect of a noise abatement program on reading ability. *Journal of Environmental Psychology*, 1(3), 215-222, September. doi: 10.1016/S0272-4944(81)80040-0
61. Swinburn, TK, Hammer, MS, & Neitzel, RL (2015). Valuing quiet: An economic assessment of U.S. environmental noise as a cardiovascular

health hazard. *American Journal of Preventive Medicine*, 49(3), 345-353, September. doi: 10.1016/j.amepre.2015.02.016.

62. Ulrich, RS, 1984. View through a window may influence recovery from surgery. *Science*, 224(4647), 420-421.
63. Ulrich, RS, Zimring, C, Zhu, X, DuBose, J, Seo, HB, Choi, YS, Quan, X, Joseph, A, 2008. A review of the research literature on evidence-based healthcare design. *HERD: Health Environments Research & Design Journal*, 1(3), 61-125, Spring. doi: 10.1177/193758670800100306
64. Swinburn, TK, Hammer, MS, & Neitzel, RL (2015). Valuing quiet: An economic assessment of U.S. environmental noise as a cardiovascular health hazard. *American Journal of Preventive Medicine*, 49(3), 345-353, September. doi: 10.1016/j.amepre.2015.02.016.
65. Florida Hospital Celebration Health, [n.d.] Imaging services: Seaside imaging. Celebration, FL: Florida Hospital Celebration Health.
66. ScentAir, [n.d.] Florida hospital. [case study] Charlotte, NC: ScentAir.
67. Tischler, L, 2005. Smells like brand spirit. *Fast Company*, 01 August.
68. Ulrich, RS, Zimring, C, Zhu, X, DuBose, J, Seo, HB, Choi, YS, Quan, X, & Joseph, A, 2008. A review of the research literature on evidence-based healthcare design. *HERD: Health Environments Research & Design Journal*, 1(3), 61-125, Spring. doi: 10.1177/193758670800100306
69. Commoner, B, 1971. *The closing circle: nature, man, and technology*. New York: Alfred A. Knopf.

CHAPTER 7 – SLEEP

1. Edison, TA, 1880. Electric lamp. (Patent number US 223,898 A). Washington, DC: United States Patent and Trademark Office, January 27.
2. New York Times, 1908. Four hours' sleep enough for anyone, says Edison. *New York Times*, 31 May, page 35.
3. Derickson, A, 2013. *Dangerously sleepy: overworked Americans and the cult of manly wakefulness*. Philadelphia: University of Pennsylvania Press.
4. Lewis, M, 2012. Obama's way. *Vanity Fair*, 11 September.
5. de Castella, T, 2013. Thatcher: can people get by on four hours' sleep? *BBC News Magazine*, 10 April.
6. Haglage, A, 2016. Donald Trump's 4-hour sleep habit could explain his personality. *The Daily Beast*, 02 April.
7. Trump, DJ, 2005. *Trump: Think like a billionaire: everything you need to know about success, real estate, and life*. New York: Ballantine Books, page xix.
8. Goldstein, AN, & Walker, MP, 2014. The role of sleep in emotional brain function. *Annual Review of Clinical Psychology*, 10, 679-708, March. doi: 10.1146/annurev-clinpsy-032813-153716 – Knutson, KL, Spiegel, K, Penev, P, & Van Cauter, E, 2007. The metabolic consequences of sleep deprivation. *Sleep Medicine Reviews*, 11(3), 163-178, June. doi: 10.1016/j.smrv.2007.01.002. – Cirelli, C, & Tononi, G, 2008. Is sleep essential? *PLoS Biology*, 6(8), e216, 26 August. doi: 10.1371/journal.pbio.0060216
9. Prather, AA, Janicki-Deverts, D, Hall, MH, & Cohen, S, 2015. Behaviorally assessed sleep and susceptibility to the common cold. *Sleep*, 38(9), 1353-1359, 01 September. doi: 10.5665/sleep.4968
10. Institute of Medicine (US), Committee on Sleep Medicine and Research, 2006. Extent and health consequences of chronic sleep loss and sleep disorders. In HR Colten & BM Altevogt, eds., 2006. *Sleep disorders and sleep deprivation: an unmet public health problem*. Washington: National Academies Press, Chapter 3. – Vgontzas, AN, Liao, D, Bixler, EO, Chrousos, GP, & Vela-Bueno, A, 2009. Insomnia with objective short sleep duration is associated with a high risk for hypertension. *Sleep*, 32(4), 491-497, April. – Spiegel, K, Knutson, K, Leproult, R, Tasali, E, & Van Cauter, E, 2005. Sleep loss: a novel risk factor for insulin resistance and Type 2 diabetes. *Journal of Applied Physiology*, 99(5), 2008-2019, November. doi: 10.1152/japplphysiol.00660.2005 – Watanabe, M, Kikuchi, H, Tanaka, K, & Takahashi, M, 2010. Association of short sleep duration with weight gain and obesity at 1-year follow-up: A large-scale prospective study. *Sleep*, 33(2), 161-167, February. – Sabanayagam, C, & Shankar, A, 2010. Sleep duration and cardiovascular disease: results from the National Health Interview Survey. *Sleep*, 33(8), 1037-1042, August. – Bagai, K, 2010. Obstructive sleep apnea, stroke, and cardiovascular diseases. *Neurologist*, 16(6), 329-339, November. doi: 10.1097/NRL.0b013e3181f097cb
11. Grandner, MA, Hale, L, Moore, M, & Patel, NP, 2010. Mortality associated with short sleep duration: the evidence, the possible mechanisms, and the future. *Sleep Medicine Reviews*, 14(3), 191-203, June. doi: 10.1016/j.smrv.2009.07.006
12. Léger, D, Guilleminault, C, Bader, G, Lévy, E, & Paillard, M, 2002. Medical and socio-professional impact of insomnia. *Sleep*, 25(6), 625-629, 15 September. – Bagai, K, 2010. Obstructive sleep apnea, stroke, and cardiovascular diseases. *Neurologist*, 16(6), 329-339, November. doi: 10.1097/NRL.0b013e3181f097cb – Garcia-Borreguero, D, Egatz, R, Winkelmann, J, & Berger, K, 2006. Epidemiology of restless legs syndrome: the current status. *Sleep Medicine Reviews*, 10(3), 153-167, June.
13. Prather, AA, Gurfein, B, Moran, P, Daubenmier, J, Acree, M, Bacchetti, P, Sinclair, E, Lin, J, Blackburn, E, Hecht, FM, & Epel, ES, 2015. Tired telomeres: poor global sleep quality, perceived stress, and telomere length in immune cell subsets in obese men and women. *Brain, Behavior, and Immunity*, 47, 155-162, July. doi: 10.1016/j.bbi.2014.12.011
14. Gruber, R, & Cassoff, J, 2014. The interplay between sleep and emotion regulation: conceptual framework empirical evidence and future directions. *Current Psychiatry Reports*, 16(11), 500, November. doi: 10.1007/s11920-014-0500-x – Boudebesse, C, & Henry, C, 2012. [Emotional hyper-reactivity and sleep disturbances in remitted patients with bipolar disorders.] [article in French] *L'Encéphale*, 38(S4), S173-S178, December. doi: 10.1016/S0013-7006(12)70096-9 – Bower, B, Bylsma, LM, Morris, BH, & Rottenberg, J, 2010. Poor reported sleep quality predicts low positive affect in daily life among healthy and mood-disordered persons. *Journal of Sleep Research*, 19(2), 323-332, June. doi: 10.1111/j.1365-2869.2009.00816.x
15. Boivin, DB, Czeisler, CA, Dijk, DJ, Duffy, JF, Folkard, S, Minors, DS, Totterdell, P, & Waterhouse, JM, 1997. Complex interaction of the sleep-wake cycle and circadian phase modulates mood in healthy subjects. *Archives of General Psychiatry*, 54(2), 145-152, February. doi: 10.1001/archpsyc.1997.01830140055010
16. Lockley, SW, Cronin, JW, Evans, EE, Cade, BE, Lee, CJ, Landrigan, CP, Rothschild, JM, Katz, JT, Lilly, CM, Stone, PH, Aeschbach, D, & Czeisler, CA; Harvard Work Hours, Health and Safety Group, 2004. Effect of reducing interns' weekly work hours on sleep and attentional failures. *New England Journal of Medicine*, 351(18), 1829 1837, 28 October. doi: 10.1056/NEJMoa041404 – Toker, A, 2006. [Interns: the relationship between sleep deprivation, working hours and performance.] [Article in Hebrew] *Harefuah*, 145(7), 502-504, 550, July. – Mansukhani, MP, Kolla, BP, Surani, S, Varon, J, & Ramar, K, 2012. Sleep deprivation in resident physicians, work hour limitations, and related outcomes: a systematic review of the literature. *Postgraduate Medicine*, 124(4), 241-249, July. doi: 10.3810/pgm.2012.07.2583.
17. Stutts, JC, Wilkins, JW, Scott, OJ, & Vaughn, BV, 2003. Driver risk factors for sleep-related crashes. *Accident Analysis & Prevention*, 35(3), 321-331, May. doi: 10.1016/S0001-4575(02)00007-6
18. Williamson, A, & Feyer, A, 2000. Moderate sleep deprivation produces impairments in cognitive and motor performance equivalent to legally prescribed levels of alcohol intoxication. *Occupational and Environmental Medicine*, 57(10), 649-655, October. doi: 10.1136/oem.57.10.649
19. Institute of Medicine (US), Committee on Sleep Medicine and Research, 2006. Functional and economic impact of sleep loss and sleep-related disorders. In HR Colten & BM Altevogt, eds., *Sleep disorders and sleep deprivation: an unmet public health problem*. Washington: National Academies Press, Chapter 4.
20. Centers for Disease Control and Prevention, 2015. Insufficient sleep is a public health problem. Atlanta, GA: Centers for Disease Control and Prevention, 03 September.
21. Gladwell, M, 2008. *Outliers: the story of success*. New York: Little, Brown.
22. Ericsson, KA, Krampe, R, & Tesch-Romer, C, 1993. The role of deliberate practice in the acquisition of expert performance. *Psychological Review*, 100(3), 363-406.
23. Kamdar, BB, Kaplan, AA, Kezirian, EJ, & Dement, WC, 2004. The impact of extended sleep on daytime alertness, vigilance, and mood. *Sleep Medicine*, 5(5), 441-448, September.
24. Mah, CD, Mah, KE, Kezirian, EJ, & Dement, WC, 2011. The effects of sleep extension on the athletic performance of collegiate basketball players. *Sleep*, 34(7), 943-950, 01 July. doi: 10.5665/SLEEP.1132
25. Hirshkowitz, M, Whiton, K, Albert, SM, Alessi, C, Bruni, O, DonCarlos, L, Hazen, N, Herman, J, Katz, ES, Kheirandish-Gozal, L, Neubauer, DN, O'Donnell, AE, Ohayon, M, Peever, J, Rawding, R, Sachdeva, RC, Setters, B, Vitiello, MV, Ware, JC, & Adams Hillard, PJ, 2015. National Sleep Foundation's sleep time duration recommendations: methodology and results summary. *Sleep Health Journal*, 1(1), 40-43. doi: 10.1016/j.sleh.2014.12.010
26. Ford, ES, Cunningham, TJ, & Croft, JB, 2015. Trends in self-reported sleep duration among US adults from 1985 to 2012. *Sleep*, 38(5), 829-832, 01 May. doi: 10.5665/sleep.4684

27. Soldatos, CR, Allaert, FA, Ohta, T, & Dikeos, DG, 2005. How do individuals sleep around the world? results from a single-day survey in ten countries. *Sleep Medicine*, 6(1), 5-13, January. doi: 10.1016/j.sleep.2004.10.006.
28. Matricciani, LA, Olds, TS, Blunden, S, Rigney, G, & Williams, MT, 2012. Never enough sleep: A brief history of sleep recommendations for children. *Pediatrics*, 129(3), 548-556, March. doi: 10.1542/peds.2011-2039.
29. He, Y, Jones, CR, Fujiki, N, Xu, Y, Guo, B, Holder, JL, Rossner, MJ, Nishino, S, & Fu, YH, 2009. The transcriptional repressor DEC2 regulates sleep length in mammals. *Science*, 325(5942), 866-870, 14 August. doi: 10.1126/science.1174443
30. Harmon, K, 2009. Rare genetic mutation lets some people function with less sleep. *Scientific American*, 13 August 13.
31. Ferrara, M, & De Gennaro, L, 2001. How much sleep do we need? *Sleep Medicine Reviews*, 5(2), 155-179, April. doi: 10.1053/smrv.2000.0138
32. Reddy, S, 2014. Why seven hours of sleep might be better than eight: Sleep experts close in on the optimal night's sleep. *The Wall Street Journal*, July 21.
33. Natale, V, Adan, A, & Fabbri, M, 2009. Season of birth, gender, and social-cultural effects on sleep timing preferences in humans. *Sleep*, 32(3), 423-426, March. – Ferrara, M, & De Gennaro, L, 2001. How much sleep do we need? *Sleep Medicine Reviews*, 5(2), 155-179, April. doi: 10.1053/smrv.2000.0138
34. Goldstein, AN, Greer, SM, Saletin, JM, Harvey, AG, Nitschke, JB, & Walker, MP, 2013. Tired and apprehensive: anxiety amplifies the impact of sleep loss on aversive brain anticipation. *Journal of Neuroscience*, 33(26), 10607-10615, 26 June. doi: 10.1523/jneurosci.5578-12.2013.
35. Takahashi, M, 2003. The role of prescribed napping in sleep medicine. *Sleep Medicine Reviews*, 7(3), 227-235, June. doi: 10.1053/smrv.2002.0241
36. Takahashi, M, Fukuda, H, & Arito, H, 1998. Brief naps during post-lunch rest: effects on alertness, performance, and autonomic balance. *European Journal of Applied Physiology and Occupational Physiology*, 78(2), 93-98, July. doi: 10.1007/s004210050392 – Hayashi, M, Ito, S, & Hori, T, 1999. The effects of a 20-min nap at noon on sleepiness, performance and EEG activity. International Journal of Psychophysiology, 32(2), 173-180, May. doi:10.1016/S0167-8760(99)00009-4 – Milner, CE, & Cote, KA, 2009. Benefits of napping in healthy adults: impact of nap length, time of day, age, and experience with napping. *Journal of Sleep Research*, 18(2), 272-281, June. doi: 10.1111/j.1365-2869.2008.00718.x
37. Strogatz, SH, Kronauer, RE, & Czeisler, CA, 1987. Circadian pacemaker interferes with sleep onset at specific times each day: role in insomnia. *American Journal of Physiology*, 253(1 Pt 2), R172-R178, July.
38. Milner, CE, & Cote, KA, 2009. Benefits of napping in healthy adults: impact of nap length, time of day, age, and experience with napping. *Journal of Sleep Research*, 18(2), 272-281, June. doi: 10.1111/j.1365-2869.2008.00718.x
39. Institute of Medicine (US), Committee on Sleep Medicine and Research, 2006. Sleep physiology. In HR Colten & BM Altevogt, eds., *Sleep disorders and sleep deprivation: an unmet public health problem*. Washington: National Academies Press, Chapter 2.
40. Cirelli, C, & Tononi, G, 2008. Is sleep essential? *PLoS Biology*, 6(8), e216, 26 August. doi: 10.1371/journal.pbio.0060216
41. Wolf-Meyer, M, 2013. Where have all our naps gone? or Nathaniel Kleitman, the consolidation of sleep, and the historiography of emergence. *Anthropology of Consciousness*, 24(2), 96-116, September. doi: 10.1111/anoc.12014
42. *Studying mystery of sleep, scientists live month in cave.* (News of the Day) Metrotone News Newsreel, 01 [?] September, 1938. – Film News of the Week, 1938. *The Sydney Morning Herald* (New South Wales), 01 September, page 28.
43. Kleitman, N, 1939, rev. 1963. *Sleep and wakefulness*. Chicago: University of Chicago Press.
44. Aserinsky, E, & Kleitman, N, 1953. Regularly occurring periods of eye motility, and concomitant phenomena, during sleep. First published in *Science*, 118, 273-274, 04 September. Reprinted 2003 in *The Journal of Neuropsychiatry and Clinical Neurosciences*, 15(4), 454-455, Fall.
45. Benington, JH, & Heller, HC, 1995. Restoration of brain energy metabolism as the function of sleep. *Progress in Neurobiology*, 45(4), 347-360. doi: 10.1016/0301-0082(94)00057-O – Horne, J, 1992. Human slow wave sleep: A review and appraisal of recent findings, with implications for sleep functions, and psychiatric illness. *Experientia*, 48(10), 941-954, 15 October. doi: 10.1007/BF01919141
46. Chow, HM, Horovitz, SG, Carr, WS, Picchioni, D, Coddington, N, Fukunaga, M, Xu, Y, Balkin, TJ, Duyn, JH, & Braun AR, 2013. Rhythmic alternating patterns of brain activity distinguish rapid eye movement sleep from other states of consciousness. *Proceedings of the National Academy of Sciences of the United States of America*, 110(25), 10300-10305, 18 June. doi: 10.1073/pnas.1217691110
47. Luyster, FS, Strollo, PJ, Zee, PC, & Walsh, JK, 2012. Sleep: A health imperative. *Sleep*, 35(6), 727-734, 01 June. doi: 10.5665/sleep.1846.
48. Xie, L, Kang, H, Xu, Q, Chen, MJ, Liao, Y, Thiyagarajan, M, O'Donnell, J, Christensen, DJ, Nicholson, C, Iliff, JJ, Takano, T, Deane, R, Nedergaard, M, 2013. Sleep drives metabolite clearance from the adult brain. *Science*, 342(6156), 373-377, 18 October. doi: 10.1126/science.1241224
49. Gallagher, J, 2013. Sleep 'cleans' the brain of toxins. *BBC News*, 17 October.
50. Jessen, NA, Munk, ASF, Lundgaard, I, & Nedergaard, M, 2015. The Glymphatic system: a beginner's guide. *Neurochemical Research*, 40(12), 2583-2599, December. doi: 10.1007/s11064-015-1581-6
51. Wulff, K, Gatti, S, Wettstein, JG, & Foster, RG, 2010. Sleep and circadian rhythm disruption in psychiatric and neurodegenerative disease. *Nature Reviews Neuroscience*, 11(8), 589-599, August. doi: 10.1038/nrn2868
52. de Souza Lopes, C, Robaina, R, & Rotenberg, L, 2012. Epidemiology of insomnia: prevalence and risk factors. In S. Sahoo, ed. *Can't Sleep? Issues of Being an Insomniac*. Rijeka, Croatia: InTech.
53. Wittchen, HU, Jacobi, F, Rehm, J, Gustavsson, A, Svensson, M, Jönsson, B, Olesen, J, Allgulander, C, Alonso, J, Faravelli, C, Fratiglioni, L, Jennum, P, Lieb, R, Maercker, A, van Os, J, Preisig, M, Salvador-Carulla, L, Simon, R, & Steinhausen, HC, 2011. The size and burden of mental disorders and other disorders of the brain in Europe 2010. *European Neuropsychopharmacology*, 21(9), 655-679, September. doi: 10.1016/j.euroneuro.2011.07.018
54. Katic, B, Heywood, J, Turek, F, Chiauzzi, E, Vaughan, TE, Simacek, K, Wicks, P, Jain, S, Winrow, C, & Renger, JJ, 2015. New approach for analyzing self-reporting of insomnia symptoms reveals a high rate of comorbid insomnia across a wide spectrum of chronic diseases. *Sleep Medicine*, 16(11), 1332-1341, November. doi: 10.1016/j.sleep.2015.07.024.
55. Saddichha, S, 2010. Diagnosis and treatment of chronic insomnia. *Annals of Indian Academy of Neurology*, 13(2), 94-102, April. doi: 10.4103/0972-2327.64628 – Katic, B, Heywood, J, Turek, F, Chiauzzi, E, Vaughan, TE, Simacek, K, Wicks, P, Jain, S, Winrow, C, & Renger, JJ, 2015. New approach for analyzing self-reporting of insomnia symptoms reveals a high rate of comorbid insomnia across a wide spectrum of chronic diseases. *Sleep Medicine*, 16(11), 1332-1341, November. doi: 10.1016/j.sleep.2015.07.024.
56. Riemann, D, Nissen, C, Palagini, L, Otte, A, Perlis, ML, & Spiegelhalder, K, 2015. The neurobiology, investigation, and treatment of chronic insomnia. *Lancet. Neurology*, 14(5), 547-558, May. doi: 10.1016/S1474-4422(15)00021-6.
57. Borbély, AA, & Achermann, P, 1999. Sleep homeostasis and models of sleep regulation. *Journal of Biological Rhythms*, 14(6), 559-570, December. doi: 10.1177/074873099129000894
58. Huang, ZL, Urade, Y, & Hayaishi, O, 2011. The role of adenosine in the regulation of sleep. *Current Topics in Medicinal Chemistry*, 11(8), 1047-1057.
59. Ribeiro, JA, & Sebastião, AM, 2010. Caffeine and adenosine. *Journal of Alzheimer's Disease*, 20(Suppl 1), S3-S15. doi: 10.3233/JAD-2010-1379
60. Brown, GM, 1994. Light, melatonin and the sleep-wake cycle. *Journal of Psychiatry & Neuroscience*, 19(5), 345-353, November. – Richardson, G, & Tate, B, 2000. Hormonal and pharmacological manipulation of the circadian clock: recent developments and future strategies. *Sleep*, 23(Suppl 3), S77-S85, May.
61. Clark, I, & Landolt, HP, 2016. Coffee, caffeine, and sleep: A systematic review of epidemiological studies and randomized controlled trials. *Sleep Medicine Reviews*, pii: S1087-0792(16)00015-0, January 30. doi: 10.1016/j.smrv.2016.01.006.
62. Ribeiro, JA, & Sebastião, AM, 2010. Caffeine and adenosine. *Journal of Alzheimer's Disease*, 20(Suppl 1), S3-S15. doi: 10.3233/JAD-2010-1379
63. Zwyghuizen-Doorenbos, A, Roehrs, TA, Lipschutz, L, Timms, V, & Roth, T, 1990. Effects of caffeine on alertness. *Psychopharmacology*, 100(1), 36-39, March. doi: 10.1007/BF02245786.
64. Kalow, W, 1985. Variability of caffeine metabolism in humans. *Arzneimittel-Forschung*, 35(1A), 319-324, February.
65. Robillard, R, Bouchard, M, Cartier, A, Nicolau, L, & Carrier, J, 2015. Sleep is more sensitive to high doses of caffeine in the middle years of life. *Journal of Psychopharmacology*, 29(6), 688-697, June. doi: 10.1177/0269881115575535

66. Drake, C, Roehrs, T, Shambroom, J, & Roth, T, 2013. Caffeine effects on sleep taken 0, 3, or 6 hours before going to bed. *Journal of Clinical Sleep Medicine*, 9(11), 1195-1200, 15 November. doi: 10.5664/jcsm.3170
67. Landolt, HP, Werth, E, Borbély, AA, & Dijk, DJ, 1995. Caffeine intake (200 mg) in the morning affects human sleep and EEG power spectra at night. *Brain Research*, 675(1-2), 67-74, March. doi:10.1016/0006-8993(95)00040-W.
68. Holzman, DC, 2010. What's in a color? The unique human health effects of blue light. *Environmental Health Perspectives*, 118(1), A22-A27, January. doi: 10.1289/ehp.118-a22
69. Czeisler, CA, Allan, JS, Strogatz, SH, Ronda, JM, Sánchez, R, Ríos, CD, Freitag, WO, Richardson, GS, Kronauer, RE, 1986. Bright light resets the human circadian pacemaker independent of the timing of the sleep-wake cycle. *Science*, 233(4764), 667-671, 08 August. doi: 10.1126/science.3726555
70. Tooley, GA, Armstrong, SM, Norman, TR, & Sali, A, 2000. Acute increases in night-time plasma melatonin levels following a period of meditation. *Biological Psychology*, 53(1), 69-78, May. doi: 10.1016/S0301-0511(00)00035-1 – Martires, J, & Zeidler, M, 2015. The value of mindfulness meditation in the treatment of insomnia. *Current Opinion in Pulmonary Medicine*, 21(6), 547-552, November. doi: 10.1097/MCP.0000000000000207
71. Johnson EO, Roehrs T, Roth T, & Breslau N, 1998. Epidemiology of alcohol and medication as aids to sleep in early adulthood. *Sleep*, 21(2), 178-86, 15 March.
72. Ebrahim, IO, Shapiro, CM, Williams, AJ, & Fenwick, PB, 2013. Alcohol and sleep I. Effects on normal sleep. *Alcoholism, Clinical and Experimental Research*, 37(4), 539-549, April. doi: 10.1111/acer.12006.
73. Park, SY, Oh, MK, Lee, BS, Kim, HG, Lee, WJ, Lee, JH, Lim, JT, & Kim, JY, 2015. The effects of alcohol on quality of sleep. *Korean Journal of Family Medicine*, 36(6), 294-299, November. doi: 10.4082/kjfm.2015.36.6.294
74. Reinberg, A, Touitou, Y, Lewy, H, & Mechkouri, M, 2010. Habitual moderate alcohol consumption desynchronizes circadian physiologic rhythms and affects reaction-time performance. *Chronobiology International*, 27(9-10), 1930-1942, October. doi: 10.3109/07420528.2010.515763
75. Arroll, B, Fernando, A, Falloon, K, Goodyear-Smith, F, Samaranayake, C, & Warman, G, 2012. Prevalence of causes of insomnia in primary care: A cross-sectional study. *British Journal of General Practice*, 62(595), e99-e103, February. doi: 10.3399/bjgp12X625157
76. de Zambotti, M, Sugarbaker, D, Trinder, J, Colrain, IM, & Baker, FC, 2016. Acute stress alters autonomic modulation during sleep in women approaching menopause. *Psychoneuroendocrinology*, 66, 1-10, April. doi: 10.1016/j.psyneuen.2015.12.017 – Zisapel, N, Tarrasch, R, & Laudon, M, 2005. The relationship between melatonin and cortisol rhythms: Clinical implications of melatonin therapy. *Drug Development Research*, 65(3), 119-125, July. doi: 10.1002/ddr.20014
77. Shochat, T, 2012. Impact of lifestyle and technology developments on sleep. *Nature and Science of Sleep*, 4, 19-31, 05 March. doi: 10.2147/NSS.S18891
78. Cohrs, S, Rodenbeck, A, Riemann, D, Szagun, B, Jaehne, A, Brinkmeyer, J, Gründer, G, Wienker, T, Diaz-Lacava, A, Mobascher, A, Dahmen, N, Thuerauf, N, Kornhuber, J, Kiefer, F, Gallinat, J, Wagner, M, Kunz, D, Grittner, U, & Winterer G, 2014. Impaired sleep quality and sleep duration in smokers – results from the German Multicenter Study on Nicotine Dependence. *Addiction Biology*, 19(3), 486-496, May. doi: 10.1111/j.1369-1600.2012.00487.x
79. Wetter, DW, & Young, TB, 1994. The relation between cigarette smoking and sleep disturbance. *Preventive Medicine*, 23(3), 328-334, May. doi: 10.1006/pmed.1994.1046 – Zhang, L, Samet, J, Caffo, B, & Punjabi, NM, 2006. Cigarette smoking and nocturnal sleep architecture. *American Journal of Epidemiology*, 164(6), 529-537, 15 September. doi: 10.1093/aje/kwj231
80. Benowitz, NL, 2009. Pharmacology of nicotine: addiction, smoking-induced disease, and therapeutics. *Annual Review of Pharmacology and Toxicology*, 49, 57-71, February. doi: 10.1146/annurev.pharmtox.48.113006.094742 – Martin, LJ, 2015. Nicotine and tobacco. In *MedlinePlus Medical Encyclopedia*. Bethesda, MD: MedlinePlus, August 29. – Mishra, A, Chaturvedi, P, Datta, S, Sinukumar, S, Joshi, P, & Garg, A, 2015. Harmful effects of nicotine. *Indian Journal of Medical and Paediatric Oncology*, 36(1), 24-31, January-March. doi: 10.4103/0971-5851.151771.
81. Benowitz, NL, 2009. Pharmacology of nicotine: addiction, smoking-induced disease, and therapeutics. *Annual Review of Pharmacology and Toxicology*, 49, 57-71, February. doi: 10.1146/annurev.pharmtox.48.113006.094742
82. McNamara, JP, Wang, J, Holiday, DB, Warren, JY, Paradoa, M, Balkhi, AM, Fernandez-Baca, J, & McCrae, CS, 2014. Sleep disturbances associated with cigarette smoking. *Psychology, Health & Medicine*, 19(4), 410-419. doi: 10.1080/13548506.2013.832782.
83. Jaehne, A, Unbehaun, T, Feige, B, Cohrs, S, Rodenbeck, A, Schütz, AL, Uhl, V, Zobe, A, & Riemann, D, 2015. Sleep changes in smokers before, during and 3 months after nicotine withdrawal. *Addiction Biology*, 20(4), 747-755, July. doi: 10.1111/adb.12151.
84. Morris, C, 2007. Late risers unite in Denmark. London: *BBC News*, 14 June.
85. B-Society, [n.d.] Who we are. [web page] Copenhagen: B-Society.
86. Adan, A, Archer, SN, Hidalgo, MP, Di Milia, L, Natale, V, & Randler, C, 2012. Circadian typology: A comprehensive review. *Chronobiology International*, 29(9), 1153-1175, November. doi: 10.3109/07420528.2012.719971
87. Roenneberg, T, Kuehnle, T, Juda, M, Kantermann, T, Allebrandt, K, Gordijn, M, & Merrow, M, 2007. Epidemiology of the human circadian clock. *Sleep Medicine Reviews*, 11(6), 429-438, December. doi: 10.1016/j.smrv.2007.07.005
88. Barclay, NL, Eley, TC, Buysse, DJ, Archer, SN, & Gregory, AM, 2010. Diurnal preference and sleep quality: same genes? a study of young adult twins. *Chronobiology International*, 27(2), 278-296, January. doi: 10.3109/07420521003663801
89. Kim, SJ, Lee, YJ, Kim, H, Cho, IH, Lee, JY, & Seong-Jin, C, 2010. Age as a moderator of the association between depressive symptoms and morningness-eveningness. *Journal of Psychosomatic Research*, 68(2), 159-164, February. doi: 10.1016/j.jpsychores.2009.06.010
90. Owens, J, 2014. Insufficient sleep in adolescents and young adults: An update on causes and consequences. *Pediatrics*, 134(3), e921-e932, August. doi: 10.1542/peds.2014-1696
91. Selvi, Y, Aydin, A, Boysan, M, Atli, A, Agargun, MY, & Besiroglu, L, 2010. Associations between chronotype, sleep quality, suicidality, and depressive symptoms in patients with major depression and healthy controls. *Chronobiology International*, 27(9-10), 1813-1828, October. doi: 10.3109/07420528.2010.516380
92. Urbán, R, Magyaródi, T, & Rigóa, A, 2011. Morningness-eveningness, chronotypes and health-impairing behaviors in adolescents. *Chronobiology International*, 28(3), 238-247, April. doi: 10.3109/07420528.2010.549599 – Adan, A, 1994. Chronotype and personality factors in the daily consumption of alcohol and psychostimulants. *Addiction*, 89(4), 455-462, April. doi: 10.1111/j.1360-0443.1994.tb00926.x – Prat, G, & Adan, A, 2011. Influence of circadian typology on drug consumption, hazardous alcohol use, and hangover symptoms. *Chronobiology International*, 28(3), 248-257, April. doi: 10.3109/07420528.2011.553018
93. Rosenberg, J, Maximov, II, Reske, M, Grinberg, F, & Shah, NJ, 2014. "Early to bed, early to rise": Diffusion tensor imaging identifies chronotype-specificity. *NeuroImage*, 84, 428-434, 01 January. doi: 10.1016/j.neuroimage.2013.07.086
94. Yu, JH, Yun, CH, Ahn, JH, Suh, S, Cho, HJ, Lee, SK, Yoo, HJ, Seo, JA, Kim, SG, Choi, KM, Baik, SH, Choi, DS, Shin, C, & Kim, NH, 2015. Evening chronotype is associated with metabolic disorders and body composition in middle-aged adults. *Journal of Clinical Endocrinology and Metabolism*, 100(4), 1494-1502, April. doi: 10.1210/jc.2014-3754.
95. Roenneberg T, Allebrandt KV, Merrow M, & Vetter C, 2012. Social jetlag and obesity. *Current Biology*, 22(10), 939-943, May 22. doi: 10.1016/j.cub.2012.03.038.
96. Wittmann, M, Dinich, J, Merrow, M, & Roenneberg, T, 2006. Social jetlag: Misalignment of biological and social time. *Chronobiology International*, 23(1&2), 497-509. doi: 10.1080/07420520500545979
97. Owens, J, Drobnich, D, Baylor, A, & Lewin, D, 2014. School start time change: An in-depth examination of school districts in the United States. *Mind, Brain and Education*, 8(4), 182-213, December. doi: 10.1111/mbe.12059
98. Roenneberg, T, Kantermann, T, Juda, M, Vetter, C, & Allebrandt, KV, 2013. Light and the human circadian clock. In A. Kramer and M. Merrow, *Circadian Clocks*. (Series: *Handbook of Experimental Pharmacology*, (217), 311-331). Berlin: Springer. doi: 10.1007/978-3-642-25950-0_13
99. Vartanian, GV, Li, BY, Chervenak, AP, Walch, OJ, Pack, W, Ala-Laurila, P, & Wong, KY, 2015. Melatonin suppression by light in humans is more sensitive than previously reported. *Journal of Biological Rhythms*, 30(4), 351-354, 30 August. doi: 10.1177/0748730415585413
100. Brainard, GC, Hanifin, JP, Greeson, JM, Byrne, B, Glickman, G, Gerner, E,

& Rollag MD, 2001. Action spectrum for melatonin regulation in humans: evidence for a novel circadian photoreceptor. *Journal of Neuroscience*, 21(16), 6405-6412, August 15. – Thapan, K, Arendt, J, Skene, DJ, 2001. An action spectrum for melatonin suppression: evidence for a novel non-rod, non-cone photoreceptor system in humans. *Journal of Physiology*, 535(Pt 1), 261-267, 15 August. doi: 10.1111/j.1469-7793.2001.t01-1-00261.x

101. Gringras, P, Middleton, B, Skene, DJ, & Revell, VL, 2015. Bigger, brighter, bluer-better? Current light-emitting devices – adverse sleep properties and preventative strategies. *Frontiers in Public Health*, 3, 233, 13 October. doi: 10.3389/fpubh.2015.00233
102. Chang, AM, Aeschbach, D, Duffy, JF, & Czeisler, CA, 2015. Evening use of light-emitting eReaders negatively affects sleep, circadian timing, and next-morning alertness. *Proceedings of the National Academy of Sciences of the United States of America*, 112(4), 1232-1237, 27 January. doi: 10.1073/pnas.1418490112.
103. Wahnschaffe, A, Haedel, S, Rodenbeck, A, Stoll, C, Rudolph, H, Kozakov, R, Schoepp, H, & Kunz, D, 2013. Out of the lab and into the bathroom: evening short-term exposure to conventional light suppresses melatonin and increases alertness perception. *International Journal of Molecular Sciences*, 14(2), 2573-2589, 28 January. doi: 10.3390/ijms14022573.
104. Burkhart, K, & Phelps, JR, 2009. Amber lenses to block blue light and improve sleep: a randomized trial. *Chronobiology International*, 26(8), 1602-1612, December. doi: 10.3109/07420520903523719 – van der Lely, S, Frey, S, Garbazza, C, Wirz-Justice, A, Jenni, OG, Steiner, R, Wolf, S, Cajochen, C, Bromundt, V, & Schmidt, C, 2015. Blue blocker glasses as a countermeasure for alerting effects of evening light-emitting diode screen exposure in male teenagers. *Journal of Adolescent Health*, 56(1), 113-119, January. doi: 10.1016/j.jadohealth.2014.08.002
105. Escofet, J, & Bará, S, 2015. Reducing the circadian input from self-luminous devices using hardware filters and software applications. *Lighting Research and Technology*, 12(9), 10 December. doi: 10.1177/1477153515621946
106. Gross, CR, Kreitzer, MJ, Reilly-Spong, M, Wall, M, Winbush, NY, Patterson, R, Mahowald, M, & Cramer-Bornemann, M, 2011. Mindfulness-based stress reduction vs. pharmacotherapy for primary chronic insomnia: a pilot randomized controlled clinical trial. *Explore: The Journal of Science and Healing*, 7(2), 76-87, March-April. doi: 10.1016/j.explore.2010.12.003
107. Meadows, G, 2015. Does sleep deprivation have any impact on our appearance? Bensons for Beds, May 18. – Oyetakin-White P, Suggs A, Koo B, Matsui MS, Yarosh D, Cooper KD, & Baron ED, 2015. Does poor sleep quality affect skin ageing? *Clinical and Experimental Dermatology*, 40(1), 17-22, January. doi: 10.1111/ced.12455.
108. Axelsson, J, Sundelin, T, Ingre, M, Van Someren, EJ, Olsson, A, Lekander, M, 2010. Beauty sleep: experimental study on the perceived health and attractiveness of sleep deprived people. *BMJ*, 341:c6614, 14 December. doi: 10.1136/bmj.c6614. – Sundelin, T, Lekander, M, Kecklund, G, Van Someren, EJ, Olsson, A, & Axelsson, J. Cues of fatigue: effects of sleep deprivation on facial appearance. *Sleep*, 36(9), 1355-1360, 01 September. doi: 10.5665/sleep.2964.
109. Lewith, GT, Godfrey, AD, & Prescott, P, 2005. A single-blinded, randomized pilot study evaluating the aroma of *Lavandula augustifolia* as a treatment for mild insomnia. *Journal of Alternative and Complementary Medicine*, 11(4), 631-637, August.

CHAPTER 8 – HEALTHCARE

1. Dignity Health, 2013. *Majority of Americans rate kindness as top factor in quality health care.* [news release] San Francisco: Dignity Health, November 13.
2. Guarneri, M, 2014. The science of connection. [editorial] *Global Advances in Health and Medicine,* 3(1), 5-7, January. doi: 10.7453/gahmj.2013.101.
3. Weil, A, 2005. Aging naturally. *Time*, 09 October. – Kluger, J, 1997. Dr. Andrew Weil: Mr. Natural. *Time*, 12 May.
4. Gupta, S, 2005. Scientists & thinkers: Andrew Weil. *Time*, 18 April.
5. Weil, A, 2016. *About DrWeil.com.* [web site]
6. Arizona Center for Integrative Medicine, 2016. About the Center. [web site] Tucson, AZ: Arizona Center for Integrative Medicine.
7. Weil, A, 2016. *Fact sheet.* DrWeil.com.
8. Specter, M, 2011. The power of nothing. *The New Yorker*, December 12.
9. Kaptchuk, TJ, 2000. *The web that has no weaver: Understanding Chinese medicine.* Chicago: Contemporary Books.
10. Feinberg, C, 2013. The placebo phenomenon. *Harvard Magazine*, January-February.
11. Program in placebo studies & therapeutic encounter (PiPS), [n.d.] [website] Boston: Beth Israel Deaconess Medical Center and Harvard Medical School.
12. Kaptchuk, TJ, Kelley, JM, Conboy, LA, Davis, RB, Kerr, CE, Jacobson, EE, Kirsch, I, Schyner, RN, Nam, BH, Nguyen, LT, Park, M, Rivers, AL, McManus, C, Kokkotou, E, Drossman, DA, Goldman, P, & Lembo, AJ, 2008. Components of placebo effect: randomised controlled trial in patients with irritable bowel syndrome. *British Medical Journal*, 336(7651), 999-1003, 03 May. doi: 10.1136/bmj.39524.439618.25.
13. Benedetti, F, 2002. How the doctor's words affect the patient's brain. *Evaluation & the Health Professions*, 25(4), 369-386, December. doi: 10.1177/0163278702238051
14. Benedetti, F, 2002. How the doctor's words affect the patient's brain. *Evaluation & the Health Professions*, 25(4), 369-386, December. doi: 10.1177/0163278702238051 – Bensing, JM, & Verheul, W, 2010. The silent healer: the role of communication in placebo effects. *Patient Education and Counseling*, 80(3), 293-299, September. doi: 10.1016/j.pec.2010.05.033.
15. Erci, B, Sayan, A, Tortumluoğlu, G, Kiliç, D, Şahin, O, & Güngörmüş, Z, 2003. The effectiveness of Watson's Caring Model on the quality of life and blood pressure of patients with hypertension. *Journal of Advanced Nursing*, 41(2), 130-139, January. doi: 10.1046/j.1365-2648.2003.02515.x
16. Thomas, KB, 1987. General practice consultations: is there any point in being positive? *British Medical Journal*, 294 (6581), 1200-1202, 09 May. doi: 10.1136/bmj.294.6581.1200
17. Derksen, F, Bensing, J, Lagro-Janssen, A, 2013. Effectiveness of empathy in general practice: a systematic review. *British Journal of General Practice*, 63(606), e76-e84, January. doi: 10.3399/bjgp13X660814.
18. Kaptchuk, TJ, Friedlander, E, Kelley, JM, Sanchez, MN, Kokkotou, E, Singer, JP, Kowalczykowski, M, Miller, FG, Kirsch, I, &, Lembo, AJ, 2010. Placebos without deception: a randomized controlled trial in irritable bowel syndrome. *PLoS ONE*, 5(12), e15591, 22 December. doi: 10.1371/journal.pone.0015591.
19. Benedetti, F, Maggi, G, Lopiano, L, Lanotte, M, Rainero, I, Vighetti, S, & Pollo, A, 2003. Open versus hidden medical treatments: the patient's knowledge about a therapy affects the therapy outcome. *Prevention & Treatment*, 6(1), June. doi: 10.1037/1522-3736.6.1.61a.
20. Luparello T, Leist N, Lourie CH, & Sweet P, 1970. The interaction of psychologic stimuli and pharmacologic agents on airway reactivity in asthmatic subjects. *Psychosomatic Medicine*, 32(5), 509-513, September. doi: 10.1097/00006842-197009000-00009
21. Benedetti, F, Maggi, G, Lopiano, L, Lanotte, M, Rainero, I, Vighetti, S, & Pollo, A, 2003. Open versus hidden medical treatments: the patient's knowledge about a therapy affects the therapy outcome. *Prevention & Treatment*, 6(1), June. doi: 10.1037/1522-3736.6.1.61a.
22. Levine, JD, Gordon, NC, Smith, R, & Fields, HL, 1981. Analgesic responses to morphine and placebo in individuals with postoperative pain. *Pain*, 10(3), 379-389, June. doi: 10.1016/0304-3959(81)90099-3 – Levine, JD, & Gordon, NC, 1984. Influence of the method of drug administration on analgesic response. *Nature*, 312(5996), 755-756, 02 January. doi: 10.1038/312755a0.
23. Cannon, WB, 1942. "VOODOO" Death. (Reprint of Cannon, WB, 1942. "Voodoo" death. *American Anthropologist*, 44 [new series], 169-181.) (Series: Voices from the Past) *American Journal of Public Health.* 92(10), 1593-1596, October 2002. doi: 10.2105/AJPH.92.10.1593
24. Cannon, WB, 1942. "VOODOO" Death. (Reprint of Cannon, WB, 1942. "Voodoo" death. *American Anthropologist*, 44 [new series], 169-181.) (Series: Voices from the Past) *American Journal of Public Health.* 92(10), 1593-1596, October 2002. doi: 10.2105/AJPH.92.10.1593
25. Sternberg, EM, 2002 Walter B. Cannon and " 'Voodoo' Death": a perspective from 60 years on. *American Journal of Public Health*, 92(10), 1564-1566, October. doi: 10.2105/AJPH.92.10.1564
26. Sternberg, EM, 2002 Walter B. Cannon and " 'Voodoo' Death": a perspective from 60 years on. *American Journal of Public Health*, 92(10), 1564-1566, October. doi: 10.2105/AJPH.92.10.1564
27. Mitsikostas, DD, Chalarakis, NG, Mantonakis, LI, Delicha, EM, & Sfikakis, PP, 2012. Nocebo in fibromyalgia: meta-analysis of placebo-controlled clinical trials and implications for practice. *European Journal of Neurology*, 19(5), 672-680, May. doi: 10.1111/j.1468-1331.2011.03528.x – Papadopoulos, D, & Mitsikostas, DD, 2010.

Nocebo effects in multiple sclerosis trials: a meta-analysis. *Multiple Sclerosis*, 16(7), 816-828, July. doi: 10.1177/1352458510370793 – Mitsikostas, D. D. (2012). Nocebo in headaches: Implications for clinical practice and trial design. *Current Neurology and Neuroscience Reports*, 12(2), 132-137, April. doi: 10.1007/s11910-011-0245-4 – Stathis, P, Smpiliris, M, Konitsiotis, S, & Mitsikostas, DD, 2013. Nocebo as a potential confounding factor in clinical trials for Parkinson's disease treatment: a meta-analysis. *European Journal of Neurology*, 20(3), 527-533, March. doi: 10.1111/ene.12014 – Mitsikostas, DD, Mantonakis, L, & Chalarakis, N, 2014. Nocebo in clinical trials for depression: a meta-analysis. *Psychiatry Research*, 215(1), 82-86, 30 January. doi: 10.1016/j.psychres.2013.10.019

28. Stathis, P, Smpiliris, M, Konitsiotis, S, & Mitsikostas, DD, 2013. Nocebo as a potential confounding factor in clinical trials for Parkinson's disease treatment: a meta-analysis. *European Journal of Neurology*, 20(3), 527-533, March. doi: 10.1111/ene.12014
Abstract: www.ncbi.nlm.nih.gov/pubmed/23145482
29. Zis, P, & Mitsikostas, DD, 2015. Nocebo in Alzheimer's disease: meta-analysis of placebo-controlled clinical trials. *Journal of Neurological Sciences*, 355(1-2), 94-100, August. doi: 10.1016/j.jns.2015.05.029
30. Rodríguez Huerta, MD, Trujillo-Martín, MM, Rúa-Figueroa, Í, Cuellar-Pompa, L, Quirós-López, R, Serrano-Aguilar, P; & Spanish SLE CPG Development Group, 2016. Healthy lifestyle habits for patients with systemic lupus erythematosus: a systemic review. *Seminars in Arthritis and. Rheumatism*, 45(4), 463-470, February. doi: 10.1016/j.semarthrit.2015.09.003.
31. Association of American Medical Colleges, 2012. *New Medical College Admission Test approved: Changes add emphasis on behavioral and social sciences.* [news release] Washington: Association of American Medical Colleges, 16 February.
32. Empathetics: Neuroscience of Emotions [training program] [n.d.] [Boston, MA]: Empathetics. http://empathetics.com/
33. Boodman, SG, 2015. How to teach doctors empathy. *The Atlantic*, 15 March.
34. Riess, H, Kelley, JM, Bailey, RW, Dunn, EJ, & Phillips, M, 2012. Empathy training for resident physicians: a randomized controlled trial of a neuroscience-informed curriculum. *Journal of General Internal Medicine*, 27(10), 1280-1286, October. doi: 10.1007/s11606-012-2063-z
35. Hickson, GB, Federspiel, CF, Pichert, JW, Miller, CS, Gauld-Jaeger, J, & Bost, P, 2002. Patient complaints and malpractice risk. *Journal of the American Medical Association*, 287(22), 2951-2957, 12 June. doi: 10.1001/jama.287.22.2951. – Levinson, W, Roter, DL, Mullooly, JP, Dull, VT, & Frankel, RM, 1997. Physician-patient communication: the relationship with malpractice claims among primary care physicians and surgeons. *Journal of the American Medical Association*, 277(7), 553-559, 19 February. doi:10.1001/jama.1997.03540310051034.
36. Hojat, M, Louis, DZ, Markham, FW, Wender, R, Rabinowitz, C, & Gonnella, JS, 2011. Physicians' empathy and clinical outcomes for diabetic patients. *Academic Medicine*, 86(3), 359-364, March. doi: 10.1097/ACM.0b013e3182086fe1. – Rakel, DP, Hoeft, TJ, Barrett, BP, Chewning, BA, Craig, BM, & Niu, M, 2009. Practitioner empathy and the duration of the common cold. *Family Medicine*, 41(7), 494-501, July-August. – Derksen, F, Bensing, J, & Lagro-Janssen, A, 2013. Effectiveness of empathy in general practice: a systematic review. *British Journal of General Practice*, 63(606), e76-e84, January. doi: 10.3399/bjgp13X660814.
37. Kim, SS, Kaplowitz, S, Johnston, MV, 2004. The effects of physician empathy on patient satisfaction and compliance. *Evaluation & the Health Professions* 27(3), 237-251, September. doi: 10.1177/0163278704267037
38. Krasner, MS, Epstein, RM, Beckman, H, Suchman, AL, Chapman, B, Mooney, CJ, & Quill, TE, 2009. Association of an educational program in mindful communication with burnout, empathy, and attitudes among primary care physicians. *Journal of the American Medical Association*. 302(12), 1284-1293, 23 September. doi: 10.1001/jama.2009.1384. – Hojat, M, Vergare, M, Isenberg, G, Cohen, M, & Spandorfer, J, 2015. Underlying construct of empathy, optimism, and burnout in medical students. *International Journal of Medical Education*, 6:12-16, 29 January. doi:10.5116/ijme.54c3.60cd. – Lamothe, M, Boujut, E, Zenasni, F, & Sultan, S, 2014. To be or not to be empathic: the combined role of empathic concern and perspective taking in understanding burnout in general practice. *BMC Family Practice*, 15, 15, 23 January. doi: 10.1186/1471-2296-15-15.
39. Jacobs, D. [n.d.] A placebo mobile app that changes your life - from Placebo Effect. [online appeal] Seattle: Placebo Effect.
40. Howick, J, Bishop, FL, Heneghan, C, Wolstenholme, J, Stevens, S, Hobbs, FD, & Lewith, G, 2013. Placebo use in the United Kingdom: results from a national survey of primary care practitioners. *PLoS ONE*, 8(3), e58247, 20 March. doi: 10.1371/journal.pone.0058247.
41. Fässler, M, Meissner, K, Schneider, A, & Linde, K, 2010. Frequency and circumstances of placebo use in clinical practice: a systematic review of empirical studies. *BMC Medicine*, 8, 15, 23 February. doi: 10.1186/1741-7015-8-15
42. Colloca, L, & Miller, FG, 2011. Harnessing the placebo effect: the need for translational research. *Philosophical Transactions of the Royal Society of London. Series B, Biological Sciences*, 366(1572), 1922-1930, 27 June. doi: 10.1098/rstb.2010.0399
43. Coghlan, ML, Maker, G, Crighton, E, Haile, J, Murray, DC, White, NE, Byard, RW, Bellgard, MI, Mullaney, I, Trengove, R, Allcock, RJ, Nash, C, Hoban, C, Jarrett, K, Edwards, R, Musgrave, IF, & Bunce, M 2015. Combined DNA, toxicological and heavy metal analyses provides an auditing toolkit to improve pharmacovigilance of traditional Chinese medicine (TCM). *Scientific Reports*, 5, 17475, 10 December. doi: 10.1038/srep17475
44. Global Wellness Institute, [n.d.] [web site] *Statistics and facts*. Miami, FL: The Global Wellness Institute.
45. Wechsler, ME, Kelley, JM, Boyd, IO, Dutile, S, Marigowda, G, Kirsch, I, Israel, E, & Kaptchuk, TJ, 2011. Active albuterol or placebo, sham acupuncture, or no intervention in asthma. *New England Journal of Medicine*, 365(2), 119-126, 14 July. doi: 10.1056/NEJMoa1103319
46. Kaptchuk, TJ, & Miller, FG, 2015. Placebo effects in medicine. *New England Journal of Medicine*, 373(1), 8-9, 02 July. doi: 10.1056/NEJMp1504023

CHAPTER 9 – RELATIONSHIPS

1. Casamento, J, 2013. Winning gold easier than motherhood - Freeman. *Daily Life*, 19 May.
2. Strogatz, SH, 1987. Human sleep and circadian rhythms: a simple model based on two coupled oscillators. *Journal of Mathematical Biology*, 25(3), 327-347. doi: 10.1007/BF00276440
3. Siffre, M, 1975. Six months alone in a cave. *National Geographic*, 147(3), 426-435, March
4. AP Archive, 1972. Synd 7-9-72 Scientist Michel Siffre emerges from cave after 5 months. [video online]
New York: Associated Press.
5. Brown, RE, & Milner, PM, 2003. The legacy of Donald O. Hebb: More than the Hebb Synapse. *Nature Reviews. Neuroscience*, 4(12), 1013-1019, December. doi: 10.1038/nrn1257
6. Loucks, EB, Berkman, LF, Gruenewald, TL, & Seeman, TE, 2006. Relation of social integration to inflammatory marker concentrations in men and women 70 to 79 years. *American Journal of Cardiology*, 97(7), 1010-1016, 01 April. – Shankar, A, McMunn, A, Banks, J, & Steptoes, A, 2011. Loneliness, social isolation, and behavioral and biological health indicators in older adults. *Health Psychology*, 30(4), 377-385, July. doi: 10.1037/a0022826 – Grant, N, Hamer, M, & Steptoe, A, 2009. Social isolation and stress-related cardiovascular, lipid, and cortisol responses. *Annals of Behavioral Medicine*, 37(1), 29-37, February. doi: 10.1007/s12160-009-9081-z – Cacioppo, JT, Ernst, JM, Burleson, MH, McClintock, MK, Malarkey, WB, Hawkley, LC, Kowalewski, RB, Paulsen, A, Hobson, JA, Hugdahl, K, Spiegel, D, & Berntson, GG, 2000. Lonely traits and concomitant physiological processes: The MacArthur social neuroscience studies. *International Journal of Psychophysiology*, 35(2-3), 143-154, March. doi: 10.1016/S0167-8760(99)00049-5
7. Barth, J, Schneider, S, & von Känel, R, 2010. Lack of social support in the etiology and the prognosis of coronary heart disease: a systematic review and meta-analysis. *Psychosomatic Medicine*, 72(3), 229-238, April. doi: 10.1097/PSY.0b013e3181d01611 – Cohen, S, Doyle, WJ, Skoner, DP, Rabin, BS & Gwaltney, JJ, 1997. Social ties and susceptibility to the common cold. *Journal of the American Medical Association*, 277(24), 1940-1944, 25 June. doi:10.1001/jama.1997.03540480040036. – Bassuk, SS, Glass, TA, & Berkman, LF, 1999. Social disengagement and incident cognitive decline in community-dwelling elderly persons. *Annals of Internal Medicine*, 131(3), 165-173, 03 August. doi:10.7326/0003-4819-131-3-199908030-00002 – Tomaka, J, Thompson, S, & Palacios, R, 2006. The relation of social isolation, loneliness, and social support to disease outcomes among the elderly. *Journal of Aging and Health*, 18(3), 359-384, June. doi: 10.1177/0898264305280993

8. Kroenke, CH, Kubzansky, LD, Schernhammer, ES, Holmes, MD, & Kawachi, I, 2006. Social networks, social support, and survival after breast cancer diagnosis. *Journal of Clinical Oncology*, 24(7), 1105-1111, 01 March. doi: 10.1200/JCO.2005.04.2846
9. Steptoe, A, Shankar, A, Demakakos, P, & Wardle, J, 2013. Social isolation, loneliness, and all-cause mortality in older men and women. *Proceedings of the National Academy of Sciences of the United States of America*, 110(15), 5797-5801, 09 April. doi: 10.1073/pnas.1219686110 – Hawkley, LC, & Cacioppo, JT, 2010. Loneliness matters: a theoretical and empirical review of consequences and mechanisms. *Annals of Behavioral Medicine*, 40(2), 218-227, October. doi: 10.1007/s12160-010-9210-8
10. Holt-Lunstad, J, Smith, TB, Baker, M, Harris, T, & Stephenson, D, 2015. Loneliness and social isolation as risk factors for mortality: a meta-analytic review. *Perspectives on Psychological Science*, 10(2), 227-237, March. doi: 10.1177/1745691614568352
11. McPherson, M, Smith-Lovin, L, & Brashears, ME, 2006. Social isolation in America: changes in core discussion networks over two decades. *American Sociological Review*, 71(3), 353-375, June. doi: 10.1177/000312240607100301
12. Euromonitor Research, 2014. *The rising importance of single person households globally: Proportion of single person households worldwide.* London: Euromonitor International, 29 June.
13. McPherson, M, Smith-Lovin, L, & Brashears, ME, 2006. Social isolation in America: changes in core discussion networks over two decades. *American Sociological Review*, 71(3), 353-375, June. doi: 10.1177/000312240607100301
14. Heinrich, LM, & Gullone, E, 2006. The clinical significance of loneliness: a literature review. *Clinical Psychology Review*, 26(6), 695-718, October. doi: 10.1016/j.cpr.2006.04.002 –Theeke, LA, 2009. Predictors of loneliness in U.S. adults over age sixty-five. Archives of Psychiatric Nursing, 23(5), 387-396, October. doi: 10.1016/j.apnu.2008.11.002
15. Linehan, T, Bottery, S, Kaye, A, Millar, L, Sinclair, D, & Watson, J, 2014. *2030 vision: the best - and worst - futures for older people in the UK.* London: Independent Age, page 25. – Press Association, 2014. *Loneliness a 'serious issue' for older people.* [news release] Republished by London: Age UK, March 14.
16. Shenk, JW, 2009. What makes us happy? *The Atlantic*, June.
17. Vaillant, GE, 2012. *Triumphs of experience: The men of the Harvard Grant Study.* Cambridge, MA: Belknap Press, page 44.
18. Vaillant, GE, 2012. *Triumphs of experience: The men of the Harvard Grant Study.* Cambridge, MA: Belknap Press, page 56.
19. Google, Inc. See the Year in Search 2015. [web site]. Mountain View, CA: Google.
20. Lee, HJ, Macbeth, AH, Pagani, JH, & Young, WS, 2009. Oxytocin: The great facilitator of life. *Progress in Neurobiology*, 88(2), 127-151, June. doi: 10.1016/j.pneurobio.2009.04.001.
21. Hurlemann, R, & Scheele, D, 2016. Dissecting the role of oxytocin in the formation and loss of social relationships. *Biological Psychiatry*, 79(3), 185-193, 01 February. doi: 10.1016/j.biopsych.2015.05.013 – Weisman, O, Zagoory-Sharon, O, & Feldman, R, 2012. Oxytocin administration to parent enhances infant physiological and behavioral readiness for social engagement. Biological Psychiatry, 72(12), 982-989, 15 December. doi: 10.1016/j.biopsych.2012.06.011
22. Hurlemann, R, & Scheele, D, 2016. Dissecting the role of oxytocin in the formation and loss of social relationships. *Biological Psychiatry*, 79(3), 185-193, 01 February. doi: 10.1016/j.biopsych.2015.05.013
23. Kosfeld, M, Heinrichs, M, Zak, PJ, Fischbacher, U, & Fehr, E, 2005. Oxytocin increases trust in humans. (Letter) *Nature*, 435(7042), 673-676, 02 June. doi:10.1038/nature03701
24. Hurlemann, R, Patin, A, Onur, OA, Cohen, MX, Baumgartner, T, Metzler, S, Dziobek, I, Gallinat, J, Wagner, M, Maier, W, & Kendrick, KM, 2010. Oxytocin enhances amygdala-dependent, socially reinforced learning and emotional empathy in humans. *Journal of Neuroscience*, 30(14), 4999-5007, 07 April. doi: 10.1523/JNEUROSCI.5538-09.2010
25. Buchheim, A, Heinrichs, M, George, C, Pokorny, D, Koops, E, Henningsen, P, O'Connor, MF, & Gündel, H, 2009. Oxytocin enhances the experience of attachment security. *Psychoneuroendocrinology*, 34(9), 1417-1422, October. doi: 10.1016/j.psyneuen.2009.04.002
26. Naber, F, van Ijzendoorn, MH, Deschamps, P, van Engeland, H, Bakermans-Kranenburg, MJ, 2010. Intranasal oxytocin increases fathers' observed responsiveness during play with their children: a double-blind within-subject experiment. *Psychoneuroendocrinology*, 35(10), 1583-1586, November. doi: 10.1016/j.psyneuen.2010.04.007
27. Feldman, R, Gordon, I, & Zagoory-Sharon, O, 2011 Maternal and paternal plasma, salivary, and urinary oxytocin and parent-infant synchrony: considering stress and affiliation components of human bonding. *Developmental Science*, 14(4), 752-761, July. doi: 10.1111/j.1467-7687.2010.01021.x
28. Light, K, Grewen, K, &Amico, J, 2005. More frequent partner hugs and higher oxytocin levels are linked to lower blood pressure and heart rate in premenopausal women. *Biological Psychology* 69(1), 5-21, April. doi:10.1016/j.biopsycho.2004.11.002
29. Handlin, L, Nilsson, A, Ejdebäck, M, Hydbring-Sandberg, E, & Uvnäs-Moberg, K, 2012. Associations between the psychological characteristics of the human-dog relationship and oxytocin and cortisol levels. *Anthrozoös*, 25(2), 215-228, June. doi: 10.2752/175303712X13316289505468 –Nagasawa, M, Mitsui, S, En, S, Ohtani, N, Ohta, M, Sakuma, Y, Onaka, T, Mogi, K, Kikusui, T, 2015.Oxytocin-gaze positive loop and the coevolution of human-dog bonds. *Science*, 348(6232), 333-336, 15 April. doi: 10.1126/science.1261022
30. Olff, M, Frijling, JL, Kubzansky, LD, Bradley, B, Ellenbogen, MA, Cardoso, C, Bartz, JA, Yee, JR, van Zuiden, M, 2013. The role of oxytocin in social bonding, stress regulation and mental health: An update on the moderating effects of context and interindividual differences. *Psychoneuroendocrinology*, 38(9), 1883-1894, September. doi: 10.1016/j.psyneuen.2013.06.019
31. Heinrichs, M, Baumgartner, T, Kirschbaum, C, & Ehlert, U, 2003. Social support and oxytocin interact to suppress cortisol and subjective responses to psychosocial stress. *Biological Psychiatry*, 54(12), 1389-1398, 15 December. doi: http://dx.doi.org/10.1016/S0006-3223(03)00465-7 – Norman, GJ, Cacioppo, JT, Morris, JS, Malarkey, WB, Bernston, GG, & Devries, AC, 2011. Oxytocin increases autonomic cardiac control: moderation by loneliness. *Biological Psychology*, 86(3), 174-180, March. doi: 10.1016/j.biopsycho.2010.11.006. – Ditzen, B, Schaer, M, Gabriel, B, Bodenmann, G, Ehlert, U, & Heinrichs, M, 2009. Intranasal oxytocin increases positive communication and reduces cortisol levels during couple conflict. Biological Psychiatry, 65(9), 728-731, 01 May. doi: 10.1016/j.biopsych.2008.10.011
32. Gamer, M, Zurowski, B, & Büchel, C, 2010. Different amygdala subregions mediate valence-related and attentional effects of oxytocin in humans. *Proceedings of the National Academy of Sciences of the United States of America*, 107(20), 9400-9405, 18 May. doi: 10.1073/pnas.1000985107 – Kirsch, P, Esslinger, C, Chen, Q, Mier, D, Lis, S, Siddhanti, S, Gruppe, H, Mattay, VS, Gallhofer, B, Meyer-Lindenberg, A, 2005. Oxytocin modulates neural circuitry for social cognition and fear in humans. *Journal of Neuroscience*, 25(49), 11489-11493, 07 December. doi: 10.1523/JNEUROSCI.3984-05.2005 – Petrovic, P, Kalisch, R, Singer, T, & Dolan, RJ, 2008. Oxytocin attenuates affective evaluations of conditioned faces and amygdala activity. *Journal of Neuroscience*, 28(26), 6607-6615, 25 June. doi: 10.1523/JNEUROSCI.4572-07.2008
33. Guastella, AJ, Mitchell, PB, & Dadds, MR, 2008. Oxytocin increases gaze to the eye region of human faces. *Biological Psychiatry*, 63(1), 3-5, 01 January. doi: 10.1016/j.biopsych.2007.06.026
34. Marsh, AA, Yu, HH, Pine, DS, & Blair, RJ, 2010. Oxytocin improves specific recognition of positive facial expressions. *Psychopharmacology*, 209(3), 225-232, April. doi: 10.1007/s00213-010-1780-4
35. Domes, G, Heinrichs, M, Michel, A, Berger, C, & Herpertz, SC, 2007. Oxytocin improves "mind-reading" in humans. *Biological Psychiatry*, 61(6), 731-733, March. doi: 10.1016/j.biopsych.2006.07.015
36. Bruhn, JG, & Wolf, S, 1979. *The Roseto Story: An anatomy of health.* Norman, OK: University of Oklahoma. –Eliot, RS, 1994. Community and heart disease: [Review of] *The power of clan: the influence of human relationships on heart disease* by Stewart Wolf and John G. Bruhn. *Journal of the American Medical Association*, 272(7), 566, 17 August. doi: 10.1001/jama.1994.03520070086048 –Egolf, B, Lasker, J, Wolf, S, & Potvin, L, 1992. The Roseto effect: a 50-year comparison of mortality rates. *American Journal of Public Health*, 82(8), 1089-1092, August.
37. Umberson, D, & Montez, JK, 2010. Social relationships and health: a flashpoint for health policy. *Journal of Health and Social Behavior*, 51(Supplement), S54-S66. doi: 10.1177/0022146510383501
38. Spiegel, D, Bloom, JR, Kraemer, HC, & Gottheil, E, 1989. Effect of psychosocial treatment on survival of patients with metastatic breast cancer. *The Lancet*, 2(8668), 888-891, 14 October. doi: http://dx.doi.org/10.1016/S0140-6736(89)91551-1
39. Holt-Lunstad, J, Smith, TB, & Layton, JB, 2010. Social relationships and mortality risk: a meta-analytic review. *PLoS Medicine*. 7(7), e1000316, 27 July. doi: 10.1371/journal.pmed.1000316

40. Holt-Lunstad, J, Smith, TB, & Layton, JB, 2010. Social relationships and mortality risk: a meta-analytic review. *PLoS Medicine*. 7(7), e1000316, 27 July. doi: 10.1371/journal.pmed.1000316
41. Uchino, BN., Cacioppo, JT., & Kiecolt-Glaser, JK, 1996. The relationship between social support and physiological processes: a review with emphasis on underlying mechanisms and implications for health. Psychological Bulletin, 119(3), 488-531, May. doi: 10.1037/0033-2909.119.3.488 –Uchino, BN, 2006. Social support and health: a review of physiological processes potentially underlying links to disease outcomes. *Journal of Behavioral Medicine*, 29(4), 377-387, August. doi:10.1007/s10865-006-9056-5
42. Willeit, P, Willeit, J, Mayr, A, Weger, S, Oberhollenzer, F, Brandstätter, A, Kronenberg, F, & Kiechl, S, 2010. Telomere length and risk of incident cancer and cancer mortality. *Journal of the American Medical Association*, 304(1), 69-75, 07 July. doi: 10.1001/jama.2010.897
43. Schutte NS, & Malouff JM, 2014. A meta-analytic review of the effects of mindfulness meditation on telomerase activity. *Psychoneuroendocrinology*, 42:45-8, April. doi: 10.1016/j.psyneuen.2013.12.017.
44. Goetz, JL., Keltner, D, & Simon-Thomas, E, 2010. Compassion: an evolutionary analysis and empirical review. Psychological Bulletin, 136(3), 351-374, May. doi: 10.1037/a0018807
45. Shultz, S, & Dunbar, R, 2010. Encephalization is not a universal macroevolutionary phenomenon in mammals but is associated with sociality. *Proceedings of the National Academy of Sciences of the United States of America*, 107(50), 21582-21586, 14 December. doi: 10.1073/pnas.1005246107 – Dunbar, RI, & Shultz, S, 2007. Evolution in the social brain. *Science*, 317(5843), 1344-1347, 07 September. doi: 10.1126/science.1145463
46. Darwin, C, 1871. *The Descent of Man, and Selection in Relation to Sex*, Volume 1. D. New York: Appleton, page 79.
47. Trinkaus, E, 1982. The Shanidar 3 Neandertha. *American Journal of Physical Anthropology*, 57(1), 37-60, January. doi: 10.1002/ajpa.1330570107
48. Dettwyler, KA, 1991. Can paleopathology provide evidence for "compassion"? *American Journal of Physical Anthropology*, 84(4), 375-384, April. doi: 10.1002/ajpa.1330840402
49. *Shame of a Nation*, 1990. ABC 20/20 [TV programme] New York: ABC News, October 5.
50. Konnikova, M, 2015. The power of touch. *The New Yorker*, 04 March. – Rosapepe, JC, 2001. *Half way home: Romania's abandoned children ten years after the revolution: A report to Americans from the U.S. Embassy, Bucharest, Romania*. Washington, DC: U.S. Agency for International Development. – Carlson, M, and Earls, F. Psychological and neuroendocrinological sequelae of early social deprivation in institutionalized children in Romania. In CS Carter, I Lederhendler, & B Kirkpatrick (eds.) *The Integrative Neurobiology of Affiliation*. Cambridge, MA: MIT Press, 1999, Chapter 24.
51. *Shame of a Nation*, 1990. ABC 20/20 [TV programme] New York: ABC News, October 5.
52. Carlson, M, & Earls, F, 1997. Psychological and neuroendocrinological sequelae of early social deprivation in institutionalized children in Romania. *Annals of the New York Academy of Sciences*, 807, 419-428, January 15. doi: 10.1111/j.1749-6632.1997.tb51936.x
53. Harlow, HF, Dodsworth, RO, & Harlow, MK, 1965. Total social isolation in monkeys. *Proceedings of the National Academy of Sciences*, 54(1), 90-97, July.
54. Blum, D, 2002. *Love at Goon Park: Harry Harlow and the science of affection*. Boston, MA: Perseus. – Gluck, JP, 1997. Harry F. Harlow and animal research: reflection on the ethical paradox. *Ethics & Behavior*, 7(2), 149-161. – Harlow, HF, 1958. The nature of love. Address of the President at the sixty-sixth Annual Convention of the American Psychological Association, Washington, DC, August 31, 1958. *American Psychologist*, 13(12), 673-685, December. doi: 10.1037/h0047884 – *Harlow's studies on dependency in monkeys*, [n.d.] [video online]
55. Carlson, M, and Earls, F. Psychological and neuroendocrinological sequelae of early social deprivation in institutionalized children in Romania. In CS Carter, I Lederhendler, & B Kirkpatrick (eds.) *The Integrative Neurobiology of Affiliation*. Cambridge, MA: MIT Press, 1999, Chapter 24.
56. Bick, J, Zhu, T, Stamoulis, C, Fox, NA, Zeanah, C, & Nelson, CA, 2015. A randomized clinical trial of foster care as an intervention for early institutionalization: long term improvements in white matter microstructure. *JAMA Pediatrics*, 169(3), 211-219, March. doi: 10.1001/jamapediatrics.2014.3212
57. Hertenstein, MJ, 2002. Touch: its communicative functions in infancy. *Human Development*, 45(2), 70-94. doi: 10.1159/000048154 – Gallace, A, & Spence, C, 2010. The science of interpersonal touch: an overview. *Neuroscience & Biobehavioral Reviews*, 34(2), 246-259, February. doi: 10.1016/j.neubiorev.2008.10.004. – National Scientific Council on the Developing Child, 2012. *The Science of Neglect: The Persistent Absence of Responsive Care Disrupts the Developing Brain*. Cambridge, MA: National Scientific Council on the Developing Child, Center on the Developing Child at Harvard University, Working Paper No. 12.
58. Field, T, 2010. Touch for socioemotional and physical well-being: a review. *Developmental Review*, 30(4), 367-383, December. doi: 10.1016/j.dr.2011.01.001 – Heinrichs, M, Baumgartner, T, Kirschbaum, C, & Ehlert, U, 2003. Social support and oxytocin interact to suppress cortisol and subjective responses to psychosocial stress. *Biological Psychiatry*, 54(12), 1389-1398, 15 December. doi: http://dx.doi.org/10.1016/S0006-3223(03)00465-7 – Coan, JA, Schaefer, HS, & Davidson, RJ, 2006. Lending a hand: social regulation of the neural response to threat. *Psychological Science*, 17(12), 1032-1039, December. doi: 10.1111/j.1467-9280.2006.01832.x
59. Nerem, RM, Levesque, MJ, & Cornhill, JF, 1980. Social environment as a factor in diet-induced atherosclerosis. *Science*, 208(4451), 1475-1476, 27 June. doi: 10.1126/science.7384790
60. Grewen, KM, Anderson, BJ, Girdler, SS, & Light, KC, 2003. Warm partner contact is related to lower cardiovascular reactivity. *Behavioral Medicine*, 29(3), 123-130, Fall. doi: 10.1080/08964280309596065
61. Cohen, S, Janicki-Deverts, D, Turner, RB, & Doyle, WJ, 2015. Does hugging provide stress-buffering social support? a study of susceptibility to upper respiratory infection and illness. *Psychological Science*, 26(2), 135-147, February. doi: 10.1177/0956797614559284
62. Boundy, EO, Dastjerdi, R, Spiegelman, D, Fawzi, WW, Missmer, SA, Lieberman, E, Kajeepeta, S, Wall, S, Chan, GJ, 2016. Kangaroo mother care and neonatal outcomes: a meta-analysis. *Pediatrics*, 137(1). doi: 10.1542/peds.2015-2238
63. Feldman, R, Rosenthal, Z, & Eidelman, AI, 2014. Maternal-preterm skin-to-skin contact enhances child physiologic organization and cognitive control across the first 10 years of life. *Biological Psychiatry*, 75(1), 56-64, 01 January. doi: 10.1016/j.biopsych.2013.08.012
64. Field, TM, Hernandez-Reif, M, Quntino, O, Schanberg, S, & Kuhn, C, 1998. Elder retired volunteers benefit from giving massage therapy to infants. *Journal of Applied Gerontology*, 17(2), 229-239, June. doi: 10.1177/073346489801700210
65. Field, T, Diego, M, & Hernandez-Reif, M, 2007. Massage therapy research. *Developmental Review*, 27(1), 75-89, March. doi: 10.1016/j.dr.2005.12.002 – Field, T, 2014. Massage therapy research review. *Complementary Therapies in Clinical Practice*, 20(4), 224-229, November. doi: 10.1016/j.ctcp.2014.07.002
66. Jones, SE, & Yarbrough, AE, 1985. A naturalistic study of the meaning of touch. *Communication Monographs*, 52(1), 19-56, June. doi: 10.1080/03637758509376094
67. Hannon, PA, Finkel, EJ, Kumashiro, M, & Rusbult, CE, 2011. The soothing effects of forgiveness on victims' and perpetrators' blood pressure. *Personal Relationships*, 19(2), 279-289. doi: 10.1111/j.1475-6811.2011.01356.x – McCullough, ME, Orsulak, P, Brandon, A, & Akers, L, 2007. Rumination, fear, and cortisol: An in vivo study of interpersonal transgressions. Health Psychology, 26(1), 126-132, January. doi: 10.1037/0278-6133.26.1.126 – Marks, MJ, Trafimow, D, Busche, LK, & Oates, KN, 2013. A function of forgiveness: exploring the relationship between negative mood and forgiving. *SAGE Open*, 3(4), October-December, doi: 10.1177/2158244013507267
68. van Oyen Witvliet, C, Ludwig, TE, & Vander Laan, KL, 2001. Granting forgiveness or harboring grudges: implications for emotion, physiology, and health. *Psychological Science*, 12(2), 117-123, March. doi: 10.1111/1467-9280.00320
69. Karremans, JC, Van Lange, PA, Ouwerkerk, JW, & Kluwer, ES, 2003. When forgiving enhances psychological well-being: the role of interpersonal commitment. *Journal of Personality and Social Psychology*, 84(5), 1011-1026, May. doi: 10.1037/0022-3514.84.5.1011 – Reed, GL, & Enright, RD, 2006. The effects of forgiveness therapy on depression, anxiety, and posttraumatic stress for women after spousal emotional abuse. *Journal of Consulting and Clinical Psychology*, 74(5), 920-929, October. doi: 10.1037/0022-006X.74.5.920 – van Oyen Witvliet, C, Ludwig, TE, & Vander Laan, KL, 2001. Granting forgiveness or harboring grudges:

implications for emotion, physiology, and health. *Psychological Science*, 12(2), 117-123, March. doi: 10.1111/1467-9280.00320 –Worthington, EL, Witvliet, CV, Pietrini, P, & Miller, AJ, 2007. Forgiveness, health, and well-being: A review of evidence for emotional versus decisional forgiveness, dispositional forgivingness, and reduced unforgiveness. *Journal of Behavioral Medicine*, 30(4), 291-302, August. doi: 10.1007/s10865-007-9105-8

70. Hannon, PA, Finkel, EJ, Kumashiro, M, & Rusbult, CE, 2011. The soothing effects of forgiveness on victims' and perpetrators' blood pressure. *Personal Relationships*, 19(2), 279-289. doi: 10.1111/j.1475-6811.2011.01356.x – Lawler-Row, KA, Karremans, JC, Scott, C, Edlis-Matityahou, M, & Edwards, L, 2008. Forgiveness, physiological reactivity and health: the role of anger. *International Journal of Psychophysiology*, 68(1), 51-58. April. doi: 10.1016/j.ijpsycho.2008.01.001
71. Carson, JW, Keefe, FJ, Goli, V, Fras, AM, Lynch, TR, Thorp, SR, & Buechler, JL, 2005. Forgiveness and chronic low back pain: a preliminary study examining the relationship of forgiveness to pain, anger, and psychological distress. *The Journal of Pain*, 6(2), 84-91, February. doi: http://dx.doi.org/10.1016/j.jpain.2004.10.012 – Rippentrop, EA, Altmaier, EM, Chen, JJ, Found, EM, & Keffala, VJ, 2005. The relationship between religion/spirituality and physical health, mental health, and pain in a chronic pain population. *Pain*, 116(3), 311-321, August. doi: 10.1016/j.pain.2005.05.008
72. Lin, WF, Mack, D, Enright, RD, Krahn, D, & Baskin, TW, 2004. Effects of forgiveness therapy on anger, mood, and vulnerability to substance use among inpatient substance-dependent clients. *Journal of Consulting and Clinical Psychology*, 72(6), 1114-1121, December. doi:10.1037/0022-006X.72.6.1114
73. Lawler, KA, Younger, JW, Piferi, RL, Jobe, RL, Edmondson, KA, & Jones, WH, 2005. The unique effects of forgiveness on health: An exploration of pathways. *Journal of Behavioral Medicine*, 28(2), 157-167, April. DOI: 10.1007/s10865-005-3665-2
74. Marks, MJ, Trafimow, D, Busche, LK, & Oates, KN, 2013. A function of forgiveness: Exploring the relationship between negative mood and forgiving. *Sage Open*, 3(4), 1-9, 13 October. doi: 10.1177/2158244013507267
75. Worthington, EL, 2006. Just forgiving: How the psychology and theology of forgiveness and justice inter-relate. *Journal of Psychology & Christianity*, 25(2), 155-168, Summer. – Worthington, EL, Witvliet, CV, Pietrini, P, & Miller, AJ, 2007. Forgiveness, health, and well-being: A review of evidence for emotional versus decisional forgiveness, dispositional forgivingness, and reduced unforgiveness. *Journal of Behavioral Medicine*, 30(4), 291-302, August. doi: 10.1007/s10865-007-9105-8
76. Zheng, X, Fehr, R, Tai, K, Narayanan, J, & Gelfand, MJ, 2014. The unburdening effects of forgiveness: effects on slant perception and jumping height. *Social Psychological and Personality Science*, 12(23), 23 December. doi: 10.1177/1948550614564222
77. Worthington, EL, van Oyen Witvliet, C, Lerner, AJ, & Scherer, M, 2005. Forgiveness in health research and medical practice. *Explore: The Journal of Science and Healing*, 1(3), 169-176, May. doi: 10.1016/j.explore.2005.02.012
78. Worthington, EL, & Wade, NG, 1999.The psychology of unforgiveness and forgiveness and implications for clinical practice. *Journal of Social and Clinical Psychology*, 18(4), 385-418, December. doi: 10.1521/jscp.1999.18.4.385
79. Worthington, EL, Witvliet, CV, Pietrini, P, & Miller, AJ, 2007. Forgiveness, health, and well-being: A review of evidence for emotional versus decisional forgiveness, dispositional forgivingness, and reduced unforgiveness. *Journal of Behavioral Medicine*, 30(4), 291-302, August. doi: 10.1007/s10865-007-9105-8
80. Worthington, EL, ed., 2005. *Handbook of forgiveness*. New York: Routledge. –Enright, RD, & Fitzgibbons, RP, 2000. *Helping clients forgive: An empirical guide for resolving anger and restoring hope*. Washington, DC: American Psychological Association. http://dx.doi.org/10.1037/10381-000
81. Kramer, AD, Guillory, JE, & Hancock, JT, 2014. Experimental evidence of massive-scale emotional contagion through social networks. *Proceedings of the National Academy of Sciences of the United States of America*, 111(24), 8788-8790, 17 June. doi: 10.1073/pnas.1320040111
82. Booth, R, 2014. Facebook reveals news feed experiment to control emotions. *The Guardian*, 29 June
83. Sy, T, Côté, S, & Saavedra, R, 2005. The contagious leader: impact of the leader's mood on the mood of group members, group affective tone, and group processes. *Journal of Applied Psychology*, 90(2), 295-305, March. doi: 10.1037/0021-9010.90.2.295 –Bono, JE, & Ilies, R, 2006. Charisma, positive emotions and mood contagion. *The Leadership Quarterly*, 17(4), 317-334, August. doi: 10.1016/j.leaqua.2006.04.008 – King, DB, Canham, SL, Cobb, R., & O'Rourke, N, 2016. Reciprocal effects of life satisfaction and depressive symptoms within long-wed couples over time. *The Journals of Gerontology Series B: Psychological Sciences and Social Sciences*, February 11. doi: 10.1093/geronb/gbv162 – Monin, JK, Levy, BR, & Kane, HS, 2015. To love is to suffer: older adults' daily emotional contagion to perceived spousal suffering. *The Journals of Gerontology Series B: Psychological Sciences and Social Sciences*, 29 September. doi: 10.1093/geronb/gbv070 – Dishion, TJ, & Tipsord, JM, 2011. Peer contagion in child and adolescent social and emotional development. *Annual Review of Psychology*, 62, 189-214, January. doi: 10.1146/annurev.psych.093008.100412 – Omdahl, BL, & O'Donnell, C, 1999. Emotional contagion, empathic concern and communicative responsiveness as variables affecting nurses' stress and occupational commitment. *Journal of Advanced Nursing*, 29(6), 1351-1359, June. doi: 10.1046/j.1365-2648.1999.01021.x –Mireault, GC, Crockenberg, SC, Sparrow, JE, Cousineau, K, Pettinato, C, & Woodard, K, 2015. Laughing matters: infant humor in the context of parental affect. *Journal of Experimental Child Psychology*, 136, 30-41, August. doi: 10.1016/j.jecp.2015.03.012
84. Gelfand, M, Shteynberg, G, Lee, T, Lun, J, Lyons, S, Bell, C, Chiao, JY, Bruss, CB, Al Dabbagh, M, Aycan, Z, Abdel-Latif, AH, Dagher, M, Khashan, H, & Soomro, N, 2012. The cultural contagion of conflict. Philosophical Transactions of the Royal Society of London. Series B, Biological Sciences, 367(1589), 692-703, 05 March. doi: 10.1098/rstb.2011.0304
85. Haw, C, Hawton, K, Niedzwiedz, C, & Platt, S, 2013. Suicide clusters: a review of risk factors and mechanisms. *Suicide & Life-Threatening Behavior*, 43(1), 97-108, February. doi: 10.1111/j.1943-278X.2012.00130.x. – Johansson, L, Lindqvist P, & Eriksson, A, 2006. Teenage suicide cluster formation and contagion: implications for primary care. *BMC Family Practice*, 7:32, 17 May. doi: 10.1186/1471-2296-7-32 –Forum on Global Violence Prevention, Board on Global Health, Institute of Medicine, & National Research Council, 2013. *Contagion of Violence: Workshop Summary; II.4, The Contagion of Suicidal Behavior.* Washington: National Academies Press, 06 February
86. Sebastian, S, 2003. Examining 1962's 'laughter epidemic.' *Chicago Tribune*, 29 July. – Hempelmann, CF, 2007. The laughter of the 1962 Tanganyika 'laughter epidemic.' *Humor: International Journal of Humor Research*, 20(1), 49-71, March. doi: 10.1515/HUMOR.2007.003
87. Christakis, NA, & Fowler, JH, 2008. The collective dynamics of smoking in a large social network. *The New England Journal of Medicine*, 358(21), 2249-2258, 22 May. doi: 10.1056/NEJMsa0706154.
88. Rosenquist, JN, Fowler, JH, & Christakis, NA, 2011. Social network determinants of depression. *Molecular Psychiatry*, 16(3), 273-281, March. doi: 10.1038/mp.2010.13
89. Fowler, JH, & Christakis, NA, 2008. Dynamic spread of happiness in a large social network: Longitudinal analysis over 20 years in the Framingham Heart Study. *British Medical Journal*, 337, a2338, 05 December. doi: 10.1136/bmj.a2338
90. Fowler, JH, & Christakis, NA, 2010. Cooperative behavior cascades in human social networks. *Proceedings of the National Academy of Sciences of the United States of America*, 107(12), 5334-5338. doi: 10.1073/pnas.0913149107
91. Johns, DM, 2011. Disconnected? *Slate*, 05 July. – Gelman, A, 2011. *Controversy over the Christakis-Fowler findings on the contagion of obesity.* [blog post] Statistical Modeling, Causal Inference, and Social Science, 10 June. – Lyons, R, 2011. The Spread of evidence-poor medicine via flawed social-network analysis. *Statistics, Politics, and Policy*, 2(1), Article 2. doi: 10.2202/2151-7509.1024
92. Hatfield, E, Cacioppo, JT, Rapson, RL, 1993. Emotional contagion. *Current Directions in Psychological Science*, 2(3), 96-99.
93. Provine, RR, 2005. Contagious yawning and laughing: everyday imitation and mirror-like behavior. *Behavioral and Brain Sciences*, 28(2), 142, April. doi: 10.1017/S0140525X05390030
94. Shalizi, CR, & Thomas, AC, 2011. Homophily and contagion are generically confounded in observational social network studies. *Sociological Methods and Research*, 40(2), (2011), 211-239. doi: 10.1177/0049124111404820
95. Christakis, NA, & Fowler, JH, 2009. *Connected: The amazing power of social networks and how they shape our lives*. London: Harper.
96. Wing, RR, & Jeffery, RW, 1999. Benefits of recruiting participants with friends and increasing social support for weight loss and maintenance. *Journal of Consulting and Clinical Psychology*, 67(1), 132-138, March. 10.1037/0022-006X.67.1.132

97. Gorin, AA, Wing, RR, Fava, JL, Jakicic, JM, Jeffery, R, West, DS, Brelje, K, Dilillo, VG; & Look AHEAD Home Environment Research Group, 2008. Weight loss treatment influences untreated spouses and the home environment: Evidence of a ripple effect. *International Journal of Obesity*, 32(11), 1678-1684, November. doi: 10.1038/ijo.2008.150
98. Buller, DB, Morrill, C, Taren, D, Aickin, M, Sennott-Miller, L, Buller, MK, Larkey, L, Alatorre, C, Wentzel, TM, 1999. Randomized trial testing the effect of peer education at increasing fruit and vegetable intake. *Journal of the National Cancer Institute*, 91(17), 1491-1500, 01 September. doi: 10.1093/jnci/91.17.1491
99. Pearson, N, Biddle, SJH, & Gorely, T, 2008. Family correlates of fruit and vegetable consumption in children and adolescents: A systematic review. *Public Health Nutrition*, 12(2), 267-283, February. doi: 10.1017/S1368980008002589
100. Fredrickson, BL, Cohn, MA, Coffey, KA, Pek, J, & Finkel SM, 2008. Open hearts build lives: positive emotions, induced through loving-kindness meditation, build consequential personal resources. *Journal of Personality and Social Psychology*, 95(5):1045-1062, November. doi: 10.1037/a0013262.
101. Masi, C, Chen, HY, Hawkley, LC, & Cacioppo, JT, 2010. A meta-analysis of interventions to reduce loneliness. *Personality and Social Psychology Review*, 15(3), 219-266, August. doi: 10.1177/1088868310377394

CHAPTER 10 – LASTING CHANGE

1. Friedman, H, & Martin, L, 2011. *The longevity project: surprising discoveries for health and long life from the landmark eight-decade study.* New York: Hudson Street Press, page xviii.
2. Greenwood, V, 2011. The Longevity project: decades of data reveal paths to long life. *The Atlantic*, March 10. – About the authors. [blurb from Friedman, H, & Martin, L, 2011. *The longevity project: surprising discoveries for health and long life from the landmark eight-decade study.* New York: Hudson Street Press.]
3. Tucker, JS, Friedman, HS, Wingard, DL, & Schwartz, JE, 1996. Marital history at midlife as a predictor of longevity: alternative explanations to the protective effect of marriage. *Health Psychology*, 15(2), 94-101, March. doi: 10.1037/0278-6133.15.2.94
4. Friedman, HS, Kern, ML, Hampson, SE, & Duckworth, AL, 2014. A new life-span approach to conscientiousness and health: combining the pieces of the causal puzzle. *Developmental Psychology*, 50(5), 1377-1389, May. doi:10.1037/a0030373 – Goodwin, RD, & Friedman, HS, 2006. Health status and the five-factor personality traits in a nationally representative sample. *Journal of Health Psychology*, 11(5), 643-654, September. doi: 10.1177/1359105306066610 – Shanahan, MJ, Hill, PL, Roberts, BW, Eccles, J, & Friedman, HS, 2014. Conscientiousness, health, and aging: the life course of personality model. *Developmental Psychology*, 50(5), 1407-1425, May. doi: 10.1037/a0031130
5. Roberts, BW, Kuncel, NR, Shiner, R, Caspi, A, & Goldberg, LR, 2007. The power of personality: the comparative validity of personality traits, socioeconomic status, and cognitive ability for predicting important life outcomes. *Perspectives on Psychological Science*, 2(4), 313-345, December. doi: 10.1111/j.1745-6916.2007.00047.x – Friedman, HS, Kern, ML, Hampson, SE, & Duckworth, AL, 2014. A new life-span approach to conscientiousness and health: combining the pieces of the causal puzzle. *Developmental Psychology*, 50(5), 1377-1389, May. doi: 10.1037/a0030373 – Kern, ML, & Friedman, HS, 2008. Do conscientious individuals live longer? a quantitative review. *Health Psychology*, 27(5), 505-512, September. doi: 10.1037/0278-6133.27.5.505.
6. Bogg, T, & Roberts, BW, 2004. Conscientiousness and health-related behaviors: a meta-analysis of the leading behavioral contributors to mortality. *Psychological Bulletin*, 130(6), 887-919, November. doi: 10.1037/0033-2909.130.6.887 – Lodi-Smith, J, Jackson, J, Bogg, T, Walton, K, Wood, D, Harms, P, & Roberts, BW, 2010. Mechanisms of health: education and health-related behaviours partially mediate the relationship between conscientiousness and self-reported physical health. *Psychology and Health*, 25(3), 305-319, March. doi: 10.1080/08870440902736964 – Walton, KE, & Roberts, BW, 2004. On the relationship between substance use and personality traits: abstainers are not maladjusted. *Journal of Research in Personality*, 38(6), 515-535, December. doi: 10.1016/j.jrp.2004.01.002 – Chuah, SC, Drasgow, F, & Roberts, BW, 2006. Personality assessment: does the medium matter? No. *Journal of Research in Personality*, 40(4), 359-376, August. doi: 10.1016/j.jrp.2005.01.006
7. Kern, ML, & Friedman, HS, 2011. Personality and pathways of influence on physical health. *Social and Personality Psychology Compass*, 5(1), 76-87, January. doi: 10.1111/j.1751-9004.2010.00331.x – Lüdtke, O, Roberts, BW, Trautwein, U, & Nagy, G, 2011. A random walk down university avenue: life paths, life events, and personality trait change at the transition to university life. *Journal of Personality and Social Psychology*, 101(3), 620-637, September. doi: 10.1037/a0023743. – Shiner, RL, & Masten, AS, 2012. Childhood personality as a harbinger of competence and resilience in adulthood. *Development and Psychopathology*, 24(2), 507-528, May. doi: 10.1017/S0954579412000120. – Taylor, SE, Repetti, RL, & Seeman, T, 1997. Health psychology: what is an unhealthy environment and how does it get under the skin? *Annual Review of Psychology*, 48(1), 411-447, February. doi: 10.1146/annurev.psych.48.1.411
8. Hampson, SE, Goldberg, LR, Vogt, TM, & Dubanoski, JP, 2007. Mechanisms by which childhood personality traits influence adult health status: educational attainment and healthy behaviors. *Health Psychology*, 26(1), 121-125, January. doi: 10.1037/0278-6133.26.1.121 – Ozer, DJ, & Benet-Martinez, V, 2006. Personality and the prediction of consequential outcomes. *Annual Review of Psychology*, 57, 401-421, January. doi: 10.1146/annurev.psych.57.102904.190127 – Poropat, AE, 2009. A meta-analysis of the five-factor model of personality and academic performance. *Psychological Bulletin*, 135(2), 322-338, March. doi: 10.1037/a0014996 – Roberts, BW, Caspi, A, & Moffitt, TE, 2003. Work experiences and personality development in young adulthood. *Journal of Personality and Social Psychology*, 84(3), 582-593, March. doi:10.1037/0022-3514.84.3.582
9. Friedman, HS, and Kern, ML, 2014. Personality, well-being, and health. *Annual Review of Psychology*, 65(1), 719-742, January. doi: 10.1146/annurev-psych-010213-115123
10. Johnston, B, Kanters, S, Bandayrel, K, Wu, P, Naji, F, Siemieniuk, R, Ball, G, Busse, J, Thorlund, K, Guyatt, G, Jansen, J, & Mills, E, 2014. Comparison of weight loss among named diet programs in overweight and obese adults. *Journal of the American Medical Association*, 312(9), 923-933, 03 September. doi: 10.1001/jama.2014.10397
11. Johnston, B, Kanters, S, Bandayrel, K, Wu, P, Naji, F, Siemieniuk, R, Ball, G, Busse, J, Thorlund, K, Guyatt, G, Jansen, J, & Mills, E, 2014. Comparison of weight loss among named diet programs in overweight and obese adults. *Journal of the American Medical Association*, 312(9), 923-933, 03 September. doi: 10.1001/jama.2014.10397
12. Hollands, G, French, D, Griffin, S, Prevost, A, Sutton, S, King, S, & Marteau, T, 2016. The impact of communicating genetic risks of disease on risk-reducing health behaviour: systematic review with meta-analysis. *BMJ*, 352, i1102, March. doi: 10.1136/bmj.i1102.
13. Norcross, JC, Mrykalo, MS, & Blagys, MD, 2002. Auld lang syne: success predictors, change processes, and self-reported outcomes of New Year's resolvers and nonresolvers. *Journal of Clinical Psychology*, 58(4), 397-405, April. doi: 10.1002/jclp.1151
14. YouGov, 2015. *63% of Brits are planning to make New Year resolutions.* London: YouGov, 16 January. – YouGov & Pier Marketing, 2014. Resolutions [data table]. London: YouGov, 15-16 December. – Marist College Institute for Public Opinion, 2014. *Holiday spending status quo ... weight loss top resolution for 2015.* [news release] Poughkeepsie, NY: Marist College Institute for Public Opinion, 18 December.
15. Norcross, JC, Mrykalo, MS, & Blagys, MD, 2002. Auld lang syne: success predictors, change processes, and self-reported outcomes of New Year's resolvers and nonresolvers. *Journal of Clinical Psychology*, 58(4), 397-405, April. doi: 10.1002/jclp.1151 Norcross, JC, & Vangarelli, DJ, 1988. The resolution solution: longitudinal examination of New Year's change attempts. *Journal of Substance Abuse*, 1(2), 127-134. doi: 10.1016/S0899-3289(88)80016-6
16. Rhodes, RE, & de Bruijn, GJ, 2013. How big is the physical activity intention-behaviour gap? a meta-analysis using the action control framework. *British Journal of Health Psychology*, 18(2), 296-309, May. doi: 10.1111/bjhp.12032.
17. Bélanger-Gravel, A, Godin, G, & Amireault, S, 2011. A meta-analytic review of the effects of implementation intentions on physical activity. *Health Psychology Review*, 7(1), 23-54, March. doi: 10.1080/17437199.2011.560095
18. Adriaanse, MA, Vinkers, CDW, De Ridder, DDT, Hox, JJ, & De Wit, JBF, 2011. Do implementation intentions help to eat a healthy diet? a systematic review and meta-analysis of the empirical evidence. *Appetite*, 56(1), 183-193, February. doi: 10.1016/j. appet.2010.10.012

19. Norberg, PA, Horne, DR, & Horne, DA, 2007. The Privacy paradox: personal information disclosure intentions versus behaviors, *Journal of Consumer Affairs*, 41(1), 100-126. doi: 10.1111/j.1745-6606.2006.00070.x
20. Carrington, MJ, Neville, BA, & Whitwell, GJ, 2014. Lost in translation: exploring the ethical consumer intention-behavior gap, *Journal of Business Research*, 67(1), 2759-2767, January. doi: 10.1016/j.jbusres.2012.09.022
21. Sheeran, P, 2002. Intention-behavior relations: a conceptual and empirical review. *European Review of Social Psychology*, 12(1), 1-36, April. doi: 10.1080/14792772143000003
22. Sheeran, P, 2002. Intention-behavior relations: a conceptual and empirical review. *European Review of Social Psychology*, 12(1), 1-36, April. doi: 10.1080/14792772143000003 – Webb, TL, & Sheeran, P, 2006. Does changing behavioral intentions engender behavior change? A meta-analysis of the experimental evidence. *Psychological Bulletin*, 132(2), 249-268, March. doi: 10.1037/0033-2909.132.2.249
23. Gollwitzer, PM, & Sheeran, P, 2006. Implementation intentions and goal achievement: a meta-analysis of effects and processes. *Advances in Experimental Social Psychology*, 38, 69-119, January. doi:10.1016/S0065-2601(06)38002-1
24. Gollwitzer, PM, & Sheeran, P, 2006. Implementation intentions and goal achievement: A meta-analysis of effects and processes. *Advances in Experimental Social Psychology*, 38, 69-119, January. doi:10.1016/S0065-2601(06)38002-1
25. Hankonen, N, Kinnunen, M, Absetz, P, & Jallinoja, P, 2014. Why do people high in self-control eat more healthily? social cognitions as mediators. *Annals of Behavioral Medicine*, 47(2), 242-248, April. doi: 10.1007/s12160-013-9535-1
26. De Ridder, DTD, Lensvelt-Mulders, G, Finkenauer, C, Stok, FM, & Baumeister, RF, 2012. Taking stock of self-control: a meta-analysis of how trait self-control relates to a wide range of behaviors. *Personality and Social Psychology Review*, 16(1), 76-99, February. doi: 10.1177/1088868311418749
27. Godinho, CA, Alvarez, MJ, Lima, ML, & Schwarzer, R, 2014. Will is not enough: coping planning and action control as mediators in the prediction of fruit and vegetable intake. *British Journal of Health Psychology*, 19(4), 856-870, November. doi: 10.1111/bjhp.12084.
28. De Ridder, DTD, Lensvelt-Mulders, G, Finkenauer, C, Stok, FM, & Baumeister, RF, 2012. Taking stock of self-control: a meta-analysis of how trait self-control relates to a wide range of behaviors. *Personality and Social Psychology Review*, 16(1), 76-99, February. doi: 10.1177/1088868311418749
29. Mann, T, 2015. *Secrets from the eating lab: the science of weight loss, the myth of willpower, and why you should never diet again.* New York: Harper Wave.
30. Baumeister, RF, Bratslavsky, E, Muraven, M, & Tice, DM, 1988. Ego depletion: is the active self a limited resource? *Journal of Personality and Social Psychology*, 74(5), 1252-1265, May. doi: 10.1037/0022-3514.74.5.1252
31. Vohs, KD, & Heatherton, TF, 2000. Self-regulatory failure: a resource-depletion approach. *Psychological Science*, 11(3), 249-254, May. doi:10.1111/1467-9280.00250.
32. Muraven, M, Collins, RL, Shiffman, S, & Paty, JA, 2005. Daily fluctuations in self-control demands and alcohol intake. *Psychology of Addictive Behaviors*, 19(2), 140-147, June. 10.1037/0893-164X.19.2.140
33. Leeman, RF, O'Malley, SS, White, MA, & McKee, SA, 2010. Nicotine and food deprivation decrease the ability to resist smoking. *Psychopharmacology*, 212(1), 25-32, September. doi: 10.1007/s00213-010-1902-z
34. Hagger, MS, Wood, C, Stiff, C. & Chatzisarantis, NL, 2010. Ego depletion and the strength model of self-control: a meta-analysis. *Psychological Bulletin*, 136(4), 495-525, July. doi: 10.1037/a0019486.
35. Hagger, MS, Wood, C, Stiff, C. & Chatzisarantis, NL, 2010. Ego depletion and the strength model of self-control: a meta-analysis. *Psychological Bulletin*, 136(4), 495-525, July. doi: 10.1037/a0019486. – Hagger, MS, 2013. *Rumours of the demise of ego-depletion are (somewhat) exaggerated.* [blog post] Perth: Health Psychology and Behavioural Medicine Research Group.
36. Haidt, J, 2006. *The happiness hypothesis: Finding modern truth in ancient wisdom.* New York: Basic Books, page 4.
37. Haidt, J, 2006. *The happiness hypothesis: Finding modern truth in ancient wisdom.* New York: Basic Books, page xi.
38. Bargh, JA, & Morsella, E, 2008. The unconscious mind. *Perspectives on Psychological Science*, 3(1), 73-79, January. doi: 10.1111/j.1745-6916.2008.00064.x.
39. Wood, W, Quinn, JM, & Kashy, DA, 2002. Habits in everyday life: thought, emotion, and action. *Journal of Personality and Social Psychology*, 83(6), 1281-1297, December. doi: 10.1037/0022-3514.83.6.1281
40. Neal, DT, Wood, W, & Quinn, JM, 2006. Habits – a repeat performance. *Current Directions in Psychological Science*, 15(4), 198-202, August.
41. Gardner, B, 2015. A review and analysis of the use of 'habit' in understanding, predicting and influencing health-related behaviour. *Health Psychology Review*, 9(3), 277-295, 07 August. doi: 10.1080/17437199.2013.876238 – Lally, P, Wardle, J, & Gardner, B, 2011. Experiences of habit formation: a qualitative study. *Psychology, Health & Medicine*, 16(4), 484-489, August. doi: 10.1080/13548506.2011.555774. – Wood, W, & Neal, DT, 2007. A new look at habits and the habit-goal interface. *Psychological Review*, 114(4), 843-863, October. doi: 10.1037/0033-295X.114.4.843
42. Lally, P, Van Jaarsveld, CH, Potts, HW, & Wardle, J, 2010. How are habits formed: modelling habit formation in the real world. *European Journal of Social Psychology*, 40(6), 998-1009, October. doi: 10.1002/ejsp.674
43. Wood, W, Witt, MG, & Tam, L, 2005. Changing circumstances, disrupting habits. *Journal of Personality and Social Psychology*, 88(6), 918-933, June. doi: 10.1037/0022-3514.88.6.918
44. Wansink, B, & Park, S, 2001. At the movies: how external cues and perceived taste impact consumption volume. *Food Quality and Preference*, 12(1), 69-74, January. doi:10.1016/S0950-3293(00)00031
45. Neal, DT, Wood, W, Wu, M, & Kurlander, D, 2011. The pull of the past: when do habits persist despite conflict with motives? *Personality and Social Psychology Bulletin*, 37(11), 1428-1437, November. doi: 10.1177/0146167211419863.
46. Wood, W, Witt, MG, & Tam, L, 2005. Changing circumstances, disrupting habits. *Journal of Personality and Social Psychology*, 88(6), 918-933, June. doi: 10.1037/0022-3514.88.6.918
47. Lally, P, Van Jaarsveld, CH, Potts, HW, & Wardle, J, 2010. How are habits formed: modelling habit formation in the real world. *European Journal of Social Psychology*, 40(6), 998-1009, October. doi: 10.1002/ejsp.674
48. Lally, P, Wardle, J, & Gardner, B, 2011. Experiences of habit formation: a qualitative study. *Psychology, Health & Medicine*, 16(4), 484-489, August. doi: 10.1080/13548506.2011.555774.
49. Lally, P, Van Jaarsveld, CH, Potts, HW, & Wardle, J, 2010. How are habits formed: modelling habit formation in the real world. *European Journal of Social Psychology*, 40(6), 998-1009, October. doi: 10.1002/ejsp.674
50. Maltz, M, 1969. *Psycho-cybernetics: a new way to get more living out of life.* New York: Prentice Hall.
51. Gollwitzer, PM, & Brandstätter, V, 1997. Implementation intentions and effective goal pursuit. *Journal of Personality and Social Psychology*, 73(1), 186-199, July. doi: 10.1037/0022-3514.73.1.186
52. Orbell, S, Hodgkins, S, & Sheeran, P, 1997. Implementation intentions and the theory of planned behavior. *Personality and Social Psychology Bulletin*, 23(9), 945-954, September. doi: 10.1177/0146167297239004 – Sheeran, P, & Orbell, S, 1999. Implementation intentions and repeated behaviour: augmenting the predictive validity of the theory of planned behaviour. *European Journal of Social Psychology*, 29(2-3), 349-369, March-May doi: 10.1002/(SICI)1099-0992(199903/05)29:2/3<349::AID-EJSP931>3.0.CO;2-Y – Adriaanse, MA, Vinkers, CDW, De Ridder, DDT, Hox, JJ, & De Wit, JBF, 2011. Do implementation intentions help to eat a healthy diet? a systematic review and meta-analysis of the empirical evidence. *Appetite*, 56(1), 183-193, February. doi: 10.1016/j. appet.2010.10.012
53. Kelly, PJ, Leung, J, Deane, FP, & Lyons, GC, 2015. Predicting client attendance at further treatment following drug and alcohol detoxification: theory of planned behaviour and implementation intentions. *Drug and Alcohol Review*, 30 September. doi: 10.1111/dar.12332
54. Mairs, L, & Mullan, B, 2015. Self-monitoring vs. implementation intentions: a comparison of behaviour change techniques to improve sleep hygiene and sleep outcomes in students. *International Journal of Behavioral Medicine*, 22(5), 635-644, October. doi: 10.1007/s12529-015-9467-1
55. Sheeran, P, & Orbell, S, 1999. Implementation intentions and repeated behaviour: augmenting the predictive validity of the theory of planned behaviour. *European Journal of Social Psychology*, 29(2-3), 349-369, March-May doi: 10.1002/(SICI)1099-0992(199903/05)29:2/3<349::AID-EJSP931>3.0.CO;2-Y
56. Luszczynska, A, 2006. An implementation intentions intervention, the use of a planning strategy, and physical activity after myocardial infarction. *Social Science & Medicine*, 62(4), 900-908, February. doi:10.1016/j.

socscimed.2005.06.043 – Prestwich, A, Lawton, R, & Conner, M, 2003. The use of implementation intentions and the decision balance sheet in promoting exercise behaviour. *Psychology & Health*, 18(6), 707-721. doi: 10.1080/08870440310001594493 – Milne, S, Orbell, S, & Sheeran, P, 2002. Combining motivational and volitional interventions to promote exercise participation: protection motivation theory and implementation intentions. *British Journal of Health Psychology*, 7(Pt 2), 163-184, May. doi: 10.1348/135910702169420 – Prestwich, A, Lawton, R, & Conner, M, 2003. The use of implementation intentions and the decision balance sheet in promoting exercise behaviour. *Psychology & Health*, 18(6), 707-721. doi: 10.1080/08870440310001594493 – Luszczynska, A, 2006. An implementation intentions intervention, the use of a planning strategy, and physical activity after myocardial infarction. *Social Science & Medicine*, 62(4), 900-908, February. doi:10.1016/j.socscimed.2005.06.043

57. Sheeran, P, & Orbell, S, 2000. Using implementation intentions to increase attendance for cervical cancer screening. *Health Psychology*, 19(3), 283-289, May. doi: 10.1037/0278-6133.19.3.283
58. Milkman, KL, Beshears, J, Choi, JJ, Laibson, D, & Madrian, BC, 2011. Using implementation intentions prompts to enhance influenza vaccination rates. *Proceedings of the National Academy of Sciences of the United States of America*, 108(26), 10415-10420, 28 June. doi: 10.1073/pnas.1103170108.
59. Adriaanse, MA, Vinkers, CDW, De Ridder, DDT, Hox, JJ, & De Wit, JBF, 2011. Do implementation intentions help to eat a healthy diet? a systematic review and meta-analysis of the empirical evidence. *Appetite*, 56(1), 183-193, February. doi: 10.1016/j. appet.2010.10.012
60. Adriaanse, MA, Vinkers, CDW, De Ridder, DDT, Hox, JJ, & De Wit, JBF, 2011. Do implementation intentions help to eat a healthy diet? a systematic review and meta-analysis of the empirical evidence. *Appetite*, 56(1), 183-193, February. doi: 10.1016/j. appet.2010.10.012
61. Gollwitzer, PM, 1999. Implementation intentions: strong effects of simple plans. *American Psychologist*, 54(7), 493-503, July. doi: 10.1037/0003-066X.54.7.493
62. Gollwitzer PM, & Sheeran P, 2006. Implementation intentions and goal achievement: a meta-analysis of effects and processes. *Advances in Experimental Social Psychology*, 38, 69-119, January. doi:10.1016/S0065-2601(06)38002-1
63. Adriaanse, MA, Vinkers, CDW, De Ridder, DDT, Hox, JJ, & De Wit, JBF, 2011. Do implementation intentions help to eat a healthy diet? a systematic review and meta-analysis of the empirical evidence. *Appetite*, 56(1), 183-193, February. doi: 10.1016/j. appet.2010.10.012
64. Holland, RW, Aarts, H, & Langendam, D, 2006. Breaking and creating habits on the working floor: a field-experiment on the power of implementation intentions. *Journal of Experimental Social Psychology*, 42(6), 776-783, November. doi: 10.1016/j.jesp.2005.11.006.
65. Zhang, Y, & Cooke, R, 2012. Using a combined motivational and volitional intervention to promote exercise and healthy dietary behaviour among undergraduates. *Diabetes Research and Clinical Practice*, 95(2), 215-223, February. doi: 10.1016/j.diabres.2011.10.006. – Parschau, L, Fleig, L, Warner, LM, Pomp, S, Barz, M, Knoll, N, Schwarzer, R, & Lippke, S, 2014. Positive exercise experience facilitates behavior change via self-efficacy. *Health Education & Behavior*, 41(4), 414-422, August. doi: 10.1177/1090198114529132
66. Adriaanse, MA, Oettingen, G, Gollwitzer, PM, Hennes, EP, De Ridder, DT, & De Wit, JB, 2010. When planning is not enough: fighting unhealthy snacking habits by mental contrasting with implementation intentions (MCII). *European Journal of Social Psychology*, 40(7), 1277-1293, December. doi: 10.1002/ejsp.730
67. Adriaanse, MA, Gollwitzer, PM, De Ridder, DTD, de Wit, JBF, & Kroese, FM, 2011. Breaking habits with implementation intentions: a test of underlying processes. *Personality and Social Psychology Bulletin*, 37(4), 502-513, April. doi: 10.1177/0146167211399102 – Verhoeven, AAC, Adriaanse, MA, Evers, C, & De Ridder, DTD, 2012. The power of habits: unhealthy snacking behaviour is primarily predicted by habit strength. *British Journal of Health Psychology*, 17(4), 758-770, November. doi: 10.1111/j.2044-8287.2012.02070.x. – Godinho, CA, Alvarez, MJ, Lima, ML, & Schwarzer, R, 2014. Will is not enough: Coping planning and action control as mediators in the prediction of fruit and vegetable intake. *British Journal of Health Psychology*, 19(4), 856-870, Novemer. doi: 10.1111/bjhp.12084.
68. Frankl, VE, 1946. *Man's search for meaning*. Translated from German by Ilse Lasch, 1959. Boston: Beacon Press. (2006 reprint of 1960 edition)
69. Noble, HB, 1997. Dr. Viktor E. Frankl of Vienna, psychiatrist of the search for meaning, dies at 92. *The New York Times*, 04 September.
70. Noble, HB, 1997. Dr. Viktor E. Frankl of Vienna, psychiatrist of the search for meaning, dies at 92. *The New York Times*, 04 September.
71. Steger, MF, 2010. Making meaning in life. *Psychological Inquiry*, 23(4), 381-385, 04 December. doi: 10.1080/1047840X.2012.720832.
72. Jim, HS, & Andersen, BL, 2007. Meaning in life mediates the relationship between social and physical functioning and distress in cancer survivors. *British Journal of Health Psychology*, 12(3), 363-381, September. doi: 10.1348/135910706X128278View
73. Martin, RA, MacKinnon, S, Johnson, J, & Rohsenow, DJ, 2011. Purpose in life predicts treatment outcome among adult cocaine abusers in treatment. *Journal of Substance Abuse Treatment*, 40(2), 183-188, March. doi: 10.1016/j.jsat.2010.10.002.
74. Kim, ES, Sun, JK, Park, N, Kubzansky, LD, & Peterson, C, 2013. Purpose in life and reduced risk of myocardial infarction among older US adults with coronary heart disease: a two-year follow-up. *Journal of Behavioral Medicine*, 36(2), 124-133, April. doi: 10.1007/s10865-012-9406-4.
75. Kim, ES, Sun, JK, Park, N, & Peterson, C, 2013. Purpose in life and reduced incidence of stroke in older adults: 'The Health and Retirement Study.' *Journal of Psychosomatic Research*, 74(5), 427-432. doi: 10.1016/j.jpsychores.2013.01.013.
76. Boyle, PA, Buchman, AS, Barnes, LL, & Bennett, DA, 2010. Effect of a purpose in life on risk of incident Alzheimer disease and mild cognitive impairment in community-dwelling older persons. *Archives of General Psychiatry*, 67(3), 304-310, March. doi: 10.1001/archgenpsychiatry.2009.208.
77. Boyle, PA, Buchman, AS, Wilson, RS, Yu, L, Schneider, JA, & Bennett, DA, 2012. Effect of purpose in life on the relation between Alzheimer disease pathologic changes on cognitive function in advanced age. Archives of general psychiatry, 69(5), 499-504, May. doi. 10.1001/archgenpsychiatry.2011.1487.
78. Steger, M, 2014. Is it time to consider meaning in life as a public policy priority? *Ewha Journal of Social Sciences*, 30(2). doi: 10.16935/ejss.2014.30.2.003
79. Zilioli, S, Slatcher, RB, Ong, AD, & Gruenewald, TL, 2015. Purpose in life predicts allostatic load ten years later. *Journal of Psychosomatic Research*, 79(5), 451-457, November. doi: 10.1016/j.jpsychores.2015.09.013.
80. Roepke, AM, Jayawickreme, E, & Riffle, OM, 2014. Meaning and health: A systematic review. *Applied Research in Quality of Life*, 9(4), 1055-1079, December. doi: 10.1007/s11482-013-9288-9
81. Bower, JE, Kemeny, ME, Taylor, SE, & Fahey, JL, 2003. Finding positive meaning and its association with natural killer cell cytotoxicity among participants in a bereavement-related disclosure intervention. *Annals of Behavioral Medicine*, 25(2), 146-155, Spring. doi: 10.1207/S15324796ABM2502_11
82. Kim, ES, Hershner, SD, & Strecher, VJ, 2015. Purpose in life and incidence of sleep disturbances. *Journal of Behavioral Medicine*, 38(3), 590-597, June. doi: 10.1007/s10865-015-9635-4.
83. Brassai, L Piko, BF, & Steger, MF, 2015. A reason to stay healthy: the role of meaning in life in relation to physical activity and healthy eating among adolescents. *Journal of Health Psychology*, 20(5), 473-482, May. doi: 10.1177/1359105315576604.
84. Kim, ES, Strecher, VJ, & Ryff, CD, 2014. Purpose in life and use of preventive health care services. *Proceedings of the National Academy of Sciences of the United States of America*, 111(46), 16331-16336, 18 November. doi: 10.1073/pnas.1414826111

Index

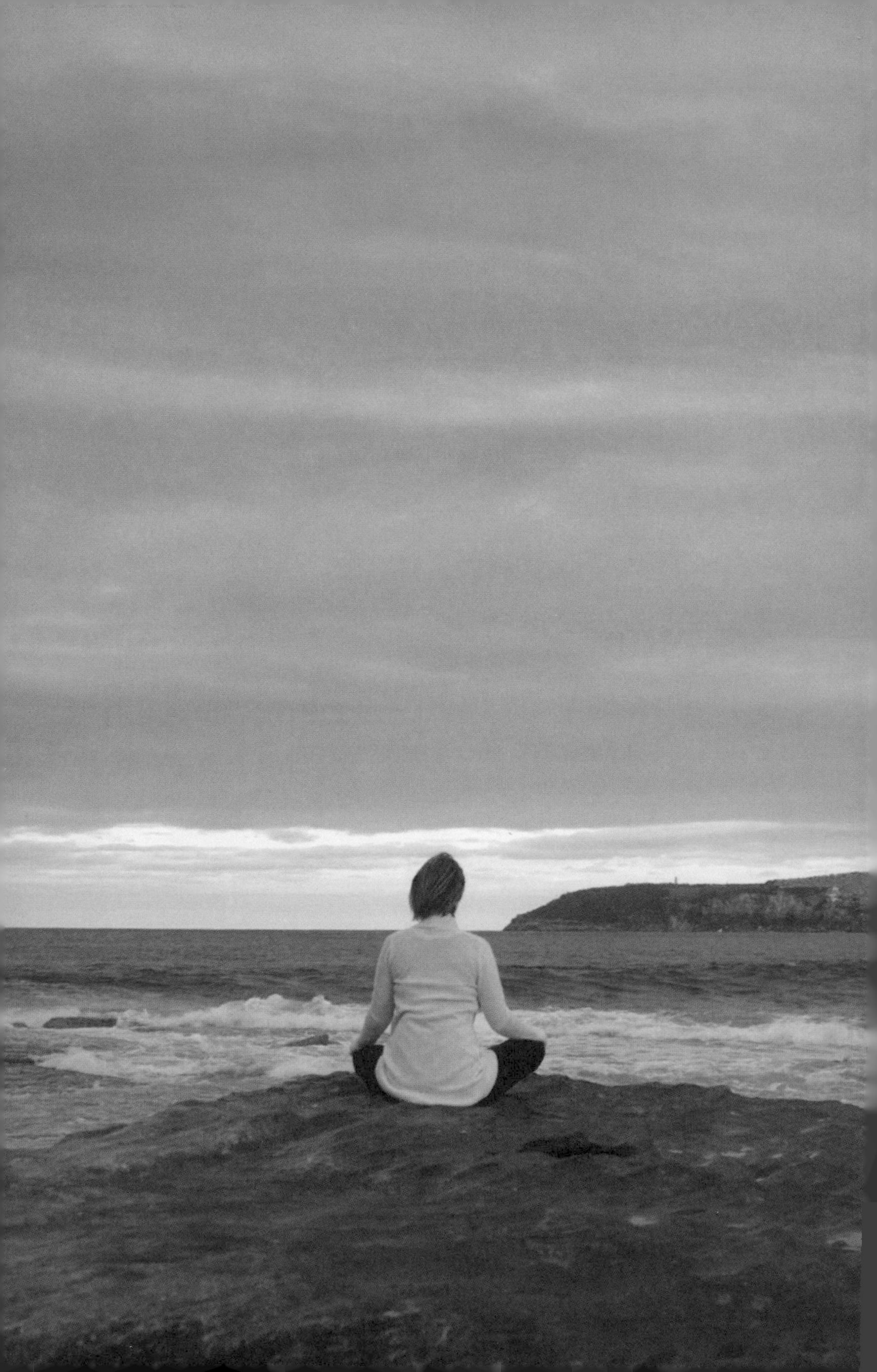